Contrace

YOUR QUESTIONS ANSWERED

Commissioning Editor: Ellen Green
Project Development Manager: Fiona Conn
Project Manager: Frances Affleck
Design Direction: George Ajayi

Contraception

YOUR QUESTIONS ANSWERED

FOURTH EDITION

John Guillebaud MA FRCSE FRCOG
Emeritus Professor of Family Planning and Reproductive Health,
University College London
Trustee of the Margaret Pyke Memorial Trust
Formerly Medical Director of the Margaret Pyke Family Planning Centre, London

CHURCHILL
LIVINGSTONE

EDINBURGH LONDON NEW YORK OXFORD PHILADELPHIA ST LOUIS SYDNEY TORONTO 2004

CHURCHILL LIVINGSTONE
An imprint of Elsevier Science Limited

First edition 1985 (Pitman Publishing Ltd)
Revised and reprinted 1989
Second edition 1993
Revised and reprinted 1994
Third edition 1999
Revised and reprinted 2001
Fourth edition 2004

ISBN 0 443 07343 0

British Library Cataloguing in Publication Data
A catalogue record for this book is available from the British Library

Library of Congress Cataloging in Publication Data
A catalog record for this book is available from the Library of Congress

Notice
Medical knowledge is constantly changing. Standard safety precautions must be followed, but as new
research and clinical experience broaden our knowledge, changes in treatment and drug therapy may
become necessary or appropriate. Readers are advised to check the most current product information
provided by the manufacturer of each drug to be administered to verify the recommended dose, the
method and duration of administration, and contraindications. It is the responsibility of the practitioner,
relying on experience and knowledge of the patient, to determine dosages and the best treatment for each
individual patient. Neither the Publisher nor the author assumes any liability for any injury and/or
damage to persons or property arising from this publication.

**ELSEVIER
SCIENCE**
your source for books,
journals and multimedia
in the health sciences

www.elsevierhealth.com

The
publisher's
policy is to use
paper manufactured
from sustainable forests

Printed in Spain

Contents

Preface

We have not inherited the earth from our grandparents – we have borrowed it from our grandchildren.

(Attributed to the ancient Chinese)

Frighteningly, since this book's first edition in 1985 we have over 1 300 000 000 more humans on the planet. An increase in 18 years that is more than the *total* population 150 years ago – of just one species sharing the planet with all other species. Population is not often *the* problem, but it is the great multiplier of many problems and threats facing our children and grandchildren: poverty, epidemics, mass migrations, violence between and within countries, unsustainable development degrading the environment, climate change, loss of biodiversity, habitat destruction, species extinctions …

Yet there are hopeful signs. With important exceptions in Africa and some regions of Asia, couples in most countries are now choosing family sizes that will lead to replacement fertility or below. This at the micro (i.e. couple) level is because we humans have contraception, that technology which gives us the edge on all other species to prevent otherwise inevitable self-destruction – as results whenever the carrying capacity of environments is exceeded.

Moreover, in comparison with the not-very-distant past, contraceptive technology is approaching closer to a 'contraceptive utopia'. If only every couple in the world could have access to the full range – a situation that is impossible (for many astoundingly bad reasons) for 350 million, or one-third of all there are – it ought, in theory, to be possible to offer a method to suit everyone. Yet even in the UK, where the choice is wider than in most countries (with recent brilliant additions, notably the LNG-IUS, Implanon™, Cerazette™, EVRA™ and, shortly, NuvaRing™), almost 200 000 pregnancies are terminated annually and, from a recent large survey (Farrow et al 2002, *see Q 5.61* in this book), it seems that almost one-third of children still owe their arrival more to chance than to caring choice.

Since the last edition, teenagers have been rightly highlighted as a group at ongoing special risk. I was invited to represent the RCOG on the independent Advisory Group to the Teenage Pregnancy Unit. This has produced two reports and is well integrated within the Sexual Health Strategy. Watchwords are 'joined-up working', confidentiality and forgetability – the last being a feature of the long-acting methods, which ought to be far more available and more often offered to teens (*see Qs 1.15 and 2.1*).

It ought not to need saying that contraception has everything to do with sex! Sexuality and communication influence crucially both strong and weak motivation for effective contraception, and we forget that whole area, and the other crucial interface of sexually transmitted infections, at our peril. Why do we so often neglect to take a simple sexual history (*see Qs 1.13 and 1.14*)? Or fail to detect psychosexual unhappiness through the hidden clues, verbal and by body language, particularly at the 'moment of truth' before, during and after a genital examination? As the NHS gets ever more stressful, we need to remind ourselves to avoid the busy doctor's knee-jerk reaction of reaching for the prescription pad.

I proudly record that I am myself an ex-GP in the NHS; during my training years I worked as a locum in places as diverse as Barnsley, Cambridge, Luton and Eltham, in south-east London. As the Preface to the first edition says, this book is intended primarily for general practitioners and family planning doctors but it will also be of value to gynaecologists and most other healthcare professionals – above all nurses, who are rightly being given an ever-increasing executive hands-on and prescribing role in this field. Primarily, the book is about how best to select and use the existing reversible birth control technology. The rather brief discussion of related subjects – notably sexually transmitted infections, psychosexual medicine, male and female sterilization, the Sexual Health Strategy, ethics and the law – does not imply that they are unimportant. See also the Further reading section!

In addition to those already acknowledged who helped with the first edition, I wish to thank Drs Elphis Christopher, Ron Kleinman, Anne MacGregor, Catherine Nelson-Piercy and Sam Rowlands; also Anne Szarewski and other colleagues at the Margaret Pyke Centre; and for their keyboard and computer skills my secretary Helen Prime and my son Jonathan. Based on her unique first hand experience as Director of Information of the UK FPA, Toni Belfield provided constructive criticisms of the whole work and is extensively quoted in Chapter 11. Dr Hilary Luscombe and Joan Walsh assisted with literature searches and lists of the topics about which questions are most commonly asked. Fiona Conn, Eleanor Flood, Ellen Green, Lucy Gardner, Miranda Bromage and Rachel Robson at Churchill Livingstone, now part of Elsevier, have all helped to turn my efforts into the completed book – in this edition paying special attention (as requested by readers) to aspects of design and indexing, so as to increase accessibility to the numerous answers.

All of these are most warmly thanked. But at all times I remain happy to be reminded of my former Deputy Ali Kubba's subtitle to this book: 'Contraception – your answers questioned!'

John Guillebaud
2003

Preface to the first edition

As its title suggests, this book is designed as a ready source of answers to the many questions which are being asked, always with interest and often with a hint of anxiety, both by the consumers and the providers of modern reversible birth control methods. I have acquired experience in answering most of them as a result of lecturing in family planning very widely, in this country and abroad, and also on the postgraduate lecture courses held regularly at the Margaret Pyke Centre. In these, upwards of 600 doctors and 200 nurses are trained each year. The book is intended primarily for general practitioners and family planning doctors, working in a developed country such as Britain, but it will also be of value to other healthcare professionals, and medical students.

The questions about each method are arranged so far as possible in a logical order. They are mostly based on the questions which doctors ask of a specialist colleague like myself, arising from their clinical experience and the questions they have been asked by patients. In a concluding section of most chapters there is an assortment of the very practical questions which are asked by patients, some of which can be demanding to the unprepared (see, for example, Qs 4.266 and 6.175 [6.96 and 9.178 in the fourth edition]).

Reasons of space have required me to concentrate almost entirely on answers to questions about the technology of reversible birth control, with little discussion of male and female sterilization and induced abortion, as well as essential subjects such as counselling, social factors affecting contraceptive use, medico-legal aspects, sexual problems and health screening. Most of these are dealt with in other texts in the Further Reading section.

For reading and commenting on sections of the text, I am most grateful to the following: Walli Bounds, Ken Fotherby, Susan Hatwell, Sam Hutt, Howard Jacobs and Pram Senanayake. Special thanks are due to my deputy at the Centre, Mr Ali Kubba, who has read and constructively criticized the whole book: but I must be held responsible for any errors that remain.

Ray Phillips and his staff of the Middlesex Hospital Department of Medical Photography and Illustration, especially Stuart Nightingale and Angela Scott, have been most helpful in the preparation of figures – apart from some separately acknowledged in the figure captions and tables. Toni Belfield contributed a list of questions which have been asked of the Family Planning Association's Information Service by the general public. My publishers have been most understanding, notably Katherine Watts and

Howard Bailey. I also acknowledge the help of Mr John Adkins, Headmaster of Egerton-Rothesay School, in providing me with a haven of quiet for much of the writing. Last, but not least, I record my thanks to my select team of typists: Margaret Bailón, Diane Berry, Sue Nickells and Georgina Tregoning.

My wife Gwyneth as usual has been enormously supportive. She and our young children have been most tolerant of their recent one-parent family status.

John Guillebaud
September 1985

How to use this book

The *Your Questions Answered* series aims to meet the information needs of GPs and other primary care professionals who care for women and men with long term medical needs. It is designed to help them work with patients and their families, providing effective, evidence-based care and management.

The books are in an accessible question and answer format, with detailed contents lists at the beginning of every chapter and a complete index to help find specific information.

ICONS

Icons are used in the book to identify particular types of information:

 highlights important information

 highlights side-effect information.

PATIENT QUESTIONS

At the end of relevant chapters there are sections of frequently asked patient questions, with easy-to-understand answers aimed at the non-medical reader. These questions are also listed at the end of the book.

EVIDENCE-BASE

The answers here are the personal opinion of the author, based wherever possible on published and sometimes unpublished evidence. When (as is not infrequent) no epidemiological or other direct evidence is available, clinical advice is always as practical and realistic as possible and is based, pending more data, on the author's judgement of other sources. These may include the opinions of expert committees and any existing guidelines. In some instances the advice appearing in this book may nevertheless differ appreciably from the latter, for reasons given in the text and since medical knowledge and practice are continually evolving advice relates to the date of publication. Healthcare professionals must understand that they take ultimate responsibility for their patient and ensure that any clinical advice they use from this book is applicable to the specific circumstances they encounter.

COMPETING INTERESTS

The author has received payments for research projects, lectures, ad hoc consultancy work and related expenses from the manufacturers of contraceptive products.

Introduction: the population explosion, sexual and contraceptive history taking and counselling – the importance of fertility control

1.1 What is the population explosion?

According to 2003 figures from the Population Reference Bureau (www.prb.org), there were 6300 million humans on the planet in June 2003 (*Fig. 1.1*). There are 42 births and 17 deaths every 10 seconds, a net gain of 25 extra people somewhere on the globe every 10 seconds. These 25 extra births beyond replacement mean that a city for 1 million people needs to be built every 5 days; only this won't be a city, it will be a slum – given that less than 2% of the new humans arrive in rich 'northern' countries.

Because of demographic momentum, most of tomorrow's parents are children who have already been born (*see Q 1.6*) and so we must expect the arrival of at least half as many again before the earliest date of stabilization. Yet even now, many of the existing millions are grossly deficient in the bare necessities of life: food, clean water, clothing, housing, healthcare, education and recreation … is it quality of life we are after, or quantity of flesh?

We will never meet human needs on this finite planet until we stabilize human numbers.

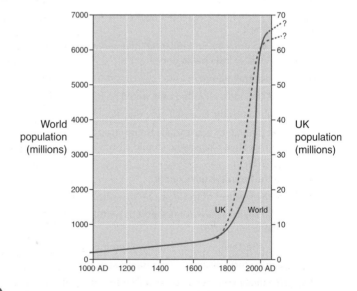

▲

Fig. 1.1 Estimated rate of population growth, AD 1750–2000. Note that the UK differs from the rest of the world mainly by having had its population explosion slightly earlier. The UK, too, was once covered by forest. Q 1.1

1.2   So how is the world doing at present?

According to United Nation (UN) figures, out of about 180 million conceptions each year at least 75 million are unwanted. This results in about 50 million abortions, of which 20 million are performed in unsafe circumstances. Around 600 000 women die each year (equalling a jumbo jet crashing every 6 hours, or one woman every minute of the day) from these pregnancies, through abortion or for lack of the basic requirements for safe delivery. An estimated 200 000 would not die if adequate services and supplies for contraception were available. They are killed by pregnancies they would have preferred not to have.

What infamous statistics! Such dreadful carnage! When you add the preventable deaths among children – as well as mothers – when births are too frequent, how is it that birth planning is so often stigmatized as anti-life! On the contrary:

Family planning could provide more benefits to more people at less cost than any other single 'technology' now available to the human race (James Grant, UNICEF Annual Report, 1992)

1.3   But isn't this primarily a problem of the 'developing' world?

Certainly. But in the 'developed' world it has been calculated that every new birth is likely to lead, in the lifetime of that individual (depending on that person's affluence and the 'greenness' of his or her technology) to up to 30–200 times more damage to the fragile environment. The environmental crisis is the consequence of multiplying per-person consumption by ever more persons. The global consequences are climate change and the relentless destruction of the habitats of other animals and plants. According to the Worldwide Fund for Nature, total extinction threatens one-quarter of all mammals, one bird species out of eight and almost one-third of terrestrial plants, and that's before considering some of the most dramatic losses occurring in the world's oceans. Moreover, as was shown by the two reports of the Brandt Commission, the developed countries of the world cannot consider themselves forever immune to events elsewhere on this small, finite planet. No wall will be high enough to stop the flood of 'economic migrants', for one thing. The rich 'north' ought to give far more and far more appropriate aid to the 'south', out of simple humanity. But even without that motivation, their own calculated self-interest should force voters, and therefore politicians, worldwide, massively to increase the aid they give to the poor countries – and the proportion of it given to reproductive health and the methods of voluntary birth control.

If we are not part of the solution, we *are* part of the problem (see www.ecotimecapsule.com, www.Optimumpopulation.org and www.peopleandplanet.net for more details).

1.4 What changes birth rates?

As shown in *Fig. 1.2*, a great deal more is necessary than simply the provision of family planning. Although all are important, some need to be highlighted:

1 Better health and fewer child deaths: it has been calculated that in rural areas of India a couple need to have five children to have a 95% chance of one son reaching maturity. But there is a vicious circle here, because child mortality is itself greater in the absence of effective family spacing, and this is now being exacerbated by the worldwide decline in breastfeeding without enough alternative contraception.

2 A better deal for women: in too many societies worldwide women remain second-class citizens and have little choice in their destiny or that of their family. They are forced by their male-dominated society in general, and their husbands in particular, as well as by their biology (*see Qs 2.1–2.10*), to have far more children than they desire. This was clearly shown by the World Fertility Survey and the Reproductive Health Surveys which, in 60 countries in the developing world, found that even in the 1980s almost 50% of married women wanted no more children. So for them at least family planning had become a perceived unmet need – we should, and could (but did not), push at an open door …

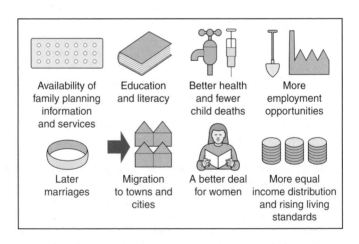

▲

Fig. 1.2 What changes birth rates? Q 1.4 (from: *The shape of things to come*. 1982, Population Concern).

3   Implicit in the whole of *Fig. 1.2* are two slogans or sayings. The first is an ancient proverb referring to the inhabitants of rural areas:

Every mouth has got two hands.

In rural poverty the hands are far more noticeable than the mouth, in that the labour and support that a child can give to its parents, especially in their old age or during disease, are far more important to them than the extra cost that might be incurred by having an extra child. It is hard for individuals to see how the macroproblems – burgeoning numbers in large tracts of the developing world leading to excessive tree-cutting, erosion and floods, desertification, salinization, habitat destruction and ultimately disaster – are in any way their business through decisions about childbearing.

Apart from the regrettable 'Big Brother' Chinese solution – enforcing one-child families – what can be done? Even the Chinese agree that this was a draconian measure forced on them mainly because they did not bring in a much less restrictive two-child policy when they had half as many people only 50 years ago. The best answer is summarized in the second slogan:

Take care of the people and the population will take care of itself.

4   Rising living standards: poverty should be eliminated. This should be done as a matter of social justice (*Fig. 1.2*) but, when coupled with (3), above, there is a vicious circle. Even if the gross domestic product (GDP) of a country like Burundi (the land of my birth) or of Rwanda, where I was brought up, does increase, the per capita GDP goes down if it is shared by more and more people. Ever more hardship results, and violence can be the outcome. When I was a child there were only 2 million Rwandans; by the time of the appalling genocide in 1994 (in which several of my playmates and friends of the 1940s were slaughtered) the population was 8 million – four people sharing the available resources where before there had been one. This has to be relevant, after all: 'the stork is the bird of war'.

1.5   Does this mean that development is the best contraceptive, so family planning doesn't matter?

Far from it; many people have misinterpreted the slogan in this way, claiming, for example, that improved child survival is a prerequisite for family planning acceptance (although experience in Bangladesh and elsewhere has disproved this). The result is that in large areas of the world, in the slums and rural areas where people actually live, the basic tools for family planning are just not available at a price that they can afford. 'Population will take care of itself' only when 'taking care of the people' includes every item in *Fig. 1.2* as part of an integrated solution. Family planning services must be provided locally, comprehensively and appropriately, as a human right, on an equal basis at least with all the other items illustrated. Instead of 'counting people' the emphasis must be 'people count', as highlighted at the UN world population conference in Cairo in 1994. The emphasis must be on reproductive health, education and empowerment for women.

At present, the proportion of aid for the developing world that is spent on the provision of voluntary birth control is around 2%. Family planning is no panacea and is not the whole answer, but it will surely provide much more than 2% of the answer!

1.6 If everything that could and should be done *was* done, what is the most likely future total world population at stabilization?

Realistically, at least 50% larger than now. Short of a cataclysm, this is a demographic certainty. Why? Because, like a supertanker, world population has so much in-built momentum. Currently, 2000 million of the world's inhabitants are under 15, and that means very nearly all of tomorrow's parents are already born. They will be responsible for a massive increase even if they have an average of only two children each. To me, this is the most frightening of all the alarming ecostatistics.

The world's population was 3 billion in 1960, when I first became aware of this problem (and, incidentally, it was this realization that drove me to make reproductive health my specialty). We now have more than two worlds of this size. And everything we must do (and are not doing nearly well enough yet) in the provision of reproductive healthcare to the world is about stopping world number 4 from coming along: world number 3 is all but inevitable! Scientists can see some chance of a passable, if perilous, future for around 9 billion humans. More than that really does risk collapse of life-support mechanisms in the ecosystem and deaths and misery on an unheard-of scale.

1.7 Is the population crisis really that bad?

A frog dropped into boiling water jumps straight out, unscathed. If this (unethical) experiment is repeated with the same water, same container, same frog and same source of heat but starting from cold, the outcome is a boiled frog. The trouble about the population, development, resources and pollution story is that it is based on numerous interconnected adverse trends rather than on catastrophic events. Very like that frog, we humans have a poor track record for reacting vigorously to serious dangers (take cigarette smoke, for instance) if they are gradual and insidious. But we must. The crisis is caused much less by wilfulness than by carelessness and ignorance. It happens through millions of people 'doing their own thing'.

All of us, rich and poor, whether clearing forests (130 000 square kilometres per year) or driving to the shops, are using technology to improve our families' material environment: oblivious to the fact that, with more and more people doing the same and continuing for long enough, the consequences for our grandchildren could be horrendous. Somehow we must – all of us – learn a 'greener' lesson. We must stop treating the fragile planet as an inexhaustible milch cow for our wants and as a bottomless cesspit for our wastes.

In the preface I quoted the saying:

> We have not inherited the world from our grandparents – we have borrowed it from our grandchildren.

I believe that our own children's children will brand this generation – living in the last quarter of the twentieth century – as the worst ever, in that it was the last to have some chance of preventing the environmental wasteland that they will have inherited, but too little was done and too late. We will be seen as having selfishly mortgaged their future for our present gain.

1.8 Should we be apologizing for damaging this 'loan from our grandchildren'?

Because I felt the need to do just that, I devised the Environment Time Capsule project. Time capsules containing objects that were environmentally relevant to the year 1994 (including 'bad' items, like a car's petrol cap, or 'good' items, like a bicycle pump and some packets of contraceptive pills and condoms), along with letters and poems written by 1000 people, mainly children, and addressed to the year 2044, were buried at strategic sites across the globe: in Mexico, UK (Kew Gardens and Ness Gardens on the Wirral, Merseyside), South Africa, the Seychelles and Australia. As well as apologizing, there was this pledge: that all those involved would work tirelessly to ensure that, hopefully, those who dug-up each time capsule in 2044 would wonder what we were on about, i.e. apologies would not be necessary! A reunion is held at Ness Gardens every year on the nearest Sunday to World Environment Day, June 5th – come along, I will be there! (see *www.ecotimecapsule.com* or my 'Personal View' in the *British Medical Journal* 1994 308:1377–1378 for more details).

1.9 In view of the urgency, and the in-built momentum of population growth, why is so little being done?

Politicians across the globe don't act because voters, faced with the challenge of less 'jam' today so that their children can inherit a tolerable world in the future, invariably vote to have at least as much jam as they currently have, and preferably more. Human perspectives are remarkably insular in terms of space, and brief in terms of time. The following sayings summarize things well: 'my car is my car, everyone else's car is traffic'; 'my visit to the seaside is my holiday, but the crowds on the beach!'; and 'my baby is my baby, everybody else's baby is overpopulation'. These attitudes are reinforced by ignorance, by apathy and by a hint of racism: 'the death of one baby in London is a tragedy; the death of millions of babies in Africa – that's a statistic'.

1.10 Is it all doom and gloom?

No, there are actually sound grounds for some optimism. Total fertility rates (average family sizes) are falling in almost every country. And there *is* enough money to tackle the problem. After all, smallpox was eradicated from the face of this planet by the equivalent amount of money that, at the time, was spent by the world's armed forces every 8 minutes. It has been estimated that the extra money required to provide adequate food, water, education, housing and health for the whole planet, including the means for each woman to control her fertility as she would choose, could be provided for as little as one month's defence spending!

1.11 Against all the odds, anything I did would be just a drop in the ocean

True, but:

The ocean is made up of drops.

As healthcare professionals, we should not underestimate our influence on those around us – our patients and our peer groups – and, through them, on the politicians. More immediately, knowledge is power. Here we come to my prime reason for writing this book: let us ensure that we are so well informed about the whole subject of contraception that we can answer the questions of the women and the men who come to us for contraceptive advice and help. In so far as we are able to influence events, the aim is simple: 'every child a wanted child'.

1.12 Is it enough to be able to answer the questions?

No – 1 g of *empathy* is worth 1 kg of *knowledge*. Moreover:

■ There are techniques to be learnt and maintained: counselling skills and practical skills in the fitting of intrauterine devices and the fitting and the training for women who wish to use female barrier methods.
■ In reproductive healthcare, the correct non-directive counselling attitude and approach are vital. Couples must decide for themselves what aspects of the list in Q 1.15 are most important in their situation. It has been well said that, in the matter of birth planning, 'we are advisers, we are the suppliers – but we are not the deciders' (*see* Q 11.14).

■ Time is always a huge constraint, so doctors should work closely with other professionals, especially (family planning trained) nurses. Appropriate delegation and teamwork ensure user-friendly services.

■ Confidentiality should feel real to all clients (*see Qs 11.5 and 11.6*).

■ Examinations of breast and pelvis should be rare (*see Q 6.3 and 6.4*) and if either is indicated, always offer a chaperone.

1.13 Given that pregnancy is a sexually transmitted condition, presumably good contraceptive counselling should always include an adequate sexual history?

Absolutely, yet many providers in a family planning context claim to be too rushed (or could they still be too embarrassed?) to do this.

If the request is for 'emergency contraception', this should be seen as a marker of risk of a sexually transmitted infection (STI) having been passed along with the sperm. Indeed, there is increasing evidence that the sperm themselves can be 'bio-vectors' of *Chlamydia* and gonococci (although no *Chlamydia* test would be positive from that act, it would need repeating about 7 days later). Remember also that 'breakthrough bleeding' in pill-takers might in fact be caused by *Chlamydia*.

1.14 What are the best questions to ask?

If asked in a matter-of-fact way and non-judgementally during the course of a consultation about periods and gynaecological symptoms, the following questions will almost never cause offence:

■ When did you last have sex?
■ Was that with your regular partner?
■ When was your last sex with anyone else?
■ Was (each) partner male or female?

Or, better yet, an initial screening query followed by more detailed probing according to the tenor and the body language of the response:

■ Have you had sex with someone different in the last 3 months? (Note how the question covers both a change of partner during 'serial monogamy' and any possible 'one-night stand' within a basically long-term relationship).

■ If Yes: did you always use condoms with a new or casual partner?

Two further questions are usually highly relevant, especially when counselling for an intrauterine method:

■ Have you ever been checked or treated for an STI? Or have you thought about having a sexual health screen?

■ Do you ever wonder whether your partner perhaps has other sexual partner(s) (of either sex)?

Exceptionally, supplementary questions become important, e.g. about oral or anal sex, or any possible abuse within a relationship. The answers given will often show how wrong our assumptions are. The young woman with multiple body piercings and tattoos might be in a mutually monogamous relationship whereas the 'pillar of society' might be having unsafe sex with multiple partners.

1.15 What are the features of the ideal contraceptive?

The list below is modified from Table 13 in my book *The pill* (see Further Reading). The ideal method would be:

- *100% effective and forgettable*: initiated by a single simple procedure and, ideally, not thereafter relying on the user's memory. Thus the 'default state' becomes one of staying contracepted, not conceiving! (At present, the two most common methods used by young people – the pill and the condom – have a completely wrong 'default state'.) For the twenty-first century, taking into account the story at the start of Chapter 2 the ideal has to be to switch off one's fertility at a certain time and then, maybe years later, to switch it on again (ideally oneself, without having to ask any provider to reverse it) when good and ready to conceive.
- *100% convenient*: including independent of intercourse.
- *100% reversible*: reversed very simply, ideally without having to ask permission or get help to stop the method.
- *100% safe*: without unwanted effects, whether fatal, dangerous or simply annoying.
- *Cheap and easy to distribute*.
- *Independent of the medical professions*: and no follow-up monitoring required.
- *Acceptable*: to every culture, religion and political view.
- *Used by or obviously visible to the woman* (whose stakes in effective contraception are obviously greatest): although an effective non-condom reversible male option would be welcome!

The ideal contraceptive must also have beneficial non-contraceptive side-effects. The most relevant in today's world has to be protection against STIs, including viruses. So far, this can only (outside of monogamy) be adequately provided by a condom (male or female) and many couples have to be advised to supplement their non-coitally related pregnancy-preventing method with a condom: the so-called 'double Dutch' approach.

Couples are almost always ignorant about established non-contraceptive benefits, such as less ovarian cancer with the pill or less blood-loss with the LNG-IUS. Because good news is not 'news', almost by definition, these advantages get no publicity.

1.16 How do the available reversible methods perform when tested against the list in Q 1.15?

Unfortunately, maximum effectiveness and independence from intercourse tend to go together and, also unfortunately, to be inversely linked with freedom from health risk. So, in practice, when counselling most couples, one can explain that there is always a dilemma, a bit of a 'Hobson's choice', as depicted in *Table 1.1*.

1.17 How is the effectiveness of any method commonly reported?

The data about efficacy, particularly of the non-medical methods, have shown extremely variable results. In clinical investigations an effort is usually made to make the (in practice very difficult) distinction between pregnancies that occurred despite the fact that the method was used correctly during every act of intercourse (method failures) and those that resulted from incorrect use or non-use on one or more occasions (user failures). This process results in estimates of the consistent use or method-effectiveness and of the actual use-effectiveness:

- Method-effectiveness rates vary because of physiological differences between individuals, notably increasing age, which diminishes fertility.
- Use-effectiveness is a function of the motivation of the study population, the acceptability of another baby, the adequacy of counselling, the difficulty of using the method, the effect of experience

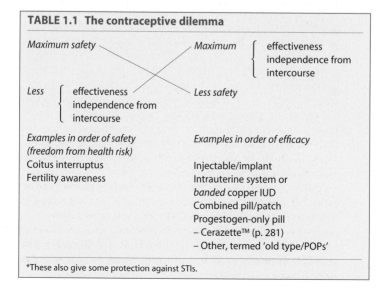

TABLE 1.1 The contraceptive dilemma

Maximum safety   *Maximum* { effectiveness / independence from intercourse

Less { effectiveness / independence from intercourse   *Less safety*

Examples in order of safety (freedom from health risk)	*Examples in order of efficacy*
Coitus interruptus	Injectable/implant
Fertility awareness	Intrauterine system or *banded* copper IUD
	Combined pill/patch
	Progestogen-only pill
	– Cerazette™ (p. 281)
	– Other, termed 'old type/POPs'

*These also give some protection against STIs.

through increasing duration of use, and other factors. Hence the findings are even more variable and it is very difficult to compare data from different studies among different populations.

■ Extended use-effectiveness is a measure of all the pregnancies occurring in a large population based on their initial intention to use a particular method. It includes individuals who abandon the method that they initially set out to use. Failure rates calculated on this basis tend to be very high indeed, even for a highly effective method such as the combined pill, because side-effects or anxiety about side-effects can lead to it being abandoned, without any effective replacement, in a large proportion of the initial users.

1.18 How are the effectiveness rates measured and expressed?

Both method- and use-effectiveness rates are usually expressed as failure rates/100 woman-years of exposure. The basis for many calculations is known as the Pearl pregnancy rate, calculated from the formula:

$$\text{Failure rate} = \frac{\text{Total accidental pregnancies} \times 1200}{\text{Total months of exposure}}$$

Every known conception must be included, whatever its outcome, when applying this formula. The figure 1200 is the number of months in 100 years. By convention, 10 months are deducted from the denominator for each full-term pregnancy and 4 months for any kind of abortion.

Trussell (of Princeton, USA) points out that the usual convention of using the same denominator (total number of months) whether the numerator is the number of method failures or user failures is wrong because it fails to account for the fact that many contraceptive users make errors and 'get away with it'. Any such method-failure rate is artificially lowered by the larger denominator. The true 'perfect use' (or 'consistent use') rate would use only the months of total compliance for the denominator. Very few studies, in which all users kept coital diaries, have had any chance of computing this true rate. Because errors in compliance are so common and vary so widely, and the likelihood of 'getting away with it' also varies, this means that standard method- and user-failure rates should ideally not be compared between populations. Yet in practice this is unavoidable (e.g. in preparing *Table 1.2*)

The risk of contraceptive failure tends to fall with the duration of use because of changes in the population under study, as women drop out for whatever reason. Long-term users obviously tend to be those who use the method efficiently and also include those of lower fertility (the more fertile ones are likely to leave the study by conceiving!) The life-table method of analysis is an attempt to overcome these problems. This takes into account all the reasons for contraceptive discontinuation, and permits the calculation of failure rates (or the rates for other events such as expulsion of an IUD) for specified intervals of use. The Pearl rate pools the data and can give only one common measurement, not compensating for drop-outs for varying reasons nor different durations of use in different studies.

1.19 What effectiveness rates can be quoted for potential users?

Vested interests (especially by advertisers) and the distinct lack of comparative studies – let alone randomized controlled trials – readily lead to misuse of the data on the effectiveness of particular techniques. Failure rates need to be interpreted by the provider to each potential user, in the context of the woman's age and factors such as the steadiness of the relationship and the frequency of intercourse (*Table 1.2*).

Note how modern intrauterine devices (IUDs) and the intrauterine system (IUS) have entirely comparable efficacy to female sterilization (*see Q 9.10*). Vasectomy is also clearly more effective than female sterilization, and injectables and implants beat the remainder (including the combined oral contraceptive [COC]) because of the user failure problem. Note the considerable overlaps: careful condom users have been known to do better than poor pill users. See also the important caveats in *Q 4.9* about the Oxford/Family Planning Association (FPA) study, which recruited an untypically good population as regards contraceptive compliance!

In interpreting *Table 1.2* to couples at counselling, it is sometimes helpful to divide 100 by the figures given for the rates. This calculation gives the number of years of regular intercourse, using the method carefully, which would be expected to lead to one conception. For example, if per 100 woman-year rates of 10 and 1 were being compared, the couple could be told that regular use of the method would give an 'evens' chance of one pregnancy by the end of 10 years or 100 years of fertility, respectively. This clearly shows the difference, although for a full understanding it is very important to add 'Of course, that one pregnancy could occur in the very first year, with betting odds of 1 in 10 or 1 in 100, respectively'.

1.20 Why is it that, as you say, most accidents are caused by humans and most humans are still caused by accidents? What can I as a prescriber do about this?

It is no good just blaming the method users. Prescribers can fail them in a number of ways, both by errors but more commonly by omissions, for example, simply not allowing enough time for basic instructions and for users to ask questions. 'You cannot make the horse drink' … but in the first place have we *properly* 'taken the horse to the water?' More on this follows in Chapter 11 (*see Qs 11.3–11.16*): we need first to be fully informed about the methods available.

Table 1.3 shows current usage of the methods in the UK.

TABLE 1.2 First-year user-failure rates/100 women for different methods of contraception

	Range in the world literature*	Oxford/FPA Study (Lancet report in 1982; all women married and aged above 25)		
		Overall (any duration)	Age 25–34 (≤2 years use)	Age 35+ (≤2 years use)
Sterilization				
Male (after azoospermia)	0–0.1	0.02	0.08	0.08
Female (Filshie clip)	0–0.5	0.13	0.45	0.08
Subcutaneous implant				
Jadelle™	0–0.1	–	–	–
Implanon™	0–0.07	–	–	–
Injectable (DMPA)	0–1	–	–	–
Combined pills				
50 µg oestrogen	0.1–3	0.16	0.25	0.17
<50 µg oestrogen	0.2–3	0.27	0.38	0.23
EVRA™ patch	0.6–0.9	–	–	–
Cerazette™ progestogen-only pill	0.7–1.1	–	–	–
Old-type POP	0.3–4	1.2	2.5	0.5
IUD (see Q9.10)				
Levonorgestrel intrauterine system (IUS)	0–0.6	–	–	–
T-SafeCu 380A™	0.3–0.8	–	–	–
GyneFIX™	0.1–1.2	–	–	–
Other >300 mm copper IUDs (Nova-T 380™, Multiload 375™, Flexi-T 300™	0.2–1.5	–	–	–
Male condom	2–15	3.6	6.0	2.9
Female condom	5–15	–	–	–

TABLE 1.2—cont'd

	Range in the world literature*	Oxford/FPA Study (Lancet report in 1982; all women married and aged above 25)		
		Overall (any duration)	Age 25–34 (≤2 years use)	Age 35+ (≤2 years use)
Diaphragm (all caps believed similar, not all tested)	6–20	1.9	5.5	2.8
Coitus interruptus	4–19	6.7	–	–
Spermicides alone	4–25	11.9	–	–
Fertility awareness	2–20	15.5	–	–
'Persona'™	6–?	–	–	–
No method, young women	80–90	–	–	–
No method at age 40	40–50	–	–	–
No method at age 45	10–20	–	–	–
No method at age 50 (if still having menses)	0–5	–	–	–

*Excludes atypical studies and all extended-use studies. For sterilization the rates in first column are estimated lifetime failure rates.

Note:
1. First figure of range in first column gives a rough measure of 'consistent use', formerly calculated as 'method-failure' rates.
2. Influence of age: all the rates in the fourth column being lower than those in the third column. Lower rates still may be expected above age 45.
3. Much better results also obtainable in other states of relative infertility, such as lactation.
4. Oxford/FPA users were established users at recruitment – greatly improving results for barrier methods (see text Qs 1.19 and 4.9).
5. The Implanon™, Cerazette™ and EVRA™ results are different. They come from pre-marketing studies in each case, giving an estimate of the Pearl 'method-failure' rate and the upper bound of the 95% confidence interval. The rates for these three products are for cautious use, a 'handle' on what consistent users might expect to achieve.

TABLE 1.3 Current use of contraception by age. From the Omnibus Survey of the Office for National Statistics – of representative adults from a random probability sample of households, surveyed between June 2001 and March 2002

Current use of contraception	Age 16–17	18–19	20–24	25–29	30–34	35–39	40–44	45–49	All 2001/02	Compare with: 1997/98
	%	%	%	%	%	%	%	%	%	%
Non-surgical										
Pill*	42	56	51	44	33	19	11	4	28	26
Minipill	4	7	6	10	6	4	6	2	5	5
Combined pill	30	43	41	31	25	13	5	2	21	19
Male condom	40	35	29	23	22	17	17	11	21	21
Withdrawal	1	–	6	4	4	4	4	2	4	4
IUD	–	–	2	3	4	5	4	3	3	4
Injection/implant	–	8	7	7	4	1	1	1	3	2
Safe period/rhythm method/Persona™	–	0	0	1	3	2	1	1	2	2
Cap/diaphragm	–	–	–	0	1	1	1	1	1	2
Foams/gels	–	–	–	–	–	0	–	–	0	0
Hormonal IUS	–	0	–	0	1	1	1	0	1	0
Female condom	–	–	0	–	0	–	–	–	0	0
Emergency contraception[†]	–	–	3	1	1	1	–	0	1	0
Total at least one method non-surgical	61	69	72	72	63	47	38	23	53	52
Surgical										
Sterilized	–	–	1	4	7	13	19	20	10	11
Partner sterilized	–	–	1	2	7	19	25	24	12	10

TABLE 1.3—cont'd

Current use of contraception	Age 16–17	18–19	20–24	25–29	30–34	35–39	40–44	45–49	All 2001/02	Compare with: 1997/98
Total at least one method	61	69	73	79	77	79	82	67	**75**	74
Not using a method										
No heterosexual relationship**	39	25	20	10	10	10	6	11	13	14
Sterile after another operation	–	–	1	2	2	3	5	9	3	4
Wants to get pregnant	–	1	0	4	5	3	1	–	2	2
Pregnant now	–	5	3	3	3	1	–	–	1	2
Going without sex to avoid pregnancy	1	1	0	0	–	0	0	1	0	1
Unlikely to conceive because of menopause	–	–	–	–	–	–	–	6	1	1
Possibly infertile	–	–	1	0	1	2	3	3	2	1
Doesn't like contraception	–	–	0	1	1	0	1	0	0	0
Other reason	–	–	1	2	2	2	2	3	2	0
Total not using a method	**39**	**31**	**27**	**21**	**23**	**21**	**18**	**33**	**25**	**26**
Base***	71	129	230	270	366	364	322	316	2068	3357

In each column, – means zero respondents and 0 means less than 0.5%. Other percentages are rounded to nearest integer.

*Includes women who did not know the type of pill used.

†Category included for the first time in the 2000/01 questionnaire.

**In 2001/02 this category was changed to 'No method used – no sexual relationship with someone of the opposite sex', prior to this the category was 'No method used – no sexual relationship'.

***Percentages sum to more than 100 as respondents could give more than one answer.

Aspects of human fertility and fertility awareness: natural birth control

2

Apparently, after God created Adam, He said to him: 'I have some news for you: two bits of good news and one bit of bad news. Which would you like to hear first?' And Adam said, 'The good news first please, God.' So God said to Adam: 'The first good news is that I am going to create for you an Organ. This Organ is called the Brain. With this gift of mine you will be able to think, and to learn, and to feel – and if you use it well you will be a good steward of all my other creatures.'

'Thank you very much', said Adam. 'What's the other good news?'

'Well', said God, 'I am going to create for you another Organ. This Organ is called the Penis. With it you will be able to give to your wife and receive back from her, much pleasure – and with my help create children to follow you, and so you will be fruitful and multiply.'

'Thank you again', said Adam. 'So, what's the bad news?'

'You will never be able to use both at the same time', said God.

BACKGROUND CONSIDERATIONS

2.1 How fertile are human beings?

Given the disjunction between brain and genitalia (in both sexes, although men are undoubtedly the worse affected …) both the devising and the practising of effective contraception are difficult (*see* Q 1.15)! We break no records in the animal kingdom but we are fertile enough to become – numerically – far and away the most successful vertebrate that this planet has ever known.

The first half of this chapter deals with physiological factors that promote conception. We first consider aspects relating to intercourse, then the sperm, the ova, fertilization and implantation.

We can at least be grateful that the fertility of average couples is not as great as the human maximum, which must have been approached by the couple described in the *Guinness book of records*:

The greatest officially recorded number of children produced by a mother is 69 by the first of the two wives of Feodor Vasilyev (b. 1707), a peasant from Shuya, 241 km east of Moscow. In 27 confinements, she gave birth to 16 pairs of twins, 7 sets of triplets and 4 sets of quadruplets. … Almost all survived to their majority.

2.2 What features of human intercourse are particularly favourable to fertility?

1 The attraction between a man and a woman is frequently powerful and mutual, and the human female is exceptional in having no breeding season and in being potentially receptive on most days of the cycle.

2 Some indication of the power of the human sex instinct is provided by the calculation (never mind the assumptions) by the World Health Organization (WHO), in the early 1990s, that intercourse takes place about 42 000 million times per year. This worked out, somewhere in the world, to over 1300 ejaculations per second … and even more by now.

3   The drive towards copulation in both sexes is in 'real-time' – now – and feels irresistible. This frustrates forward planning and the successful use of intercourse-related methods of contraception. And men are the worst culprits – they omit to tell their partners important nuisance details (e.g. that the condom split!) and sometimes tell the most flagrant lies (whether about their undying love or their HIV status).

4   Some women report that maximum desire coincides with the most fertile phase, when there is an abundance of oestrogenic mucus, which is very favourable to sperm survival; whereas minimum desire is often in the premenstrual 'safe' phase.

5   The outpouring of vaginal transudate described by Masters and Johnson raises the pH of the vagina so that it becomes favourable to sperm.

6   There is evidence that, at least in some women, there is a negative pressure in the uterus at orgasm. This might (though never proved) promote physical aspiration of sperm into the cervix and uterus. Sperm are certainly found in the cervix within 90 s of ejaculation.

2.3   How do the mechanics of intercourse interfere with the efficacy of vaginal methods of contraception?

1   The ballooning of the whole upper two-thirds of the vagina, also described by Masters and Johnson, leads to:
   (a)   an increased risk of sperm passing over the rim of a diaphragm or other cervical cap
   (b)   the risk of displacement of any cervical device into a fornix.

2   The penile thrusts themselves lead to:
   (a)   the potential to dislodge all forms of female barrier, particularly in certain positions of intercourse
   (b)   if a vaginal spermicide is used, it is probable that the spreading effect of intercourse means that there is ultimately too little spermicide around the external os of the cervix at ejaculation. This might in part explain how spermicides have usually appeared far more effective in vitro than in vivo (*see* Q 4.63).

2.4   What are the relevant facts about cervical mucus?

Cervical mucus is only the most obvious component of the genital tract mucus and fluid, which extend right through the cavity of the uterus and both tubes. Under the influence of unopposed oestrogen in the follicular phase it becomes increasingly fluid and receptive to sperm, with a marked Spinnbarkeit. It helps to capacitate sperm and provides an optimum environment for them to proceed to the upper tract. The ability to promote sperm survival for prolonged durations varies from woman to woman and from cycle to cycle, as does the length of time within the cycle that ovulatory mucus is present.

The characteristics of mucus change abruptly under the influence of progesterone, even though the corpus luteum continues to secrete oestrogens. The mucus rapidly becomes impenetrable and hostile to sperm. Women can be taught to feel the change from the earlier, slippery 'ovulatory' mucus to the sticky mucus of the luteal phase. But before ovulation, WHO (1983) found 'a substantial' probability of pregnancy if intercourse occurs (even) in the presence of sticky mucus.

2.5 What other changes occur at the cervix during the cycle?

Continuing research into birth planning by methods of fertility awareness has shown that women can be taught to detect the changes occurring in the size of the external cervical os, and also in its position relative to the introitus. The cervix starts low and feels firm, then rises appreciably during the follicular phase, until around ovulation it reaches peak height from the introitus with maximum softness and sufficient dilation to admit a finger tip. The cervix then descends and narrows rapidly early in the luteal phase, becoming once more closed, firm and closer to the vulva. It is reported that daily autopalpation of these cervical changes can assist in the detection of the return of fertility towards the end of lactation (*see Q 3.36*).

2.6 What are the most important physiological facts about sperm that promote conception?

All of us whose work involves family planning rapidly develop an enormous respect for these little swimmers! There is great individual variation between men, and between individual sperm within the same man's ejaculate. Sperm counts and quality have fallen in some areas, attributed to oestrogenic chemical pollutants in the environment: is Nature biting back, against the species that is multiplying like there were no tomorrow? (*see Chapter 1*).

Yet there is still an overkill of numbers produced by most men. From the point of view of preventing pregnancy we have to consider the very best sperm with regard to motility, survival and fertilizing ability, rather than those exhibiting average or lesser qualities.

2.7 How many sperm are present, and what are the implications?

Spermatogenesis proceeds in normal men at rates of the order of 1000 per second from each testicle! With a count of say 80 million/mL being not unrepresentative, it would not be unusual for there to be 350 million sperm in the 3–5 mL of a typical ejaculate. If each sperm could find an egg this would be enough to populate most of North America! One per cent of this number (enough to people Costa Rica or New Zealand) might very well cause a pregnancy (*see Q 2.9*). Yet this would be contained in the hardly visible volume of less than 0.05 mL. This has obvious implications for coitus interruptus (*see Q 3.7*) and also for any lack of care when using the condom (*see Q 3.20*). In contraceptive terms, semen is a dangerous fluid!

2.8   What is the extreme limit of sperm survival in genital tract mucus, and what are the implications?

This has proved very difficult to study directly because the studies themselves are liable to alter what is being observed. It seems clear that sperm *normally* survive no more than about 6 h in the vagina, because its pH reverts to its normal low value after intercourse. However, motile sperm have been found even in the vagina up to 16 h after intercourse and survival in the cervical, uterine and tubal fluid appears very variable. Survival depends on features of the sperm themselves, the seminal fluid and to what degree the oestrogenic mucus approaches the ideal – in that woman or in that particular cycle.

In the past, most authorities talked in terms of average survival times of about 3–4 days. However, with so many millions ejaculated one must be concerned not with average sperm survival but 'lunatic fringe' sperm survival! It is the duration of the ability to fertilize of the first centile of the sperm (i.e. the most vigorous 3 million or so) that is the relevant figure. This is not known but direct and indirect studies suggest that this can certainly exceed 6 days. On some rare occasions in some rare couples, particularly where the woman produces good mucus for an unusually long time, it might even reach 7 days. Mucus assessment (*see Qs 2.4 and 2.25*) should theoretically give more advance warning of ovulation than usual in those very cases, but it can fail to do so.

The main implication is the likely ineffectiveness, in long-term use by most couples, of the *first* phase of the so-called 'safe period' (*see Q 2.17*).

2.9   How can it be that 1% of a man's ejaculate (i.e. about 3 million sperm) could cause a pregnancy, when men with that number of sperm/mL are usually infertile?

This question implies a common misunderstanding of the nature of semen analysis in an infertility clinic. For a start, an excessively high count can actually be associated with male subfertility. Also, when there is a low count this might be acting as a marker for other much more important features of the sperm that are causing the subfertility, such as poor motility, frequent abnormal forms or the presence of antibodies. Paucity of sperm tends to go along with them being pretty poor individuals and this does not apply when 3 million good sperm from a fertile man are deposited at the cervix.

Evidence for the above comes from routine sperm counts in men having vasectomies who have fathered children. Counts less than 2 million/mL are not uncommon; and in a study of late recanalization reported from Oxford, it appeared that a man with counts of only 500 000 and 750 000/mL (with motility demonstrated) was responsible for his wife's pregnancy.

2.10   What are the relevant physiological facts about ova?

1   More often than expected by many couples, ovulation occurs early. Many women claiming 28-day menstrual cycles really sometimes have 26-day cycles, and some can feature fertile cycles as short as 21 or 22 days in length (*see* Q 2.15 for the implications).

2   Ovum fertilizability is short – practically the only physiological fact so far discussed that helps contraception. From in vitro fertilization research, maximum ovum survival is believed to be 24 h but successful fertilization appears to be unlikely beyond 12 h. This means that if a pregnancy is desired, the best chance of successful fertilization is when that fragile ovum arrives at a tube that is already populated with adequate numbers of vigorous, motile sperm.

2.11   Can human females be like rabbits, ovulating on intercourse?

I think the answer to this question, which is often asked, can (fortunately) be a fairly definite 'no'. First, there is no need to postulate any such mechanism when one adds together the data mentioned above concerning sperm survival and the frequent occurrence of ovulation earlier than usual. Intercourse can be fertile almost any time, not excluding during the menses, if sperm can survive for up to 7 days and ovulation can be unexpectedly early or late.

A second and more important reason for rejecting this hypothesis is the fact that, were it to be true, newly married women would have shorter menstrual cycles than women who were abstaining from intercourse (such as nuns). Such a shortening of the mean duration of menstrual cycles has not been observed.

2.12   After fertilization, how much preimplantation wastage occurs?

Here we have another fact that, fortunately, reduces the size of the contraceptive task. Assessments of postfertilization wastage vary considerably but a good modern estimate would be around 30–40%. There are frequently chromosomal abnormalities but local factors affecting the receptivity of the endometrium to the blastocyst are also important. These can be enhanced by contraceptive methods (*see* Q 10.7).

2.13 Putting the above physiological facts together, how long is the fertile window in each cycle?

First, forget the traditional myth that this is mid-cycle! Recent in vivo and in vitro studies, which form the basis of the physiology described in the last ten questions, clearly indicate that the fertile phase both starts and finishes earlier and is also longer than is often assumed. The latest work would imply that, under optimal conditions for sperm survival, the potentially fertile phase is not less than days 7–14 (i.e. the whole of the second week of a 4-week cycle). If ovulation takes place on day 14–15 a further 1-plus days needs to be added to allow for maximum ovum survival, i.e. in all there is a potential fertile window from day 7 to day 15 of a hypothetical, normal cycle. Given that the luteal phase is relatively fixed, such that ovulation occurs 12–16 days before the next menses starts, the start day of the fertile window alters if the cycle is longer or shorter than 28 days.

2.14 How was the Barrett and Marshall study designed? What is the risk of conception on each day of the cycle (*Fig. 2.1*)?

In brief, 241 previously fertile women who had been fully trained to keep basal body temperature (BBT) charts also kept a careful record of every act of intercourse. Whether conception took place in a given cycle was also known. Some were attempting to conceive, others to avoid pregnancy. All the data on 1898 cycles and 6015 acts of coitus were fed into a computer and, for each woman, the day of BBT shift, and hence presumed ovulation, was identified in a standard way for that cycle.

The analysis gave figures for the percentage risk of conception for intercourse on each day of the cycle relative to the BBT shift, and these have been charted to produce *Fig. 2.1* (in which 0 represents the BBT shift). The continuous line joins the points for which the data were sufficient for an estimate of percentage risk of conception to be made; the dotted lines are approximate projections down to the horizontal axis.

2.15 What are the main observations from *Fig. 2.1*?

1 As just shown, the fertile window, when percentage risk of conception exceeds 0%, lasts in many fertile cycles for at least 8 days, 7 of which precede the moment of ovulation – as predicted from sperm and ovum survival studies (*see* Q 2.13). Recent work by Wilcox et al (published in the *New England Journal of Medicine* in 1998), suggests a slightly

Fig. 2.1 The risk of conception on different days of the menstrual cycle. Q2.1 (based on data from Barrett and Marshall (1969), redrawn from Population Studies 1969 23:455–461, Table 2). See also Qs 2.14–2.16.

shorter fertile window of 7 days but I prefer to retain the 1 day's extra margin. The congruence of this recent work with that of Barrett and Marshall in 1969 is remarkable.

2   Peak fecundability occurs well before ovum release, again congruent with the notion that it is best for the sperm to be waiting in the tubes in advance of ovulation.

3   The first 'infertile' phase of the cycle is shown to be short, even in a woman who never ovulates earlier than day 14. As it is well known that very many women do occasionally ovulate earlier in the cycle, in a 24-day cycle intercourse any later than day 3 might, on the basis of these data, sometimes result in conception!

4   The good news from *Fig. 2.1* is that the second phase is potentially a very 'safe period', dependent only on the reliability of ovulation detection. There is, normally, only one ovum and it is fertilizable for a predictable, short time. This is quite unlike the first phase, which is beset by problems: the millions of sperm, the capriciousness with which enough of them might just survive on occasion for as much as a week, coupled with the possibility of a random, early ovulation. So far, no means have been devised of predicting ovulation accurately, far enough ahead, to eliminate the risk of sperm survival up to the point of fertilization.

2.16 And when in any given cycle will the fertile window occur?

In practice, no one knows – outside of research situations. Even women who believe they have 'regular cycles' can produce much shorter or longer ones 'out of the blue', perhaps every 2 years or so. Given the variability of the day of ovulation that this implies (14 ± 2 days before the unknown first day of the next menses), women need to understand that the 8-day fertile window can therefore 'move': it might start unpredictably even before the last days of a period, or contrariwise involve the whole of the third week should it be going to be a 5-week cycle.

Ideally, school sex and relationships education (SRE) should routinely include these 'new' facts. And clinicians need to note the implication that emergency contraception can rarely be refused because the exposure day was one of 'zero conception risk'.

2.17 How does the variable onset of the fertile window influence the efficacy of the two infertile phases identified in natural family planning (NFP)?

In my view, with any combination of present technologies, all users of natural family planning (NFP) ought to be informed that the second infertile phase is the more effective of the two. Good results can be obtained by optimally trained and motivated couples when both phases are used. But, in my view, a woman who feels that she must avoid pregnancy should have otherwise unprotected sex only in the postovulatory phase. The first phase is primarily suitable for those who are delaying a wanted pregnancy ('spacing'). The one exception to this recommendation might be a woman with very regular longish menstrual cycles (never less than 28 days) who is good at detecting mucus and cervical changes. She should abstain in each cycle from the first day of detection of mucus or from 21 days before her shortest cycle would end, whichever comes earlier, to identify the first potentially fertile day (*see Q 2.18*).

However, the capriciousness of sperm survival under occasional optimal conditions still means that, whatever methodology based on fertility awareness is used, the preovulatory phase will always be 'in a different ball-park' of potential efficacy than the postovulatory phase.

2.18 Why have family planning specialists traditionally decried NFP methods? What should be their attitude now?

The bad reputation of these methods followed from the high failure rate of the old calendar/rhythm approach, coupled with a lack of awareness of the fundamental difference in effectiveness potential between the first and the second infertile phases, however they might be determined. That lack of awareness is still common today among both the opponents and the proponents of the methods.

The correct attitude today should be a very positive one to this choice for couples, with accurate information and advice about the appropriateness of the choice in each case. The website *www.fertilityuk.org* is invaluable educationally and – along with the UK FPA – also provides the names of local NFP teachers for potential NFP users.

2.19 Although not recommended as the sole method, what calculations are required for the calendar/rhythm method?

1 The woman should define the shortest and longest menstrual cycle over the previous six (preferably 12) cycles.

2 She should subtract (preferably) 21 days from the length of the shortest cycle to derive the first day of the fertile phase. This allows 14, 15 or 16 days for the length of the luteal phase plus 7, 6 or 5 days for maximum sperm survival. Sadly, although this is more cautious by one day than the 20 days advised in standard NFP teaching, in any particular cycle these durations might come to more than 21 days! But in the identification of the start of the fertile phase, this particular calculation is an important additional safeguard (to the first appearance of any mucus, *see Q 2.24*).

3 Subtract 10 from the longest cycle observed to derive the last day of the fertile phase, so allowing 11 days for minimum length of a fertile luteal phase and 1 day for the duration of ovum fertilizability.

Even with good compliance this method has a high failure rate. Compliance is also difficult, because few women have regular menstrual cycles so the amount of abstinence required becomes intolerable to many couples. The 'Standard Days' method (*see Q 2.38*) shortens this abstinence time at the price of a higher failure rate.

2.20 How are the phases of the fertility cycle defined (*Fig. 2.2*)?

1 The first infertile phase starts on day 1 of the menses and ends with the earliest time that any sperm could survive to cause a pregnancy. It varies in length, depending on the rapidity of the follicular response to the pituitary hormones.

2 The true fertile phase (or fertile window) extends from the end of phase 1 until that time following ovulation when the ovum is incapable of being fertilized. Its duration is therefore the sum of the maximum number of days of sperm survival (say 7 days) and the maximum duration of fertilizability of the ovum (say 24 h). In practice, the identified fertile phase tends to be longer than this, because the clinical indicators of fertility are not 100% accurate.

3   The second infertile phase extends from the end of the fertile phase until the onset of the next menstruation. This phase has a mean duration of 13 days with a range, in likely fertile cycles, of about 11–15 days. It is often called the 'absolute' infertile phase because significantly delayed superovulation 'never' occurs in the human. (If two or more eggs are released this is believed to be nearly always within the same 24 h.) Provided ovulation is accurately determined and sufficient time is allowed for the ovum to succumb, conception is close to impossible in this phase.

2.21 How can the phases be determined, in practice?

We must distinguish carefully between:

1   The biological events that delineate the phases – these are clear-cut and defined in Q 2.20. But they are not the same as:
2   The biological indicators of the events, which can be further classified into:

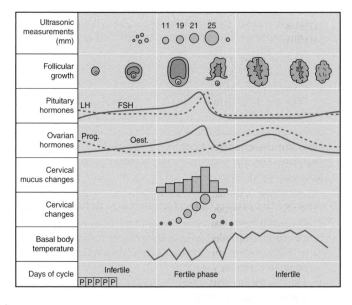

Fig. 2.2 The relationship during the cycle of serial ultrasound measurements, hormonal control and clinical indicators of fertility. Q 2.20 (reproduced courtesy of the late Dr A. Flynn, Birmingham Maternity Hospital, Queen Elizabeth Medical Centre, Birmingham). See also Q 2.19.

(a) biophysical methods (e.g. serial ultrasonic monitoring of follicular growth, changes in vaginal, ovarian or hand blood flow, etc.)
(b) biochemical methods, which detect the change in concentration of the sex steroids or their metabolites in body fluids such as urine or saliva
(c) clinical indicators, such as BBT, mucus and cervical changes. The accuracy of these indicators of the events at (1) varies, and must also be distinguished from:
3 The quality of the teaching of the couple, which result in the woman and her partner accurately detecting the indicator. And finally, after detection and recording of the indicator, we have to consider:
4 The compliance of the woman and of her partner, which is a problem with **all** methods with 'user' involvement.

The importance of (3) and (4) was well shown in a celebrated study, which apparently showed that the pregnancy rate was higher when charts of clinical indicators were interpreted by the woman's husband than when the woman decided when it was 'safe' to have intercourse!

2.22 What are the major clinical (patient-identifiable) indicators of fertility?

1 Changes in the cervical mucus (*see Qs 2.4 and 2.24*).
2 Changes involving the cervix itself (*see Q 2.5*).
3 Changes in the BBT (*see Q 2.23*).
4 With the aid of technology, other indicators in body fluids (e.g. Persona™)

2.23 How are the changes in the BBT used?

The biphasic nature of the temperature cycle is caused by metabolites of progesterone, hence this can only be used to detect the onset of the second infertile phase. A woman must measure her temperature under basal conditions after a period of sleep, without getting out of bed, having a drink or smoking a cigarette. The shift of temperature is small (0.2–0.4°C), hence a special expanded-scale mercury thermometer should be used or, better still a modern, direct-reading, electronic version. The temperature may be taken orally or vaginally or in the auditory meatus, sticking to the same orifice for any given cycle.

The results are plotted daily on a special chart. To detect the shift a cover line is drawn 0.05°C over the lower phase temperatures, of which there should be a minimum of six. The second infertile phase is held to begin on the morning of the third consecutive high temperature after the temperature shift; each being a minimum of 0.2°C higher than those six earlier temperatures, covered by the line drawn as just described.

2.24 What are the difficulties of BBT assessment?

Some women have problems with using and reading thermometers, and with keeping interpretable charts. All should be taught to identify factors such as mild infection or drugs which can misleadingly raise the temperature prematurely before ovulation in what is actually going to be a relatively long cycle.

2.25 How are the mucus changes used to detect the fertile and infertile phases?

At every micturition the woman is instructed to observe the quantity, colour, fluidity, glossiness, transparency and stretchiness of the mucus. The most fertile characteristics of the mucus over the entire day are charted each night. The woman fills in either a colour (green for dry, yellow for mucus and red for bleeding) or writes in a description of the mucus seen.

The peak mucus day can only be identified retrospectively, and corresponds closely with the peak secretion of oestrogen in the blood. This is the last day during which the mucus is clear, wet, slippery and with an elastic quality allowing it to be stretched for several centimetres before it breaks, like raw egg white. After ovulation, the rise in progesterone causes – within a day – a profound change in the amount and characteristics of the mucus. If present at all it resembles the opaque, sticky and tacky postmenstrual type. The peak mucus day can hence be identified. Allowing 2–3 days for ovulation to be completed and 1 day for ovum fertilizability, the second infertile phase is defined as beginning on the evening of the *fourth* day after the peak mucus symptom.

Changes in the cervix itself (*see Q 2.5*) can be used to check on the other indicators, although this is not essential.

2.26 What practical problems can confuse mucus assessment?

1 The most frequent is the effect of intercourse, or of sexual excitement without intercourse. Both the fluid of sexual arousal and semen can mimic the sensations and the features of ovulatory mucus. Careful teaching can help the woman to distinguish the latter but if in doubt she should presume possible fertility. Unprotected intercourse is usually only allowed on alternate days to allow mucus assessment. To identify the first potentially fertile day, the calculation at *Q 2.19* (shortest cycle less 20, or better, 21) must have priority over mucus observations. WHO (1983) has reported that in almost 20% of cycles no mucus at all was observed at the vulva until 3 days or less before the peak day. Therefore mucus of any type must equate to potential fertility: sticky mucus is not reliably 'infertile'.

2 Spermicidal jellies and lubricants can similarly cause confusion, particularly if the diaphragm is used during the fertile phase.
3 Mucus assessment is impossible during bleeding – a problem in some short menstrual cycles.
4 Vaginal infections and discharges can cause difficulty, notably thrush and its treatments, which tend to 'dry' the mucus.

2.27 What are the minor clinical indicators of fertility?

These tend to be specific to individual women or to occur only in some ovulatory cycles. When present they can be helpful in confirming the major signals. Among them are:

1 Ovulation pain (Mittelschmerz): ultrasound scan studies show that this regular unilateral (rarely bilateral) pain occurs 24–48 h before ovulation, not at the event itself. It is probably caused as the ovarian tissue is stretched by the rapidly growing follicle.
2 A midcycle 'show' of blood.
3 The onset of breast symptoms, acne and other skin changes, and variations in mood and sexual desire.

The second infertile phase can be held to start 5 days after Mittelschmerz ends, provided this matches the findings on a woman's temperature/mucus chart (*see Q 2.28*).

2.28 Combining indicators is obviously more effective, but what should be done if different clinical indicators give variable results?

Basically, go on the latest result. So, when identifying the second phase, for example, the woman should be instructed to act only on the *latest* of the signals being used. For example, if peak mucus plus 4 days would suggest that intercourse was 'safe' on a Thursday evening, but only two higher temperatures had been recorded, intercourse would be deferred until the third higher temperature was recorded the following (Friday) morning.

For those who are 'spacing' rather than limiting pregnancy, and therefore wish to rely on both infertile phases, the following summary rule is helpful:

■ The fertile time starts 20 or 21 days before the woman's shortest cycle would end or earlier when any secretions are detected
■ It ends after at least three higher temperatures have been recorded all *after* the peak mucus day.

2.29 What about Persona™ – the Unipath Personal Contraceptive System?

Charting mucus and temperatures and other symptoms is obviously rather a hassle. Persona™ is an innovative product, first marketed in 1996, consisting of a series of disposable test sticks and a hand-held computerized monitor. As instructed by a yellow light on the monitor, the test sticks are dipped in the user's early morning urine samples and transferred to a slot in the device. There the levels of both estrone-3-glucuronide (E-3-G) and luteinizing hormone (LH) are measured by a patented immunochromatographic assay, utilizing an optical monitor (*Fig. 2.3*). As soon as the first significant rise in the E-3-G level is detected the fertility status is changed to 'unsafe' and a red light replaces the green one on the monitor. After subsequent detection of the first significant rise of LH, the end of the fertile period is not signalled by a green light until four further days have elapsed, to allow for the time to ovulation and then demise of the ovum.

The system initially requests 16 tests in the first cycle, dropping to eight thereafter. Utilizing data on the individual's previous six menstrual cycles as well as the current one, it is sensitive to cyclical changes so that the number of 'red' days varies. In the first few months there are typically 12–15 red days, falling later (according to the manufacturer's brochure) to as low as 6 to 10 days among users with the most regular cycles but rising if urine tests are missed or subsequent to an unusually long or short cycle.

▲

Fig. 2.3 Persona™ (Unipath Personal Contraceptive System). Q 2.29 (from Kubba et al 1999 *Contraception and office gynecoloogy: choices in reproductive healthcare* p. 45. London, WB Saunders. With permission).

Given the facts about potential sperm survival (*see Q 2.8*), the group given only six infertile days must include those at a higher risk of follicular-phase method failures (*see also Qs 2.30 and 2.31*).

2.30 Who can use Persona™? And what are the short- and long-term contraindications?

Persona™ is usable if cycle lengths are between 23 and 35 days, and can accommodate variations of up to 10 days within this range. It should not be used:

1. if the woman has experienced menopausal (vasomotor) symptoms
2. while breastfeeding or soon after childbirth
3. after recent use of any hormonal contraception, including all pills and injectables
4. during a cycle in which tetracycline is used (itself, *not* any of its relatives, e.g. doxycycline) as this can result in an enhancement of the LH signal from the urine.

If numbers (2) and (3) apply (including a single use of hormonal emergency contraception), the user is advised to wait for two natural consecutive cycles, each of 23–35 days, and initiate use of Persona™ only when the third menses start.

The main contraindication, of course, relates to suitability of the method to the lifestyle of the couple, and often too little thought is given to the man's views. If he is going to come home drunk on a Saturday night and (maybe only metaphorically) kick the Persona™ across the bedroom whatever light it shows, this is hardly the right method! Much attention also needs to be paid to explaining its known failure rate even with correct use (*see Q 2.31*).

2.31 What is the failure rate of Persona™ as currently marketed?

Efficacy information from the European trials by the manufacturer suggests a first-year failure rate in consistent users of around 6 per 100 woman-years. This is a best estimate, and is thought by Trussell (*Q 1.18*) to be optimistic, for 'perfect use' of Persona™.

The best results using multiple-index fertility awareness are as good, so the main advantage of this device is that of user-friendliness. However, this failure rate is considerably higher than would be acceptable to those accustomed to the efficacy of the injectable or even the COC. The device usually signals a shorter fertile period than the 10–12 days' abstinence typically demanded by the multiple index methods.

Couples should be reminded that they might well themselves be among the (at least) 6% in whom the method fails, and that this equates to a 1 in 17 chance of pregnancy in the next year.

2.32   What if that 1 in 17 risk of conception is not acceptable?

Then there is a useful combination option. Indeed, in my opinion this should always have been on offer – it should have been described in the instructions with this product. Given the higher in-built risk of intercourse before ovulation (because of those capricious sperm! *see Qs 2.8 and 2.16*), I recommend the following combination method, for a monogamous couple wanting high efficacy:

- from day 1 until the red light first appears: *use condoms*
- throughout the 'red' phase: *abstain*
- after the second 'green' phase starts: *unprotected sex.*

I would confidently give a low failure rate of 1–3% if this advice were followed accurately; and the scientists involved in the testing of Persona™ confirm that this was achieved in the trials by those who relied solely on the second 'green' phase.

EFFECTIVENESS

2.33   What is the efficacy of multiple-index NFP or Persona™?

If the second infertile phase only is relied on, provided during the fertile phase there is complete abstinence (*NOT* condom use, because condoms are often used inadequately!), highly acceptable method-failure rates of 1–3/100 woman-years are easily obtainable. In fairness, it should be reported that similar excellent method-failure rates have sometimes been reported for the use of multiple-index methods even where intercourse has been permitted in the first, preovulatory, phase. This is partly because the most highly fertile couples tend to drop out of, or never enter, the studied population. And as Trussell (*see Q 1.18*) has also pointed out, rates as low as 1–3/100 woman-years are not relevant for average potential users of NFP; there is no doubt that it is extremely unforgiving of less-than-perfect use, which – let's face it – is *normal* use of any method for most normal people. (Contrast the pill: most people forget pills from time to time but the difference is that they are much more likely to get away with it.)

ADVANTAGES AND INDICATIONS

2.34   What are the advantages of methods based on fertility awareness?

1   First and foremost, they are completely free from any known physical side-effects for the user.
2   They are acceptable to many with certain religious and cultural views, not only Roman Catholics. According to strict interpretations, they are

used rightly when the intention is family spacing, with the possibility of conceiving retained.

3   The methods are under the couple's personal control (abstinence is always available!).

4   The methods readily lend themselves, if the couple's scruples permit, to the additional use of an artificial method such as a barrier at the potentially fertile times – always with acceptance of that method's failure rate, which is always higher than abstinence!

5   Once established as efficient users, after proper teaching, no further expensive follow-up of the couple is necessary.

6   Understanding of the methods can help any couple, with or without any subfertility, when they come to try to conceive.

PROBLEMS AND DISADVANTAGES

2.35 What are the problems of natural family planning methods?

1   Interestingly enough, the majority of established users believe the method is helpful to their marriage/relationship, rather than a cause of stress – but conflicts and frustrations are also reported.

2   Several studies, including the 1993 WHO study, have shown no hint of an increase in the incidence of birth defects among failures, due to ageing gametes, and this postulated risk can now be discounted.

BREASTFEEDING AS NATURAL BIRTH CONTROL

2.36 Can fertility awareness predict the return of fertility after lactation?

Full breastfeeding, in which the baby takes no fluids other than from its mother, is a highly efficient natural contraceptive. The most important factor is the frequency and duration of suckling. In practice, therefore, the return of fertility is a prolonged process, during which spurious attempts at follicular growth and ovulation occur over weeks or months before actual ovulation. Moreover, the first ovulation often antedates the first vaginal bleed. The cervical mucus pattern at this time is not always sufficient to help the woman distinguish false alarms from genuine ovulation. If artificial contraception is acceptable to her, she will simply have to begin to use it from the very first mucus sign of ovarian follicular activity.

For those who wish to continue the natural methods, workers in Birmingham have found that marked changes in the cervix (i.e. softening in consistency, widening of the external os and elevation of position) occur only in the days immediately preceding the first true ovulation. The reliability of the cervix as an additional indicator at this time requires further testing (see Q 2.5).

See *Q 11.53* for the problems of identifying the infrequent ovulations of women approaching the menopause.

2.37 Can breastfeeding (lactational amenorrhoea method, LAM) alone be a satisfactory method?

Very much so, and no method could be more natural. A consensus statement from a conference in Bellagio, Italy, is summarized in *Fig. 2.4*. If all three facts apply – amenorrhoea since the lochia ceased, baby not yet 6 months old, and total breastfeeding (or very nearly so) – the risk of conception by 6 months is only 2%. This compares favourably with other accepted methods of birth control. Hence it can be presented just like any other method to a woman – provided there is the usual caveat, that she is not promised that she will not be one of those 2% for whom the method fails.

However, for even greater efficacy and peace of mind many women will prefer to use the progestogen-only pill in addition to their breastfeeding (*see Qs 7.54 and 7.55*).

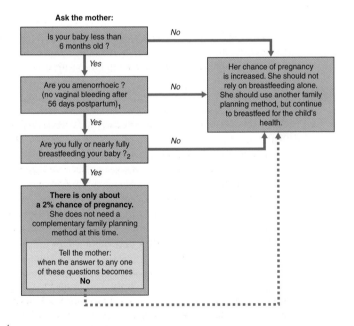

▲

Fig. 2.4 Use of the lactational amenorrhoea method (LAM) during the first six postpartum months. Q 2.37. *Notes:* 1. Spotting that occurs during the first 56 days is not considered to be menses. 2. 'Nearly full' breastfeeding means that *very* occasional non-breastfeeds are given.

2.38 What of the future? Are there any developments that could make fertility awareness methods more acceptable?

Most of these are suggested in *Fig. 2.2*. One (Persona™) has already arrived in the UK.

1 *Ultrasound*: ultimately, the relative price of ultrasound machines might fall so low, and their user-friendliness increase to such a degree, that women could simply plug them in to their television sets. Follicular growth, rupture and corpus luteum formation could then be monitored by the woman and her partner themselves!

2 *Home kits*: more realistically, a number of new home kits are being devised based on the cyclic changes in the hormones of the menstrual cycle, or their metabolites and other substances in body fluids. The most useful fluids are urine, saliva and breast milk; but biochemical changes in the mucus are also being studied.

3 *Other approaches*:

(a) The *Rovumeter*: this device simply measures the daily amount of cervicovaginal fluid aspirated from the posterior vaginal fornix by the woman into a sterile, disposable, calibrated, plastic aspirator. Volume changes are more objective than the usual mucus awareness approach, and can apparently be used for family planning purposes.

(b) New possibilities might arise by serendipity, such as occurred at King's College Medical School, London, where researchers studying Raynaud's phenomenon found that normal women (as well as those with Raynaud's) gave different measurements at different phases of their menstrual cycle. It appears that oestrogen tends to increase the reactivity of the arteries of the hand and that progesterone tends to relax the vessels, producing a localized increase in blood volume. Appropriate daily measurements in the hand could – in theory – therefore be used both to predict and to detect the woman's fertile period. No device for possible home use has yet appeared, however.

(c) *Standard Days Method* (Arevalo et al. *Contraception* 2000; 60:357–360) This is the calendar method reinvented for simplicity, using a ring of beads with different colours, one bead for each day of the cycle. Days 8–19 inclusive are those signalled for 'no unprotected sex'. Proponents claim that although no adjustments are made for cycles shorter or larger than 28 days (*Q 2.19*) this is balanced by easier compliance. It should not be used by women who record two cycles outside the range of 26–32 days in any one year.

Male methods of contraception

3

COITUS INTERRUPTUS

3.1 What is coitus interruptus?

This is well described by its most common euphemism: 'withdrawal' (in time, before ejaculation, ensuring that all sperm are deposited outside the vagina). There are many other terms, notably 'being careful' and also local idioms such as 'getting off at Fratton instead of going through to Portsmouth' (used in Hampshire, but with many regional equivalents!). These have often misled interviewers into thinking that no contraceptive method is being used.

3.2 What is the history of the method?

Coitus interruptus is doubtless the earliest form of birth control. It is mentioned in Genesis, the only explicit mention of contraception in the Bible:

Then Judah said to Er's brother Onan, 'Go and sleep with your brother's widow. Fulfil your obligation to her as her husband's brother, so that your brother may have descendants.' But Onan knew that the children would not belong to him, so whenever he had intercourse with his brother's widow he let the semen spill on the ground, so that there would be no children for his brother. What he did displeased the Lord and the Lord killed him also. (Genesis 38:8–10)

Although this text is widely quoted as implying that withdrawal is itself sinful, and by extension that other 'artificial' methods that prevent the sperm meeting the egg are also wrong, according to most commentators the sin was not in the method at all; it was Onan's failure to comply with the Levirate Law and perform his family duty that was sinful.

Although Islamic societies and numerous Imams are basically pronatalist, the Koran describes a more liberal attitude to withdrawal and, by inference, to other methods of contraception. In the Tradition of the Prophet we find:

A man said, 'O Prophet of God! I have a slave girl and I practise coitus interruptus with her. I dislike her becoming pregnant, yet I have the desires of men. The Jews believe that coitus interruptus constitutes killing a life in miniature form'.
The Prophet (Mohammed) replied, 'The Jews are liars. If God wishes to create it, you can never change it.'

Right up to the second half of the twentieth century, withdrawal remained a major and often the primary method of contraception. As late as 1947 the Royal Commission on Population in England found that amongst recently married couples with contraceptive experience, 43% used withdrawal as the sole method of birth control, the proportion rising to 65% in social class V. Studies in developing countries showed its use, at least on some occasions, by more than half of all couples in Jamaica, Puerto Rico and Hungary in the 1960s.

3.3 What is the effectiveness of coitus interruptus?

High failure rates alleged by early family planners have been quoted and requoted by subsequent generations of writers. Yet the evidence contradicts that view. In 1949 the Royal Commission (see above) reported that:

No difference has been found between users of appliance and users of non-appliance methods as regards the average number of children.

Withdrawal was by far the most popular of the non-appliance methods and the pregnancy rate was found to be a creditable 8/100 woman-years of exposure. A study in Indianapolis revealed a Pearl failure rate of only 10, compared with an average rate of 12 for all other methods, and amongst high-income couples the rate was precisely the same as for the diaphragm.

Some older readers of this book might, like me, have met couples who have two well-spaced children both in their teens and claim that withdrawal has been their regular and sole method. So it obviously works for some.

3.4 What are the advantages of coitus interruptus?

Chiefly, that the method is free of charge, requires no prescription, is always available and cannot be left at home when the couple go on holiday. Moreover, it does not cause nausea or weight gain! Its use has been associated with some of the lowest birth rates in history, for example in eastern Europe after the Second World War. It is obviously acceptable to many users.

3.5 What are the disadvantages?

Obviously intercourse is incomplete, and many find the method very unsatisfying to both partners. Yet no significant adverse effects have ever been demonstrated among those who do choose to use it. It seems to be assumed without discussion that there would be an inevitable lack of satisfaction of the woman, compounded by anxiety that her partner would not withdraw 'in time'. Psychological problems are assumed to follow. Yet in a survey of nearly 2000 British women questioned in 1967–68, only 31% of 311 who had discontinued use of the method did so because they found it unpleasant, and only 4% because they believed it harmful to health. By contrast, 54% of 381 former condom users gave up the method because they found it unpleasant to use.

Even among those professionally engaged in family planning, this method is unjustifiably overlooked, condemned or ridiculed. Marie Stopes stated that it was 'harmful to the nerves as well as unsafe'.

3.6 Why has the method been so neglected?

One reason, perhaps, is that it has no manufacturers to advertise its virtues. Also, because it has the reputation of being unsatisfying and ineffective, there is a feeling that it should certainly not be promoted. But it is unfortunate that many unplanned pregnancies among young people having intercourse unexpectedly are probably caused by the conventional teaching of doctors and nurses. Withdrawal is often not even attempted when it might have been, because the message that it is 'ineffective' has been so well conveyed. We must remember the old slogan:

Any method of family planning is better than no method, though some methods are better than others.

While encouraging the use of more modern methods, we should remember that – for many – this one works, and that it is a very great deal better than nothing 'in an emergency'.

3.7 Aren't there sperm in the pre-ejaculate?

Yes there are, sometimes. In 1931 Abraham Stone asked several medical friends to examine preorgasmic secretions for sperm. He finally collected 24 slides from 18 individuals. Two showed many sperm, two contained few, and one an occasional sperm. Stone correctly reported that the figures were 'insignificant for a definite conclusion'. The chances of such sperm causing fertilization must be low, although not negligible (*see Q 2.9*).

A much more probable cause of failure results from the partial ejaculation of a larger quantity of semen that can occur a short while before the final male orgasm; or withdrawal during the latter rather than before it starts. Hence the suggestion for those who want to continue using the method that they might use a spermicide as well (*see Qs 3.9, 3.18*).

3.8 Should a couple always be discouraged from using coitus interruptus?

The answer has to be 'no', even outside emergency use. We must remember the basic teaching of psychosexual medicine, that there are innumerable methods of giving and receiving sexual pleasure, which couples should feel free to devise for themselves. Why should they not be able to choose to use coitus interruptus, possibly along with oral sex and other forms of mutual pleasuring (most of which carry no conception risk), if that is their agreed choice and provides for them a mutually sexually satisfying life?

3.9 How do you counsel couples who volunteer that coitus interruptus is their usual method?

Clearly, other options should always be discussed. If, however, a couple finds all alternatives unacceptable, then I always just offer as an option the additional use of spermicide (a pessary, or perhaps Delfen™ foam). This should cope satisfactorily with any small deposit of sperm before withdrawal (but *see also Q 3.18*).

3.10 Your conclusion?

Like Malcolm Potts (to whom I am indebted for much of this section) who, with Peter Diggory, wrote in his 1983 book *Textbook of contraception practice*, I conclude:

Coitus interruptus is like … a buffalo cart; there are better methods of transport and better methods of contraception, but for a great many people it represents a practical solution to an everyday problem.

THE CONDOM: BACKGROUND AND MECHANISM

3.11 What is the definition of a male sheath/condom?

A condom is a closed-ended, expansile, tubular device designed to cover the erect penis and physically prevent the transmission of semen into the vagina. It is traditionally made of vulcanized latex rubber, which is as thin as possible while maintaining adequate strength, and often lubricated to minimize 'loss of sensitivity' during intercourse, which is perhaps the method's chief disadvantage. It is also a method for use by (often) the least well-motivated of the partners: hence the renewed interest in female-controlled condoms, as well as more effective spermicide/virucides (*see Qs 4.55–4.58 and 4.61*).

3.12 What is the method's history?

This apparently dates back to Roman times, when animal bladders were used chiefly to prevent the spread of sexually transmitted disease. In folklore, the invention was much later, by Dr Condom, reputedly a physician at the court of Charles II. However, it is doubtful whether Dr C. even existed. Much more probably, the word 'condom' was derived from the Latin (*condus*: a receptacle), as a euphemism for an item already well known. The earliest published description is that of the Italian anatomist Gabriel Fallopio, who in 1564 recommended a linen sheath moistened with lotion – again in order to protect against veneral infection. Only in the eighteenth century do we find condoms described specifically to prevent pregnancy. Condoms were then made from the caeca of sheep or other animals. Similar 'skin condoms' are still available but they have always been expensive and hence beyond the means of ordinary couples. They are also not recommended for safer sex to prevent virus transmission.

It was the process of vulcanization of rubber, first carried out by Hancock and Goodyear in 1844, that revolutionized the world's contraception, as well as its transport.

3.13 How acceptable and how frequently used is the condom method?

An estimated 44 million couples now use the condom worldwide, but with striking geographical differences. Japan accounts for more than a quarter of all condom users in the world. Seventy-five percent of couples who use any contraceptive in that country use this method, generally purchased by the woman, and there has not been a major shift in usage since the arrival of the pill in 1999 in that country for the first time. By contrast, and despite the massive problem of HIV/AIDS, condom use remains low in Africa, the Middle East and Latin America, which together account for an estimated 10% of worldwide use.

It has been calculated that if world condom usage for safer sex were at the appropriate level to control the HIV/AIDS epidemic, 24 billion should be used each year; yet the estimated figure (2003) has not yet reached 10 billion.

3.14 What is the acceptability and usage of the condom in the UK?

For many, 'spoilt' by modern non-intercourse-related alternatives, it must be admitted the method remains completely unacceptable for sustained use. There is an undeniable change of sensations reported, especially by men, although this sometimes has the benefit of prolonging intercourse.

In most recent surveys, approaching 20% of all couples use the condom. Estimates are always approximate because many couples use the sheath as an occasional alternative, if not in addition to other methods, but it continues to be the second most prevalent method within each 10-year cohort, during the reproductive years.

'Double Dutch', the shorthand phrase for using the condom to reduce infection risk at the same time as another more effective contraceptive, is believed to be increasing in prevalence: but not as fast as it should be …

3.15 How can the image of the condom as a method be improved?

In the past, condoms had a very poor image. AIDS has changed all that – or has it? There are still widespread misconceptions about efficacy and reduced sensitivity. For centuries, condoms were associated with prostitution and extramarital intercourse. Even today, as he purchases his condoms a married man might sense that the retailer assumes they surely cannot be for intercourse with his wife. Removal of this unfortunate image is unlikely as long as the media maintains double standards: there is widespread portrayal of intercourse on television, for example, yet it is still perceived as against morality or good taste to mention the condom in the storyline.

THE CONDOM: EFFECTIVENESS

3.16 How effective is the condom method?

Method-failure rates can be less than 2 pregnancies/100 couple-years. These are based on selected populations where there has been no sexual contact whatever without the rubber intervening, the only failures being caused by condoms bursting due to a manufacturing defect (some bursts and most cases of condoms slipping off are user errors, *see Q 3.20*). As successful use depends so very much on the motivation and care taken by the couple, failure rates do vary widely: from a low of 0.4/100 woman-years in the north of England in 1973 to a high of no less than 32/100 woman-years in Puerto Rico in 1961. A large population-based US study of 'single' women in the 1980s documented between 8 and 11 failures per 100 woman-years. In four UK studies the range was more relevant to the careful user, from 3.1 to 4.8/100 woman-years.

As usual, failures are more frequent with the young and inexperienced, and among couples who wish to delay rather than prevent pregnancy. Among such, average use leads to at least 10% conceptions in the course of 1 year: a one in ten chance (and we do such couples a disservice if this information is withheld from them). Older couples use the method better, perhaps because of diminished fertility and (though not always!) a lower frequency of intercourse, as well as more careful use. For example, in the Oxford/FPA study a pregnancy rate of only 0.7/100 couple-years was reported among women aged 35 and older, as compared with a rate of 3.6/100 couple-years for women aged 25–34 (in both cases the partner having been before recruitment a condom user for more than 4 years).

3.17 Why are so many men so bad at using condoms (at all, or well)?

Clearly, it has a lot to do with themselves not getting pregnant! A report from two university campuses in Georgia (published in the *Journal of the American Medical Association* 1997i 278:291–292), just about says it all:

Among 98 male students aged 18–29 (mean age 22.4 years) who participated in a standardized interview about their use of condoms, 50% reported ever experiencing condom breakage.

Among these 49 men, 15 (30%) had at some time failed to disclose knowledge of a broken condom to their female sex partner, nine of them many times! Overall, 13.2% of condom breakage episodes were never revealed to the partners! The reasons given were (N = number of individuals out of the 15):

- unwillingness to interrupt intercourse because orgasm was approaching (N = 6)
- wanting to avoid being blamed for the break (N = 5)
- desire to minimize anxiety of the partner about the break (N = 4).

I was rendered quite speechless when I first learned of this study. Its implications, for example for emergency contraception, are devastating!

3.18 How important is additional spermicide use to condom effectiveness?

Theoretically, this should increase contraceptive protection but it has never been proved to do so. As the pregnancy rate among consistent users is already very low, it would require an enormous study to prove an extra degree of protection – a study that will never be done.

More importantly, the only such additional spermicide currently available in the UK is nonoxynol-9. This is an irritant to the vaginal mucosa (lesions have been shown colposcopically) and now a number of studies show that it increases rather than diminishes HIV transmission (*see* Q 4.67 for the implications for female methods of contraception).

> The most common spermicide (nonoxynol-9 or nonoxynol-11) causes damage to the vaginal epithelium in very frequent use. This affects recommendations about virus transmission prevention but not those about routine contraception (*see* Q 4.67).

3.19 Are spermicidally lubricated condoms therefore yesterday's products?

Yes, indeed there are strong recommendations by WHO and other bodies to have nonoxynol-9 (N-9)-lubricated condoms removed from the market, along with N-9 vaginal lubricants (*see* Q 4.67). We badly need substitutes for this, ideally usable as regular microbicides as well as spermicides.

3.20 What common errors in condom use can result in pregnancy?

Particularly when the combined oral contraceptive (COC) has to be stopped after many years, and condoms are used as an alternative, most couples have no idea just how 'dangerous' a fluid semen will now become. It is important to stress that the 4–5 mL of an average man's ejaculate can easily contain 300 or 400 million sperm, and hence a minute proportion of this volume from a fertile man might cause a pregnancy. Common unrecognized errors include:

1 *Genital contact*: the condom is put on just before ejaculation – but often not in time to catch the first fraction of sperm.
2 *Loss of erection*: perhaps due to overexcitement or anxiety, so the condom slips off unnoticed before ejaculation. Another cause of slippage is mentioned in Q 3.22.
3 *Leakage on withdrawal*: when the penis is flaccid.
4 *Later genital contact*: with sperm already on the glans and in the urethra

of the penis (from earlier intercourse) before a new condom is applied.

5 *Damage to the condom*: (*see* Q 3.21).

3.21 What can cause condom breakage, aside from manufacturing defects?

1 *Mechanical damage*: e.g. by sharp fingernails, especially during attempts to force it on the wrong way, which result in rolling it up tighter rather than unrolling it (an easy mistake when excited!).

2 *Chemical action*: it is still not widely enough known that vegetable and mineral oil-based lubricants, and the bases for many prescribable vaginal products, can seriously damage and lead to rupture of rubber. Baby oil, for example, often suggested as part of sex play, destroys over 90% of a condom's strength after only 15 min contact! There are many common vaginal preparations that should be regarded as unsafe to use with condoms and diaphragms, and there might be others (*Table 3.1*). Here is a definite advantage of plastic condoms!

3.22 What instructions should be given to couples planning to use rubber male condoms?

1 *Use only good-quality condoms.*

2 *Avoid any chemical or physical damage*: do not use oil-based lubricants such as Vaseline™ or baby oil. Use jelly such as KY™ or Sensilube™ (*see* Q 3.21). Plastic condoms are unaffected by chemicals.

3 *Put the condom on the penis before any genital contact whatever*: if there is

---

TABLE 3.1 Vaginal and rectal preparations that should be regarded as unsafe to use with condoms or diaphragms

Arachis oil enema	Lomexin*
Baby oil	Nizoral
Canestan*	Nystan cream (pessaries OK)
Cyclogest	Ortho-Gynest (Ovestin ? OK)
Dalacin cream	Petroleum jelly (Vaseline)
E45 (and similar)	Premarin cream ? OK
Ecostatin	
Gyno-Daktarin	Sultrin
Gyno-Pevaryl (Pevaryl ? OK)	Witepsol-based products

Note: Some suntan oils and creams, bath oils and massage oils are similarly not 'condom–friendly'. But water-based products such as 'KY jelly', also ethylene glycol, glycerol and silicones are not suspect.
*According to the BNF (March 2003)

no teat, make room for the semen by pinching the end of the sheath as it is applied. (Otherwise there is the theoretical risk of semen tracking up the shaft of the penis and either escaping or causing the condom to slip off.)

4 *After intercourse, withdraw the penis before it becomes too soft*: holding the base of the condom during withdrawal and taking care not to spill any semen.

5 *Use each condom once only*: inspect it for damage/possible leaks before disposal.

6 Most importantly, if the condom ruptures or slips off, on any potentially fertile day, obtain emergency (postcoital) contraception (*see Chapter 10*).

THE CONDOM: ADVANTAGES AND INDICATIONS

3.23 What are the advantages of the condom method?

The advantages are many:

1 easily obtainable, relatively cheap or free from NHS clinics
2 free from medical risks
3 highly effective if used consistently and correctly
4 no medical supervision required
5 protects against most sexually transmitted infections including viruses
6 possible protection against cervical neoplasia and invasive carcinoma
7 offers visible evidence of use (particularly to the woman, who has the greatest motivation to avoid pregnancy)
8 involves the male in sharing contraceptive responsibility, although with some men this can be a definite disadvantage
9 can sometimes increase the woman's pleasure by prolonging intercourse
10 minimizes postintercourse odour and messiness of vaginal semen, for those who perceive these as problems.

3.24 In what situations can the condom be particularly indicated?

1 Where couples are unable or unwilling to make use of formal family planning services.
2 During short-term contraception (e.g. while waiting to start oral contraceptives).
3 Where intercourse takes place only infrequently and unpredictably.
4 For protection against sexually transmitted infections, notably HIV.
5 With the agreement of the man (although this is not always obtainable) for the prevention of cervical neoplasia, particularly when this has already been treated (*see Q 3.26*).

Items (4) and (5) are indications that might apply even if the main birth control method being used is an IUD, a hormone or sterilization (of either sex).

3.25 Against which sexually transmitted infections does the condom provide protection?

A major benefit from the woman's point of view is the reduced risk of upper genital tract disease (pelvic infection, with its serious threat to her future fertility). Consistent condom use is protective against gonorrhoea and *Trichomonas vaginalis*, the spirochaete of syphilis, *Chlamydia* and similar bacterial and protozoal organisms. It obviously provides little or no protection against infestations such as scabies and lice.

Most importantly, the rubber or plastic can provide a useful barrier – when intact – to viruses, including HIV, the far more infectious hepatitis viruses, herpes simplex types I and II and human papilloma virus (HPV).

Whereas fertilization is possible only during about eight days per cycle, viruses can be transferred at any time. As we have seen, condom conceptions are not uncommon. So the method can only provide relative protection ('safer sex'). Bilateral (two-sided) monogamy has much going for it! (see pages 23–31 of my handbook for women, *The Pill* – details in Further Reading).

3.26 What evidence is there that the condom can be protective or even therapeutic against cervical cell abnormalities?

In a UK case–control study the relative risk of developing severe cervical dysplasia decreased with duration of condom or diaphragm use, whereas it increased with duration of oral contraceptive (OC) use. After 10 years the relative risk for women using any barrier method was 0.2, compared to 4.0 for the pill users. Many other studies confirm their protective effect.

In a US study, as many as 136 out of 139 women with cervical cell abnormalities who received no treatment apart from their partners adopting use of the condom showed complete reversal of the condition. Unfortunately there was no control group, and the findings need confirmation.

THE CONDOM: PROBLEMS AND DISADVANTAGES

3.27 What are the possible disadvantages of the method?

There are few, really, but they are enough to put many people off:

1 Use is coitus-related and interrupts the spontaneity of intercourse.
2 Decreased 'sensitivity', especially for the male (although this is now much less with modern products).

3 Not uncommonly, especially in older men, the short time it takes to don the condom is enough for them to lose their erection sufficently for penetration to fail. Failure can then lead to a vicious cycle of 'performance anxiety' and the outcome of a regular self-fulfilling prophecy of failure. In one case of my own, in his early 60s with a partner in her 30s for whom hormonal methods were contraindicated, the answer proved to be sildenafil (Viagra™) to enhance erection and so enable this chosen contraceptive to be successfully used. This could be valid grounds for prescribing such products (though not on the NHS).

4 Perceived as acting as a barrier in psychological as well as physical terms.

5 Perceived to be messy, rubber has a distinctive odour that is hard to mask (an advantage of plastic).

6 They can slip off or rupture.

7 Few users appreciate how very small leaks of semen can cause a pregnancy (*see Q 2.7*).

8 A high degree of motivation and extremely meticulous use are required for long-term avoidance of pregnancy; these characteristics are possessed by a few men!

3.28 What are the possible unwanted effects of the condom?

Very few, it is difficult to imagine how death might occur – inhalation?

1 *Allergy*: some 'allergies' (in both sexes) are excuses. But irritation is not uncommon and true allergy to residues left in the rubber after the manufacturing processes does exist. This is less of a problem with modern rubbers but the solution is generally found by transferring to a plastic condom (*see Q 3.32*).

2 The method obviously fails to protect against disorders linked to the normal/abnormal menstrual cycle, such as menorrhagia, premenstrual syndrome, functional ovarian cysts, endometriosis and carcinoma of the ovary and endometrium. These can therefore be described not so much as side-effects of the condom, but more as 'side-effects of not using the pill' (*see Q 5.56*).

3.29 How can the disadvantages be minimized?

By using ultrathin and lubricated condoms, innovative materials, colours, scents, textures and shapes, and perhaps by involving the female more in the selection of specific brands and in their actual use. For example, if a condom (whether or not brightly coloured or ribbed) is applied by the woman as part of foreplay, this can counter the 'interruption' disadvantage, and even heighten eroticism. Or a female condom could be tried, for variety.

THE CONDOM: PRESENT AND FUTURE DESIGNS

3.30 Are there any condoms that are not recommended?

So-called American Tips, which are designed to fit only over the glans penis, have a bad reputation for slipping off during use. Also not approved are some 'fun' condoms available from sex shops, which do not conform to BSI kitemark specifications.

3.31 How are rubber condoms manufactured?

In a highly automated process, condom-shaped metal or glass moulds are dipped into latex solution, from where they pass to a drying oven. After a second immersion in latex, the moulds pass into another heated air chamber for drying and vulcanization. The finished product is usually rolled off the mould by nylon brushes and then subjected to quality control testing. Each of the millions produced is tested electronically for pin-holes; and samples are put through a water test for holes and also now an air inflation test to bursting point. The international standard (ISO 4074) permits only 7/200 samples to rupture after inflation with 15 L of air.

3.32 Does the future perhaps lie with plastic condoms?

Very likely, in my view. They have no smell and are good heat conductors, non-allergenic and unaffected by any chemicals in common use. One version, Avanti™, has been on the UK market since 1966. It is well lubricated and ultrathin, which many men find preferable. But despite using polyurethane, a material with good intrinsic strength, its thinness means it is at least as likely as (and in one US study more likely than) a good rubber condom to rupture in use.

A new polyurethane product is now CE-marked and has been on the market since 1998 in the Netherlands and 2001 in the UK: Ez-on™. It is the first baggy or loose-fit male condom. Each has a patented soft flange at the open end, with which it is 'pulled on like a sock' (either way, it is 'bidirectional', unlike all rubber condoms there is no wrong way to put it on) over the erect penis – which it then firmly but comfortably grasps at its base. Importantly, the loose-fit ensures that the major part of the shaft and all the glans of the penis feel free within the well-lubricated sac. In its present version it has only moderate tensile strength, which is odd because there is no need for its walls to be especially thin. Quotes from some acceptability trials suggest that it allows more 'normal' sensations during penetrative intercourse for the male partner and has 'no disadvantages compared with rubber condoms' for the female. However, in our own study at the Margaret Pyke Centre it ruptured at least as often as the other two condoms with which it was compared (Avanti™ and Durex Gossamer™) although it was the 'preferred' type by one-third of participants. No specific efficacy data are yet available.

Clients can be informed that Ez-on™ condoms are available from CS Supplies, Brighton BN42 4zz; tel. 01273 231028 (*see Qs 4.55–4.58* for the female condom). Though not studied specifically their efficacy is presumed to be similar to other male condoms.

PATIENT QUESTIONS

QUESTIONS FREQUENTLY ASKED BY USERS

3.33   My main problem with condoms is that I am afraid I will get less hard while I am putting one on.

You are unusual in actually voicing what is a very common fear. It could well stop being a problem as you get more used to it and with your partner's involvement (maybe putting it on for you) and her being relaxed, reassuring and laid-back about it.

In just a few cases, you could ask for Viagra™ or Cialis™ to maintain your erection and enable your chosen method to be used, especially where this is the only acceptable method to you both (*see Q 3.27*). (This would have to be a private prescription.)

3.34   The condoms keep breaking – why is this?

There are several possible explanations (*see Q 3.21*). Are you allowing any oily chemicals to come into contact with them? Sometimes you or your partner could be causing damage with fingernails while it is being put on. Waiting until she is more aroused and lubricated before penetration might help, or the use of KY Jelly™. Otherwise you could try a different brand, larger and /or thicker – discuss with your pharmacist.

Perhaps surprisingly, none of the available plastic condoms has been shown to be any better with respect to rupture than the strongest rubber ones.

3.35   Do I have to use a spermicide with the condom?

No – indeed WHO is opposed to the main one (nonoxynol-9) being used at all. It might do more harm than good (*see Qs 3.18 and 3.19*). If a condom fails it is much more relevant to arrange emergency contraception (*see Chapter 10*) than to rely on any amount of spermicide in the vagina.

3.36   Some condoms have ribs, bumps and so on – are these contraceptives safe?

If they are tested to the standards of the BSI or DIN (the German equivalent), the answer is yes. Beware of those that are not so approved.

3.37 If a condom breaks or slips off, is there anything you can do to avoid a possible pregnancy?

Yes, preferably in the next 24 h, but certainly within the next 5 days, make sure you obtain emergency contraception (*see Chapter 10*).

3.38 I seem to be developing an allergic rash from the condom – is there one specially made that overcomes this problem?

It is best for a doctor to examine your penis in case, for example, your 'allergy' is caused by something else, such as thrush. If you are using a spermicidally lubricated condom, you could try one without the spermicide. Otherwise the best bet now would be plastic condoms such as Avanti™ or Ez-on™ (*see Q 3.32*). Natural skin condoms, which are available by mail order, are porous and not recommended.

3.39 Do condoms have a shelf-life?

Yes: It is usually stated to be a long one of about 5 years but it is important to realize that rubber ones can deteriorate more rapidly in abnormal conditions, such as in the tropics – and anywhere if exposed to strong ultraviolet light (*see Q 3.21*).

3.40 Can I use the condom more than once?

This is not recommended – it was feasible with the old-style reusable types.

3.41 Why can't you get condoms free from your family doctor?

Why indeed? This is an excellent method of contraception that, in my view, should certainly be available from all GPs, as it is from clinics. One day perhaps?

3.42 Can you throw a condom away down the toilet?

From the environmental point of view it is better to use a dustbin.

3.43 My partner feels very dry; is there a lubricant you can safely use with the condom?

Sometimes dryness indicates a psychosexual problem you might need to address together (*see Appendix 2*).

Some of the dryness might be overcome by better sex technique – particularly by more foreplay so increasing arousal fluid. If she has any soreness or itching she should be checked for thrush or allergy. Otherwise use a water-based lubricant (*see Qs 3.21 and 3.22*) not containing spermicide. See also Qs 4.52 and 4.53.

3.44 I tend to put the condom on just before I 'come' – is this OK?

No! You are not alone in doing this, but it is probably the commonest reason that intact condoms 'fail'. See Qs 2.6–9, 3.7.

Vaginal methods of contraception

OCCLUSIVE CAPS: SELECTION OF USERS AND DEVICES

OCCLUSIVE CAPS: INITIAL FITTING. TRAINING AND FOLLOW-UP ARRANGEMENTS

THE (NEAR) FUTURE IN VAGINAL CONTRACEPTION

QUESTIONS ASKED BY USERS ABOUT VAGINAL CONTRACEPTION

PQ PATIENT QUESTIONS

OCCLUSIVE CAPS

4.1   Why should we try to avoid the terms 'female or vaginal barriers'?

Although these are convenient, ideally I wish we could find better terms to use. They should preferably be avoided in discussions with prospective users because sexual intercourse has to do with closeness, and one can reinforce wrong feelings and fantasies about the method being a 'barrier'.

4.2   What terminology will you be using? What types are available?

To avoid confusion, I will use the term 'occlusive caps' for all the standard female barriers. This has two subgroups, namely the diaphragm and the cervical/vault caps, with the vimule being here considered as a modified vault cap (*Fig. 4.1*). FemCap™, a silicone cap, is now also on the NHS Drug Tariff.

4.3   What is the method's history?

It is a very ancient method, with descriptions dating back to 1850 BC; the Petri papyrus describes a spermicidal pessary made partly of crocodile dung. A section of the Talmud from the second century AD recommended a moistened sponge in the vagina before coitus. Rubber occlusive pessaries did not appear until the nineteenth century, in Germany, and the first diaphragm was popularized by Mensinga, the pseudonym of a German

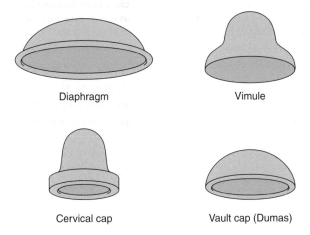

Diaphragm   Vimule

Cervical cap   Vault cap (Dumas)

Fig. 4.1 Diaphragm and cervical vault caps. Q 4.2.

physician Dr C. Hasse. The development of vulcanized rubber enabled him to produce a thinner and more pliable device incorporating a flat watch spring in the rim. It became known as the Dutch cap because of the publicity given to it by the Dutch neo-Malthusians.

The occlusive pessary was referred to in the famous manual *The wife's handbook*, published in 1887; for mentioning it, the author – Arthur Allbutt – was struck off the British Medical Register. Because of this kind of opposition, occlusive pessaries became readily available only in the 1920s. Then, to quote Malcolm Potts, 'diaphragms and caps were to family planning what the steam locomotive was to transportation; they were the first in the field, brought emancipation to millions, and for a long time had no rivals'. Ultimately they were overtaken by a new technology; yet the methods have only two major problems: some lack of independence from intercourse and relative lack of effectiveness. If these could be overcome, there could be a large-scale return to vaginal methods.

4.4 How popular are vaginal methods worldwide?

The diaphragm reached the peak of its popularity around 1959, when it was reported that the method was used by about 12% of couples practising contraception in the UK. Usage declined rapidly with the advent of the pill and now less than 1% of contracepting women use the method in the UK. In most developing countries prevalence of use is too low to measure, and is likely to remain so until vaginal barriers are devised that do not require medical fitting or special training in use, and do not pose storage and supply problems and above all, effectively prevent HIV transmission.

4.5 How important is medical attitude and training to the acceptability of vaginal methods?

Crucially, it has been well said that often the biggest 'barrier to the barriers' is the medical profession, and sometimes (although less so) the nursing profession. Many women introduced for the first time to the diaphragm at the age of 35–40 express surprise at its ease and convenience. They often complain that doctors and nurses had earlier damned the method with exceedingly faint praise.

This is a highly practical subject. The right attitude and skills can only be acquired by observing and being taught by unhurried and experienced professionals: in my experience family planning trained nurses are usually best! (*see Qs 4.33–4.49*).

4.6 What is the mode of action of the diaphragm and cervical/vault caps?

The diaphragm lies diagonally across the cervix, the vaginal vault and much of the anterior vaginal wall. As the vagina is known to 'balloon' during intercourse (*see Q 2.3*), a sperm-tight fit between the diaphragm and the vaginal wall is impossible. On a theoretical basis, the main functions of the diaphragm are:

1 acting as a carrier of the spermicide to the most important site, namely the external os, and prevent the spreading effect of intercourse (*see Q 2.3*)
2 holding sperm away as a barrier from the receptive alkaline cervical mucus, long enough for them to die in the acid vagina
3 preventing the mucus from entering the acid vagina and thereby providing a film within which the sperm can swim to the external os, and possibly
4 preventing physical aspiration of sperm into the cervix and uterus.

Some authorities question the importance of the spermicide (*see Q. 4.7*).

Cervical/vault caps and FemCap™ are meant to stay in place by suction, which makes it possible that the barrier effect is more important to their contraceptive action than is the case with the diaphragm.

4.7 How important is the use of spermicide with occlusive caps?

This has been questioned, particularly by the Australian Family Planning Association, and especially for the cervical/vault caps, which act by suction. It is a fact that with no type of occlusive cap has there ever been a proper controlled trial. This should compare (preferably by random allocation) women who follow the full routine of instructions concerning the use of spermicide (*see Q 4.44*), in every detail, with women who use exactly the same method carefully and after the same fitting routine but without any spermicide at all. Such a study has been performed at the Margaret Pyke Centre and although the power of our study was not great enough to show statistical significance, the spermicide-using group did achieve better results. We do badly need better spermicides, however, without the tissue toxicity of nonoxynol-9 (*see Q 4.67*).

OCCLUSIVE CAPS: EFFECTIVENESS

4.8 How effective is the diaphragm?

Table 1.2 (p. 14) quotes an overall failure rate for the diaphragm of 4–20 per 100 woman years, a surprisingly wide range, perhaps. As usual the lower failure rate relates to older women, whose conscientiousness in regularly using the method efficiently is of greatest importance.

Professor Trussell of Princeton, NJ, has made a special study of contraceptive failure rates. The first-year pregnancy rates were much higher in parous women if they used the cervical cap (ranging up to over 25%, even with 'perfect use'!). Parous diaphragm 'perfect users' had similar rates to nulliparae, however, although still in the range of 4–8% in the first year.

This, it should be noted, is an order of magnitude higher than the best rates obtainable by conscientious COC use.

Table 4.1 relates the failure rates to an indicator of motivation recorded in the Oxford/FPA study, namely whether or not the woman considered her family to be complete. As clearly shown, the failure rate tended to be higher when the family was not felt to be complete, implying less careful use of the diaphragm when another baby would be acceptable (i.e. 'spacers').

4.9 Are the diaphragm failure rates of the Oxford/FPA study a good indication of the rates to be expected in routine family planning practice?

No.

1 At recruitment, every woman was aged 25–39 years, married, a white British subject, and had to be already a current user of the diaphragm of at least 5 months standing.
2 The women were basically 'middle class' and were probably unusually well motivated and careful.
3 Younger and more fertile women having intercourse more frequently must be expected to have a higher failure rate, even if the method were properly fitted and always used.

The most important factor is the recruitment in the Oxford/FPA study of established users only. By 5 months the most fertile and least careful women, along with those with anatomical problems interfering with the effectiveness of the method, would not have been available for recruitment – by virtue of already becoming pregnant! All studies show the highest failure rates in the first few months of use. Even using the data of *Table 4.1*, faced with an 'Oxford/FPA-type' woman under 35 one can only quote a failure rate of around 5–6/100 woman-years for the first year of use. This is about the best to be expected, with a rate of around 10 expected for most young unmarried women of average motivation (all these rates include user failures).

TABLE 4.1 Diaphragm failure rates per 100 woman-years according to age, duration of use and completeness of family

Duration of use	Age 25–34			Age 35+		
	≤ 2years	2–4 years	4 years+	≤2 years	2–4 years	4 years+
Family complete	6.1	3.5	2.3	2.1	1.6	0.7
Family not complete	5.3	4.3	2.4	4.5	2.0	1.3

Source: Oxford/FPA Study, 1982

4.10 What failure rates can be given for cervical caps?

These are considered later (*see Qs 4.27–4.32*). Available effectiveness data are sparse, but Trussell's review in the book *Contraceptive technology* (1998, 17th edn) gives a best estimate of 9% at 1 year of use for nulliparous 'perfect users': possibly acceptable for 'spacers'. His quoted rate of 26% for parous women suggests to me that this is no longer a method to be recommended for most in that group of potential users. FemCap's™ failure rate in consistent users (pre-marketing trial) was 10.5/100 women years.

4.11 In summary, what factors promote the effectiveness of the diaphragm and similar vaginal methods?

The following questions need to be asked:

1　Is she an established user or starting the method from scratch?
2　What is her age?
3　What is her frequency of intercourse?
4　What is her motivation for obsessionally careful and regular use? In particular, is she really trying to avoid a pregnancy or just to delay one?
5　Is she at all uncomfortable about handling her own genitalia? This important factor is not at all linked with intelligence.
6　Are there any anatomical problems on examination? (*see Qs 4.22, 4.30, 4.31, 4.35*).
7　During initial training, is she good at inserting the device and particularly at checking that the cervix is covered?

4.12 What common errors in the use of occlusive caps can result in pregnancy?

The most common is failure to use at intercourse on one or more occasions in the cycle of conception. Women often report minor errors in use of the spermicide. It is not at all clear how important these are, especially as they are frequently reported also in non-conception cycles.

During use, the most important error is failure to make a secondary check after insertion that the cervix is correctly covered.

Clinicians' errors include: wrong selection of users, poor fitting (with regard to size, choice of flat spring, coil or arcing diaphragm or other cap) and poor teaching.

OCCLUSIVE CAPS: ADVANTAGES AND BENEFICIAL EFFECTS

4.13 What are the advantages of occlusive caps?

1　Effective if used with care by older women similar to those of Table 4.1.
2　Much more independent of intercourse than the male condom (*see Q 4.14*).
3　In general, neither partner suffers any loss of feeling.

4 The method is under a woman's control and needs only to be used when required.
5 Aesthetically useful for intercourse during uterine bleeding but not left in situ longterm during mensus (*see Qs 4.73, 4.84*).
6 No proven systemic effects.
7 Some definite non-contraceptive benefits (*see Q 4.15*).

4.14 Are occlusive caps necessarily intercourse-related methods?

No. In counselling, this is a most important point to explain. It is perfectly in order to insert any rubber or silicone barrier many hours ahead of intercourse. Beyond 3 h it is advisable to add extra spermicide before intercourse (*see Qs 4.44 and 4.49*) but certainly not having to insert the cap itself just before intercourse helps compliance. As keeping the cervical mucus out of the vagina could be one of the most important mechanisms (*see Q 4.6*), it could even be that insertion well ahead of intercourse actually increases effectiveness, although this has not been established.

4.15 What are the beneficial medical effects?

1 Protection against some sexually transmitted infections (STIs), including the agents causing pelvic inflammatory disease. However, the method does not protect against HIV and some other sexually transmitted viruses.
2 Reduction in the risk of cervical intraepithelial neoplasia (CIN), *see Q 4.17*.

These are most important benefits in the modern world.

4.16 How are occlusive caps protective against STIs?

In two ways:

1 Partly by providing a mechanical barrier that reduces the chance of organisms reaching the cervix and upper genital tract. However, this will not fully protect against the viruses or non-viral diseases (e.g. syphilis) that can form lesions of the vagina or vulva.
2 The associated spermicide is also relevant. Spermicides tend also to be 'germicides', a benefit unfortunately largely cancelled in the case of nonoxynol-9 by its irritant effects (*Qs 4.66–4.67*).

4.17 What is the evidence for at least some protective effect against cervical neoplasia?

In the Oxford/FPA study, the rate per 100 woman-years for oral contraceptive (OC) users was 0.95 and for intrauterine device (IUD) users 0.87. For diaphragm users, however, the rate was 0.23 after adjustment for age at first coitus, number of partners and smoking patterns. Another Oxford study showed a steady decline in the relative risk of severe cervical neoplasia for users of all types of barrier method from 1 down to 0.2 after 10 years. This benefit is believed to be mainly because of reduced transmission of the oncogenic types of HPV. However, diaphragm users might also be protected by their own sexual lifestyle and that of their partners.

OCCLUSIVE CAPS: MAIN PROBLEMS AND DISADVANTAGES

4.18 What are the disadvantages of occlusive caps?

1 Although not necessarily coitus-related, they involve a woman handling her genitalia, some forward planning and a slight loss of spontaneity.
2 Loss of cervical and some vaginal sensation (unnoticed by most).
3 Can occasionally be felt in use by the woman's partner, although not by her if properly fitted.
4 Require fitting by trained personnel and (except FemCap™, Q 4.76) a period of training in use, usually 1 week, during which another method must be used.
5 Definitely less effective than hormonal contraception or the IUD, especially under age 35 (Table 4.1).
6 Perceived as being 'messy' due to the spermicide.
7 Capable of producing some local adverse effects (*see* Q 4.19).

4.19 What are the possible adverse medical effects?

1 Increased risk of urinary tract infections and symptoms. This problem seems to apply only (and not often) to the diaphragm (*see* Q 4.51).
2 A small minority of women develop vaginal irritation and allergy due either to the rubber (not FemCap™) or more commonly to the spermicide.
3 Pressure effects due to the rim of the occlusive cap itself, leading rarely to vaginal abrasions or ulcers (*see* Q 4.54).

There are also a few unresolved safety issues, considered later (*see* Qs 4.67–4.74).

An excipient used in Cyclogest™ (progesterone) pessaries can damage rubber. If a cap-user is given this unproven form of treatment for the premenstrual syndrome, she should be advised to use the rectal route of administration (*see also* Q 3.21 for other substances that can damage rubber).

OCCLUSIVE CAPS: SELECTION OF USERS AND DEVICES

4.20 What are the conditions for the successful use of occlusive caps?

In the main, the answer depends on favourable answers to the questions about the woman herself, listed at Q 4.11. In addition, experience plus a positive attitude by the providers, ideally both a doctor and a nurse, are of paramount importance. Skilful fitting, knowledge of when to suggest a cervical/vault cap instead, and above all really satisfactory teaching of the woman, are vital factors.

4.21 What are the indications for use of occlusive caps?

1 The woman's choice.
2 As an alternative to medical methods (hormones, IUDs) for a woman who can accept reduced efficacy in return for getting rid of the side-effects of the medical method.
3 The need for contraception on an intermittent yet predictable basis.
4 For protection against pelvic infection or recurrence of cervical neoplasia. This can be worth suggesting even if another method is in use as the main contraceptive.

4.22 What are the contraindications to the diaphragm?

These include:

1 aversion to touching the genital area
2 congenital abnormalities such as a septate vagina
3 most forms of uterovaginal prolapse
4 inadequate retropubic ledge on examination
5 poor vaginal or perineal muscle tone
6 inability to learn the insertion technique
7 lack of hygiene or privacy for insertion, removal and care of the cap
8 acute vaginitis – treat first
9 recurrent urinary infections – indication for vault or cervical cap
10 past history of cap-induced vaginal trauma
11 true allergy to rubber
12 past history of toxic shock syndrome – although this not proved related to occlusive caps
13 virgo intacta – sheath use is commonly advised first, until the vagina is 'ready'. But well-motivated tampon-users can receive a small diaphragm, with refitting planned to follow 1 month's regular use.

Items (3), (4), (5) and (9) do not always contraindicate cervical/vault caps or FemCap™ (*see Qs 4.32 and 4.76*) and an arcing diaphragm could solve (6).

4.23 What is the structure of a diaphragm?

This is the most commonly used occlusive cap. It consists of a thin latex rubber hemisphere, the rim of which is reinforced by a flexible flat or coiled metal spring (*Fig. 4.2*). The sizes, measuring the external diameter, range from 50 to 100 mm in steps of 5 mm.

4.24 What types of diaphragm are available?

1   *The flat-spring diaphragm*: has a firm watch spring and is easily fitted, remaining in the horizontal plane on compression. It is suitable for the normal vagina and is often tried first.

2   *The coil-spring diaphragm*: has a spiral coiled spring. This makes it softer than the flat-spring.

3   *The arcing-spring diaphragm*: combines features of both the above and consists of a rubber dome with a firm double metal spring. It exerts strong pressure on the vaginal walls but its main characteristic is that when compressed it forms an arc, directing the posterior part of the diaphragm downwards and away from the cervix during insertion. This can be an advantage (*see Q 4.26*).

4.25 What are the indications for the coil-spring diaphragm?

Because it exerts slightly less pressure, it can be more comfortable for some women than the flat-spring. The reduced pressure makes it seem to the woman about a half-size smaller than the equivalent flat-spring diaphragm.

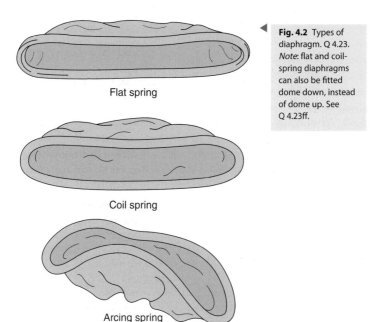

Flat spring

Coil spring

Arcing spring

Fig. 4.2 Types of diaphragm. Q 4.23. *Note*: flat and coil-spring diaphragms can also be fitted dome down, instead of dome up. See Q 4.23ff.

This can be useful because half-sizes (2.5-mm increments) are no longer available for any diaphragm.

4.26 For whom might the arcing-spring diaphragm be indicated?

This is the most widely used type of diaphragm in some countries. Some women find it more difficult to handle during insertion because of its non-horizontal shape when squeezed.

Its main positive indication is in cases where the length or direction of the cervix, or the woman's own technique, are resulting in a tendency to squeeze the diaphragm into the anterior fornix (*see Q 4.40 (7)*).

4.27 What types of cervical/vault caps are available?

1 *The cervical cap*: this is shaped like a thimble (*see Fig. 4.1*) and is designed to fit snugly over the cervix. The most common variety is the cavity rim cap with an integral thickened rim incorporating a small groove. This is intended to increase suction to the sides of the cervix. The available internal diameters of the upper rim are 22, 25, 28 and 31 mm. Other varieties are available outside the UK. *FemCap*™ is a silicone rubber cervical cap with a unique brim (see Fig. 4.6).

2 *The vault cap*: this rubber cap is shaped like a bowl with a thinner dome through which the cervix can be palpated. It covers, but does not fit closely to, the cervix. Five sizes are available ranging from 55 to 75 mm in 5-mm steps.

3 *The vimule*: this is a variation of the vault cap with a hat-shaped prolongation of the dome to accommodate longer cervices. There are three sizes: small (45 mm), medium (48 mm) and large (51 mm).

4.28 What is the mode of action of cervical/vault caps?

They all operate by suction, not by spring tension like the diaphragm. Otherwise the mode of action – and the uncertainties about spermicides – are the same as for the diaphragm (*see Qs 4.6 and 4.7*).

4.29 What indications and advantages do the cervical/vault caps share?

1 They share the advantages of the diaphragm but are suitable for patients with poorer muscle tone and some cases of uterovaginal prolapse.

2 They are generally not felt by the male partner.

3 There is no reduction of vaginal sensation.

4 They are unlikely to produce urinary symptoms.

5 Fitting is unaffected by the changes in the size of the vagina, either during intercourse or as a result of changes in body weight.

4.30 What are the conditions necessary to fit a cervical cap?

1 The cervix must be easily felt.
2 The cervix must be healthy, not torn.
3 The cervix must not point backwards, and ideally should point down the axis of the vagina.
4 The cervix must be straight sided.

4.31 What conditions are necessary for fitting a vault cap?

1 The cervix must be easily felt.
2 The cervix must be fairly short, although it can be quite bulky if it does not protrude too much into the vaginal vault.

4.32 In what circumstances would you recommend a trial of the vault or vimule caps?

The vault cap is under used. It can be very useful where there are contraindications to the diaphragm (*see Q 4.22*), particularly absence of the retropubic ledge, poor muscle tone and a history of recurrent cystitis. It is a little easier for the woman to fit and remove than the cervical cap and the precise contour and direction of the cervix are much less important but it cannot be used if the cervix is not rather *short*.

Where there is a choice I would recommend a trial of the vault cap or (for longer cervices) the new FemCap™ (*Q 4.76*) ahead of the cervical cap. The vimule is rarely used – its sole indication is to accommodate a cervix that is long enough to prevent suction being exerted in a woman for whom a vault cap would otherwise be selected.

OCCLUSIVE CAPS: INITIAL FITTING, TRAINING AND FOLLOW-UP ARRANGEMENTS

4.33 What aspects are important in the initial counselling?

The factors in *Qs 4.9 and 4.11* should be explored very carefully with the woman, particularly determining that the method is socially and psychologically acceptable to her, and in particular that she will be a regular conscientious user. She must also, in fairness, be told that the method has a moderately high failure rate despite ideal fitting and compliance with every detail of the instructions as to use.

4.34 How is the fitting performed?

In a sensitive and unhurried way. The practical aspects cannot be learnt from books. Apprenticeship is necessary in two aspects: fitting technique and instruction of the woman.

4.35 What points are noted in the initial examination?

1 The apparent health and direction of the uterus and cervix. Tenderness must be absent.
2 The type of retropubic ledge. This can be more fully assessed with a practice diaphragm in position.
3 Assessment of the vaginal musculature and tone, including the perineal muscles.
4 If the diaphragm is chosen, the distance from the posterior fornix to the posterior aspect of the symphysis is measured, as shown in *Fig. 4.3*.

Cervical cytology and other screening procedures are performed according to local practice.

To measure for diaphragm size
Hold index and middle fingers together and insert into vagina up to the posterior fornix. Raise hand to bring surface of index finger to contact with pubic arch. Use tip of thumb to mark the point directly beneath the inferior margin of the pubic bone and withdraw fingers in this position.

To determine diaphragm size
Place one end of rim of fitting diaphragm or ring on tip of middle finger.
The opposite end should lie just in front of the thumb tip.
This is the approximate diameter of the diaphragm needed.

▲

Fig. 4.3 Procedure for estimating the size of practice diaphragm to be tried Q 4.35 (reproduced courtesy of Janssen Cilag Pharmaceutical Ltd, Diaphragm Teaching Aid). See Q 4.35ff.

4.36 Successful fitting of the diaphragm – what are the steps?

1 The woman should have emptied her bladder and an initial choice of practice diaphragm is made based on the distance measured at the first examination (*Fig. 4.3*).

2 With the index finger inside the rim, compress the practice diaphragm between the thumb and remaining fingers. Separate the labia and insert the diaphragm downwards and backwards to the posterior fornix, tucking the anterior rim behind the symphysis pubis.

3 Check that the cervix is covered.

4 Insert a finger tip between the anterior rim of the cap and the symphysis:
   (a) if the cap is too small, a wider gap will be felt, or the whole diaphragm might be found to be in the anterior fornix
   (b) if the cap is too large it projects anteriorly/inferiorly and might cause immediate discomfort (or become uncomfortable or distorted later, after wearing).

5 The woman should be asked to stand and walk a few steps. On re-examination, anterior protrusion might be due to a small cystocele or a poor retropubic ledge. In this event, a vault or possibly a cervical cap should be tried.

4.37 Which way up should diaphragms be fitted?

This really does not matter. It might be slightly easier to remove a flat-spring type if it is inserted dome upwards and the patient is instructed to hook her index finger under the anterior rim. However, this is a non-problem anyway if she simply uses both index and middle fingers to grasp the rim. The arcing diaphragm forms the correct shape (with its leading edge pointing downwards) more readily if it is initially held dome upwards. This requires careful demonstration.

4.38 What are the important points when teaching the prospective user?

Thorough teaching that generates confidence in the user is essential for success. A three-dimensional plastic model helps but a short video is better still. Unless the doctor is a woman, a female nurse usually takes over at this stage (if she did not do the initial fitting). She must be very encouraging and able, without embarrassment on either side, and in secure privacy, to supervise closely all aspects of the learning process.

4.39 Successful teaching – how important is the position the woman should adopt?

This important aspect is often overlooked by the trainer. Unless instructed to the contrary, many women automatically adopt a half-standing, half-squatting position when inserting the diaphragm or when checking that it is correctly located over the cervix. This should be discouraged, as it makes it almost impossible for the fingers to reach the cervix. It might explain some so-called 'cap failures', caused solely because the woman was unable to check that the device was correctly positioned. The two best positions are:

1 Standing with one foot resting on a chair – a right-handed woman should raise her left leg and vice versa (*Fig. 4.4*).
2 Squatting right down on the ground.

Other positions are possible according to the woman's choice.

4.40 Successful teaching (diaphragm) – what are the steps?

1 In her own preferred position (as described in Q 4.39), teach the woman to locate her cervix. Most women prefer to use one finger but it is an error to insist on this. Even 'short-fingered' women can learn to feel their cervix if taught to use both index and middle fingers.
2 The instructor then inserts the cap for the patient, allowing her to feel her cervix covered with thin rubber.
3 The patient then removes the diaphragm for herself, either by hooking it out or (and this needs stressing) the use of two fingers each side of the anterior rim. If this is found difficult, practising with a slightly too large diaphragm might be all that is necessary to boost confidence.
4 The woman should feel again for the cervix to emphasize the different feel when it is uncovered.
5 She should then be taught to insert the diaphragm as described above and shown in steps 6–8 of Fig. 4.4. The instructor should emphasize that the direction of insertion is similar to that for a tampon – primarily backwards.
6 The woman should then examine herself to check that the cervix is covered by the soft rubber dome. It is absolutely vital to explain that the fact that a diaphragm fits snugly behind the symphysis and feels comfortable is no guarantee of correct insertion.
7 If the woman repeatedly inserts the diaphragm into her anterior fornix, the following useful tips come from the Sister-in-Charge (as in the 1980s she was called) at the Margaret Pyke Centre:
   (a) the woman lies on her back and holds the diaphragm in her left hand (if right-handed). She then uses her right hand to separate the labia and guide insertion, vertically. Alternatively, and in any convenient position (*see* Q 4.39), she inserts the diaphragm halfway only, then the half that is still outside is pressed towards the symphysis while completing the insertion.
   (b) the use of an arcing diaphragm. When held dome down, compression between middle finger and thumb, with the index

1. Apply two strips, each approximately 1 inch long of either contraceptive jelly or cream to both sides of the diaphragm.

2. Rub a small amount of this around the inside and outside of the rim with your finger tip.

3. Get comfortable and relax. A suitable position to insert your diaphragm would be to stand, prop one leg up on a chair (left leg if you are right-handed and vice versa). Keep the other knee slightly bent.

4. Alternatively, you may wish to squat with your knees wide apart.

5. An easier position, once you have become familiar with inserting your diaphragm, may be to lie on your back with your knees up.

Fig. 4.4 Instructions for prospective users of the diaphragm. Q 4.39 (reproduced courtesy of Janssen Cilag Pharmaceutical Ltd, Diaphragm Teaching Aid).

6. To insert your diaphragm fold it in half by pressing the middle of the opposite sides together between the thumb and forefinger of one hand. You may find it helpful to place your index finger in the dome between your thumb and fingers to help prevent it springing away.

If you have been given an arcing spring diaphragm hold it with the arc pointing downwards to ensure that the cervix will be covered.

7. Hold the lips of your vagina apart with your other hand. Gently slide the folded diaphragm into your vagina, placing your index finger on the rim to guide it. Aim towards the small of the back as if inserting a tampon. You may feel the rim pass over the cervix.

8. Use the index finger to push the front rim up behind the pubic bone.

9. To check if the diaphragm is in place insert your index finger into your vagina and touch the dome. You should feel the cervix underneath. Move your index finger to the front of the diaphragm and make sure it is firmly in place behind the pubic bone. Finally check that the back rim is behind the cervix.

10. Do not remove your diaphragm for 6 hours after intercourse. Put your index finger in your vagina and hook it behind the rim of the diaphragm under your pubic bone. Gently pull the diaphragm down and out. You may find it useful to bear down slightly especially if it is well tucked up behind the pubic bone. The diaphragm should not be left in place for more than 24 hours.

▲

Fig. 4.4—cont'd

finger between to steady it, produces a downwards bend (*see Fig. 4.2* and Q *4.26*). This helps the posterior rim to pass below the cervix and so into the posterior rather than the anterior fornix. Occasionally, with either diaphragm design, the woman's partner might be able to learn to insert it for her.

The use of an introducer is rarely much help, in our experience at MPC.

4.41 How are cervical and vault caps fitted?

1 The correct size allows the rim of the chosen cap to touch the fornices with no gap, comfortably to accommodate the cervix (the cervical cap and FemCap™ being the only ones that truly fit it) and to show evidence of a suction effect.

2 To insert the chosen cap, the rim is compressed between thumb and first two fingers and guided along the posterior vaginal wall towards the cervix. The cap is allowed to open by removing the thumb, and then is pushed over the cervix with the fingertips. A final check is made to ensure that the cervix is palpable through the cap and that there is no gap above the rim.

3 Cervical and vault caps are removed by inserting a fingertip above the rim and then easing the cap downwards, before removal with the index and middle fingers. FemCap™ has a useful removal strap (*Fig. 4.6*).

4.42 Successful teaching – what instructions for vault and cervical caps?

Feeling for the cervix, insertion and removal are taught as just described for the fitting. The important point is that if the right sort of woman has been chosen for these caps (which are a little more tricky to use than the diaphragm), she rapidly develops her own technique both for insertion and removal. Provided this is shown to result in correct location, she should be encouraged to continue.

The correct size for vault and vimule caps is that which fits snugly into the vaginal vault and covers the cervix without exerting pressure upon it.

Further practical details about fitting these smaller suction caps are best learnt in the practical, clinical situation aided by the relevant FPA leaflet and manufacturer's leaflet.

4.43 Successful teaching – what is the training 'timetable' for any type of occlusive cap?

It is usual and preferable to provide the woman with a practice cap for the first week, during which she should use an alternative contraceptive. This enables her to increase her confidence in the techniques of insertion and removal, and to test whether the method is comfortable during all normal activities. She should be informed with the aid of the most recent edition of the FPA's leaflet of all the 'rules' (*see Q 4.44*) before she leaves after the first visit. The same points should again be run through at the return visit, before she starts to rely on the method.

4.44 Successful teaching – what actual instructions are given at the first visit? see *Fig. 4.4.*

The wording that follows is addressed to a particular woman and relates specifically to the diaphragm (*see also Q 4.49*):

1 Always use the recommended spermicidal cream or jelly. Apply two strips, each of 2.5 cm (1 inch), to each side of the diaphragm. It is unnecessary to smear the surfaces too much but you might also want to put some on the leading part of the rim.

2 Put your diaphragm in place (*see Fig. 4.4*), using the position and technique you found most comfortable when you were fitted. This could be at any convenient time before lovemaking.

3 If you are having a bath, you should put your diaphragm in after rather than before it (*see Q 4.86*).

4 Most important: check the position of your diaphragm with either your index finger or with index and middle finger, as you prefer. The important thing is that you check that the diaphragm covers your cervix. This feels a bit like a rounded nose with a single nostril, upwards and backwards somewhere near the top of your vagina. You should get used to the particular way your cervix points, which could be forwards, backwards or straight downwards. Check that the rubber on your diaphragm actually covers the cervix – do not rely just on it feeling comfortable.

5 Should lovemaking take place more than 3 h after you put the cap in, either insert more cream or jelly or foam with an applicator, or use a spermicidal pessary or film pushed well up with the finger. You need to allow about 10 min for pessaries to disperse in the vagina before your partner actually deposits semen there.

6 If you have intercourse more than once, more spermicide should be added beforehand, leaving the diaphragm in place.

7 You should leave your diaphragm in place for at least 6 h after the last intercourse. It can be kept in longer but should be removed once a day for cleaning. FemCap™ is licensed to be retained for 48 h in all

8 It is no problem if your period starts while the diaphragm is in place. Also it is quite possible to get pregnant during your period. So continue to use your diaphragm for any intercourse, especially towards the end or just after a period, when many people think they can get away without using it.

9 After removal, the diaphragm (or cap) can be washed in warm water with mild toilet soap. It should then be dried and stored in its box in a cool dry place. Do not use heat, solvents, disinfectants, detergents or any mineral- or vegetable-oil-containing oils or lubricants (*see Q 3.21*) because these might damage the rubber or the silicone of FemCap™.

10 Inspect your cap regularly for holes by holding it up to the light.

> Although you have been given the cap with spermicide, everything is just for practice during the first week. Wear it during the day to make sure it stays in place. You should not be able to feel it if it is the right size and in the right position. Report any discomfort or other problems when, after 1 week, you return to the clinic or surgery. You should come with it in position so that the doctor or nurse can do a proper check.

4.45 What should take place at the second visit?

1 Any discomfort or problems should be identified.

2 If there are problems, a change in the size of the cap or use of a different spermicide might be recommended.

3 Repetition of the instructions above is important before the woman actually begins to rely on her method.

4 A final warning about the danger of risk-taking might be useful, coupled with a reminder about the availability if ever needed of postcoital contraception (*see Chapter 10*).

4.46 What extra instructions are given for users of cervical/vault caps?

1 A usual recommendation is to one-third fill the bowl of cervical, vault or vimule caps with spermicidal jelly. None is used on the rim for fear of impairing suction.

2 With these caps, an extra measure of spermicidal jelly or a pessary should be added on the vaginal side before the first as well as subsequent acts of intercourse after insertion.

4.47 What arrangements are made for routine subsequent follow-up?

1 After the first two visits it is usual to see the patients at 3 months and then at least annually. (Six-monthly visits used to be recommended but this is probably unnecessarily frequent.) The most important thing is that the woman feels free to return more frequently if difficulties occur.

2 Reassessment of the fitting is particularly required:
   (a) after full-term delivery
   (b) after any unplanned pregnancy, whether ending in a termination or miscarriage (chiefly to assess possible improvements in fitting or the user's technique)
   (c) after having vaginal surgery
   (d) after the woman loses or gains more than 3 kg in weight.

4.48 What is the scientific basis for the rules and regulations about use of occlusive caps, as in *Qs 4.44–4.47* above?

Rather weak: many assumptions, some of them fundamental ones, have never been tested in proper controlled trials, namely that:

1 Spermicides add significantly to the effectiveness of occlusive caps. Actually this has now been tested with a good study design at the Margaret Pyke Centre but the statistical power was insufficient for a conclusive result (*see Q 4.7*). In practice, spermicide use is advised with all the products, including newer ones like FemCap™.
2 Fitting the largest diaphragm that the woman finds comfortable will improve its effectiveness.
3 Extra spermicide should be used at each intercourse.
4 Extra spermicide should be used if intercourse is delayed for more than 3 h after placement of the cap.
5 The spermicide should be applied both to the top and under surface of the diaphragm. (Again this is advised for FemCap™.)
6 The shortest safe time after intercourse that any occlusive cap can be removed is 6 h (based on assumptions about the spermicidal effects of the acid vagina).
7 Gain or loss of as little as 3 kg in weight would influence the effectiveness of occlusive caps.

4.49 What variations in the instructions given to patients are worth considering?

Numerous variations are accepted practice in different countries around the world. In Australia, use of spermicide at all with occlusive caps is often left to the patient's choice. The rationale for this is the high rate of user-failure in that country and the belief that increased compliance is likely when 'messy' spermicides are avoided. This view, however, is a minority one. Pending more data, most authorities feel that spermicides should be used but that all possible efforts should be made to reduce the problems of non-compliance with which they are associated. In addition two variants seem reasonable, both with respect to the diaphragm:

1   Application of spermicide to the superior surface only of the diaphragm. This is the norm in the US and is also becoming more usual in the UK (about an 8-cm [3-inch] strip of cream or jelly from the tube being applied).
2   Increasing to 6 h the interval after placement of the diaphragm and before intercourse after which further spermicide is advised.

Other minor variations are also permitted by various family planning authorities.

OCCLUSIVE CAPS: MANAGEMENT OF SIDE-EFFECTS AND COMPLICATIONS

4.50   What should be done if the partner can feel the diaphragm during intercourse?

1   Check the size – a larger or smaller variety might be needed.
2   Re-teach the patient. The couple might already have decided not to use certain positions (e.g. for rear entry vaginal intercourse they might use the condom instead).
3   Change from a flat- to a coiled-spring diaphragm.
4   Change to a vault or perhaps a cervical cap.
5   Change the method.

4.51   Why are urinary tract infections more common in diaphragm users, and how should they be managed?

1   The fact that urinary tract infections develop more frequently is believed to be caused mainly by the pressure of the rim on the urethra and bladder base, predisposing to urethritis and cystitis.

2   Some work has also suggested that use of the diaphragm and other occlusive caps with spermicide alters the vaginal flora so as to promote infections. Vaginal cultures from cap users grow *Escherichia coli* more often than those from relevant controls.

It would appear that the first explanation is the more important because the following actions usually help, especially item (2):

1   change to a smaller size of diaphragm
2   change to a vault cap (or cervical cap or FemCap™).

The woman is also advised to empty her bladder both before and just after intercourse.

4.52   What are the possible causes of the complaint of 'vaginal soreness'?

1   There might be an incidental infection such as trichomoniasis or thrush (or urethritis, *see* Q 4.51 above).

2 Inflammatory reactions, abrasions or even frank ulcers can also be caused by local pressure.

3 Allergy is possible, either to the spermicide or to chemicals in the rubber of the occlusive cap.

4.53 How should vaginal soreness be managed?

1 *Examine the patient*: particularly her vulva and the whole vaginal surface. If there is widespread erythema and multiple vesicles or scaling, suspect allergy. Allergy cannot easily be treated by change of spermicide (*Table 4.2*)! For true rubber allergy the polyurethane female condom or FemCap™ are good options.

2 *Take swabs for possible infections*: if there is a discharge with a slightly fishy odour, it is useful to test the pH, using test paper with a pH range of 4–6. A result > 4.5 suggests either bacterial vaginosis (BV) or trichomoniasis, both of which are treatable with metronidazole. For BV, clindamycin (Dalacin™) 2% cream can also be used – but beware its possible adverse effects on rubber (*see Q 3.21*).

4.54 What should be done if actual abrasions or ulcers are seen?

I have personally only seen one severe case, in an arcing diaphragm user, but they have been described in users of other diaphragms, vimules and cervical caps.

In our case the ulcers were posterolateral on each side, 2–3 cm long and about 0.5 cm wide and deep, and very indurated. At first a carcinoma of the vagina was suspected! However, complete recovery followed non-use of the diaphragm (which was size 85 and fitted correctly) and abstinence from intercourse for 3 weeks. No other treatment was required.

TABLE 4.2 Spermicides available in the UK (from BNF March 2003)		
Name	**Manufacturer**	**Active ingredients**
Foams		
Delfen™ foam	Janssen-Cilag Pharmaceutical Ltd	Nonoxynol-9 12.5%
Creams		
Ortho-creme	Janssen-Cilag Pharmaceutical Ltd	Nonoxynol-9 2%
Jellies		
Durex Duragel™	SSL International	Nonoxynol-9 2%
Gynol II™	Janssen-Cilag Pharmaceutical Ltd	Nonoxynol-9 2%
Pessaries		
Ortho-forms	Janssen-Cilag Pharmaceutical Ltd	Nonoxynol-9 5%

All these products have vehicles that do not have adverse effects on rubber (see Q 3.21).

The woman concerned had met a new partner and intercourse had been unusually vigorous and frequent, with the diaphragm left in place for long periods of time. Cases reported from the US had similarly worn the diaphragm or vimule cap for three or more days in succession. This rare complication is also said to be more likely if the diaphragm is too large, and might be related to variations in individual anatomy (*see Q. 4.85*).

> Regrettably, the 'Today'™ and Protectaid™ contraceptive sponges – products that were found to be very user-friendly and popular among women whose fertility could be expected to be low – were removed from the UK market (solely for commercial reasons). But there are plans to reintroduce Today™ during 2004 (see www.todayswomencare.com).

FEMALE CONDOMS

4.55 What is the new female condom, first marketed during 1992?

Various designs have been proposed, including the bikini condom with its integral latex pouch, from the US and, more recently, the Janesway panty-condom, with a latex pouch attached to frilly knickers! Neither of these has reached the market to date.

The most successful product is Femidom™ (Reality™ in the US), which was first devised in Denmark. Made of polyurethane and preloaded with an efficient silicone lubricant, the currently marketed version is 17 cm long. Both brands have a large (70 mm) diameter outer ring attached at the opening, designed to prevent it advancing beyond the vulva. A 60-mm diameter loose ring at the inner closed end aids its retention within the vagina and is also squeezed like a diaphragm for insertion. The whole device thus forms a well-lubricated secondary vagina (*Fig. 4.5*).

4.56 What advantages are claimed for female condoms?

1   Over-the-counter method not requiring fitting by any outsider.
2   Under the woman's control.
3   Insertable before intercourse, like the diaphragm.
4   Does not require an erect penis at outset.
5   Male sensations are usually reported as feeling more normal than intercourse with a male rubber condom.
6   Odour free.
7   A better barrier against STIs, including viruses, than any intravaginal method can provide.
8   Worth suggesting if local soreness makes sex uncomfortable or during menses or postpartum lochia.

Fig. 4.5 Femidom™. Q 4.55.

9   Shown to be less likely than the male condom to rupture in use.
10   Not damaged by any common chemicals.

Its use-effectiveness (13.5 conceptions per 100 women at 6 months in one US trial) is probably broadly similar to the male condom (*see Table 1.2*).

4.57   Are there any problems?

Users report several in-use problems:

1   Prominence during foreplay.
2   The potential for the penis to become wrongly positioned (between the sac and the vaginal wall). Users should be warned about this risk.
3   It is rather noisy in use: prompting the suggestion to 'have the music on!'

4.58   What is the place of Femidom™ in the range of methods?

Reports about its acceptability are mixed. It was given qualified approval as a method by about half the users in the first study by the Margaret Pyke Centre. These people tried it up to ten times but used a different method for contraception. Among 106 volunteers of the same Centre's trial of Femidom™ as the sole contraceptive, more than half found it unacceptable. However, 9 of the 11 users who continued for 1 year, and most of 20 who had to stop using it solely because supplies ran out, would have wished to continue long term. As the first female-controlled method with high potential for preventing HIV transmission it must surely be welcomed to the range of contraceptive options. Further development of new variants will hopefully make it more acceptable and use-effective.

A proportion of users ring the changes along with male condoms according to choice, i.e. having 'his' night followed by 'her' night!

SPERMICIDES

4.59 What are spermicides?

These substances chemically immobilize or destroy sperm. They are one of the oldest and simplest forms of fertility control and make a useful contribution, chiefly to increase the efficacy of other methods.

4.60 What is the mode of action of spermicides?

They have two main components: a relatively inert base and an active spermicidal agent. Hence they operate both physically and biochemically, forming a partial barrier and also immobilizing sperm. The base materials vary in their physical characteristics, the best being water soluble. The active ingredients are of five main types:

1   surface-active agents, of which the most widely used worldwide is nonoxynol-9. Indeed, due to commercial pressures this has now become the only spermicide still on the UK market – resulting in real difficulties for users of occlusive caps who develop soreness or irritation (*see Q 4.67*) or an allergy to it
2   enzyme inhibitors
3   bactericides
4   acids
5   local anaesthetics and other membrane-active agents.

4.61 What types are available?

All the spermicides currently used in the UK are listed in Table 4.2. Regrettably there is very little real choice.

With the arrival of the HIV/AIDS problem we are now suffering from neglect of this field by a generation of scientists: far too little research has been done to devise better substances, more effective and safer not only as spermicides but also potentially as microbicides (*see Qs 4.66 and 4.67*).

4.62 How are spermicides used?

To be effective, the products should disperse quickly yet remain in sufficient concentration at the cervix to exert their action at the end of intercourse. Aerosol foams such as Delfen™ seem to be preferable in this respect. The products listed can be inserted just before intercourse, with the important exception of pessaries and the foaming tablets available outwith the UK. These should be inserted at least 10 min before ejaculation to allow sufficient time for dispersal.

4.63 How effective are spermicides used alone?

Spermicides are far more effective in vitro than they ever prove to be in vivo (*see Q 2.3* for a full discussion). There are greater variations in reported effectiveness for spermicides than for almost any other birth control method. The limits range from less than 1 to over 30 pregnancies/100 woman-years! In a study of almost 3000 well-motivated women attending six family planning clinics in the US, who received the proper instructions and follow-up, Bernstein documented a pregnancy rate of only 4/100 woman-years. Trussell indicates a 'perfect use' rate of 6% in the first year.

4.64 Are spermicides recommended for use alone as contraceptives?

General teaching in the UK has been that spermicides are not effective enough for use alone. Delfen™ foam and, when available, spermicide-impregnated sponges such as Today™, are believed to be more effective than the other available presentations. They are user-friendly, non-greasy and essentially unobtrusive, non-coitally-related. They can be a very useful choice under certain conditions, mainly where reduced fertility and good compliance are both expected:

1   Women's natural fertility can be low because of:
    (a) *Age*: fertility declines, most steeply after the age of 45 but less so in those with continued regular cycling (*see Qs 11.33 and 11.34*). Hence Delfen™ foam or a sponge can be very appropriate, as well as acceptable, from the age of 45 if irregular cycles with some vasomotor symptoms are occurring (and even more so after 50), through until 1 year after the menopause. This may be especially acceptable as an alternative to condoms during cyclical HRT, which alone is not adequately contraceptive.
    (b) *Lactation*: the method could be used until uterine bleeding begins to return at weaning.
    (c) *Secondary amenorrhoea* (*see Q 5.65*): although if the woman is hypo-oestrogenic the COC or HRT might be preferable.
2   Spermicide via foam or a sponge can also be used as an adjunct to other methods of birth control, such as the IUD or coitus interruptus.

3   It can also be used for those who are planning their first child fairly soon, or who are spacing their family.
4   It would certainly be better than nothing for women who are unable or unwilling to use any other more effective method.

4.65   What are the advantages and disadvantages of spermicides?

These are summarized in *Table 4.3*.

4.66   Do spermicides protect against sexually transmitted infections?

In vitro studies have shown that most spermicides can kill sexually transmitted pathogens. Nonoxynol has some activity against the organisms causing gonorrhoea, *Chlamydia*, *Trichomonas vaginalis*, genital herpes and even HIV. However, in vivo, none of this promise has been confirmed with respect to the risk of HIV/AIDS virus transmission, and the virucidal effect is completely nullified by tissue toxicity affecting the vaginal mucosa (*see Q 4.67*).

There is at last much research in progress to produce vaginal microbicides that would be active against HIV and other STIs, a subject that was well reviewed in an article by Stone (*Nature reviews. Drug Discovery* 2002 1:977–985).

TABLE 4.3   Advantages and disadvantages of spermicides

Advantages	Disadvantages
1 Easy availability	1 Perceived to be messy
2 Freedom from major health risks	2 Not highly effective in general use
3 No medical intervention/ supervision necessary	3 Are coitus-dependent and thus inconvenient to use
4 Need only be used when required	4 Waiting period of 10 min before some products effective
5 Allow the female to be in control of contraception	5 Not effective if inserted more than too far ahead
6 Provide some genital lubrication	6 Can cause local heat (foaming tablets), irritation or allergy
7 Are a valuable adjunct to other methods	7 Evidence of damage by nonoxynol-9 to the vaginal mucosa *and* increased risk of HIV transmission, in frequent use. This makes nonoxynol useful primarily with diaphragm and caps alone (Q 4.67 & 3.19) and greatly increases urgency to develop a better product
8 Possible protection against some sexually transmitted diseases – and research proceeds to enhance this benefit through innovative microbicidal compounds released vaginally	

VAGINAL CONTRACEPTION: UNRESOLVED SAFETY ISSUES

4.67 Is it true that nonoxynol sometimes seems capable of damaging the vaginal epithelium? How might this affect HIV transmission?

The answers are 'Yes' and 'adversely'. A first-line study in Nairobi prostitutes of nonoxynol (N–9) containing spermicides as a possible aid to safer sex reported 'soreness' as a frequent complaint. This was at first thought to be linked in part with trauma from very frequent coitus but subsequent studies have shown that frequent use of the product itself is the main factor. When used on average four times a day for 14 days, nonoxynol-9 released from pessaries caused erythema and colposcopic evidence of minor damage to the vaginal skin. Worse than that, Van Damme et al. in 2002 found in a randomly controlled trial a higher incidence of HIV in N–9 users than in placebo-using controls. This study and others reviewed and referenced by Wilkinson et al 2002 *The Lancet infectious diseases* 2:613–617 prompted the WHO to issue new recommendations (www.who.int) including:

1. N–9 should **not** be used for STI or HIV prevention.
2. Women at high risk of HIV should not use N–9 at all.
3. Women who have multiple daily acts of intercourse should be advised against N–9 use.
4. Women at low risk of HIV and having sex at a 'normal contraceptive frequency' (not defined by WHO but presumed to be no more than once per 24 h) may use N–9, e.g. with the female barrier method.
5. Condoms should in future not be lubricated with N–9-containing lubricants (*see Qs 3.18–3.19*).

However, pending the development of more alternatives, for the time being it is considered good practice to continue to recommend nonoxynol in the products listed in Table 4.2 for normal contraceptive use (less frequently than four times a day!), whether alone or with diaphragms or cervical caps. Nonoxynol-9 should no longer be used in the lubricants of condoms, however (*see Qs 3.18 and 3.19*).

The Margaret Pyke Trust continues to be actively involved with other bodies in urgent and previously neglected research into new and better substances for vaginal use as virucides and spermicides.

Pending their availability, the products listed in Table 4.2 are the only spermicidal options for use with all the female barriers.

4.68 Are spermicides absorbed and is there therefore a risk of systemic effects?

Yes, most substances in the vagina can be absorbed into the circulation. Hence it is impossible to say that any method that uses a spermicide is entirely free of the risk of systemic harmful effects. These could be by toxicity to vital organs, idiosyncrasy, or through carcinogenesis or teratogenesis. There have been some reports suggesting an association with unwanted effects (*see Qs 4.69 and 4.70*) following spermicide absorption, but the overall picture remains a reassuring one.

4.69 What is the evidence that standard spermicides might have toxic effects after absorption?

In 1979 it was suggested from animal experiments that nonoxynol-9 might have hepatotoxic effects and cause changes in serum lipids. However, controlled studies of the blood chemistry of women using spermicides have not demonstrated any significant changes, although long-term data are not available. Certainly no obvious harm has ever been reported among long-term users of vaginal contraceptives.

4.70 What is the evidence about teratogenesis?

Exposure to the spermicide early in pregnancy, or fertilization of an ovum by a sperm damaged by the spermicide, might in theory increase the rate of malformations. In 1981, one study reported an increase in various unrelated fetal abnormalities among the children of women who could have used spermicides around the time they became pregnant. This study has been criticized because of flaws in the study design and more recent studies have completely failed to show the risk. Present opinion is that spermicides do not have any detectable teratogenic effect in ordinary use.

4.71 Are there reports of an increase of neoplasia in women using vaginal contraception?

No – neither as a consequence of systemic absorption, nor because of any effect of spermicide or rubber on the vaginal or cervical epithelium. A few women who are sensitive to spermicides could develop hyperkeratosis of the cervix or vagina. This has not been shown to result in neoplasia. Indeed, it is very likely that barrier methods are protective against cervical neoplasia (*see Q 4.17*).

4.72 Can vaginal contraception promote infection?

Concern arises from the above story concerning HIV transmission (*Q 4.67*) coupled with evidence that *Staphylococcus aureus*, some streptococci and *E. coli* tend to proliferate in the presence of a diaphragm or a cervical cap at the expense of the usual protective lactobacilli, which can be adversely affected by the nonoxynol-9 spermicide. This could promote bacterial vaginosis and has already been mentioned as a possible factor in the increased risk of urinary infections. It might also be relevant to toxic shock syndrome (TSS), although there is no proof that vaginal contraception increases that risk, which is primarily associated with prolonged use of tampons. Once again, a low frequency of N–9 use appears to be advantageous.

4.73 Can the diaphragm or other caps cause toxic shock syndrome?

Possibly yes. There is some positive evidence from Schwartz et al 1989 *Rev Infect Dis II (Suppl 1)* 543–588. However, any added risk is probably greater (though still tiny) from use of tampons by those diaphragm users.

4.74 What is the overall safety of vaginal contraceptives?

Even allowing for the unresolved safety issues above, potential users can be told that all these methods are still believed to be medically safer than the hormonal methods. However, honesty is necessary, and it would be wrong to say that any method that uses an absorbable spermicide is completely free from systemic effects.

In assessing safety it is also important to remember that unwanted pregnancies are overall more frequent among users of any of these methods. One then has to consider the potential health hazard to the mother of the resulting unwanted pregnancies.

THE (NEAR) FUTURE IN VAGINAL CONTRACEPTION

4.75 What innovative spermicides and microbicides are being studied?

Inhibitors of the sperm's own enzymes, principally acrosin, show promise, and several surprising drugs (like propranolol) that are normally used for non-contraceptive indications have aroused interest because of their effect on the sperm membrane and motility. Derivatives of natural products such as gossypol have also been screened. Another approach is to develop agents that directly alter cervical mucus both chemically and physically.

However there is now special interest in microbicides for preventing vaginal transmission of all kinds of STIs but especially HIV. These are well reviewed in Stone 2002 *Nature Reviews* 1:977–984. Progress is slow but at least four promising new substances entered Phase III trials during 2003 – substances which, unlike N–9, are nonirritant to the vaginal epithelium. More research is also urgently required into better carrier (base) materials and systems.

4.76 What is the state of research into occlusive caps?

1 *Disposable spermicide-coated diaphragms*: designed to overcome the perceived 'messiness' of any vaginal contraceptive that requires separate application of the spermicide. No further progress has been reported.

Fig. 4.6 FemCap™ Q 4.76 (from Kubba et al 1999 *Contraception and office gynecoloogy: choices in reproductive healthcare* p. 124. London, WB Saunders. With permission).

2   *New sponges*: with different spermicides, or combinations of spermicide or microbicides should be useful, judging by the high acceptability of the sponge method in the trial by the Margaret Pyke Centre (*Q 4.64*).

3   *New cervical caps*: there was great interest in the mid-1980s in the so-called custom-fitted cervical cap, made from a mould of the user's cervix. Although trials of this Contracap™ gave a quite unacceptable failure rate, the objective remains attractive – of a non-coitally-related appliance designed to be left in place in the upper vagina for long periods of time. Lea's Shield™ and FemCap™ are US inventions and preliminary results with the latter, which does not require fitting like a diaphragm but must still be used with a spermicide, are reasonably promising (*Fig. 4.6*). FemCap™ is a small reusable cap made of silicone rubber, available from FP Sales of Oxford (see MIMS). It is available on the NHS Drug Tariff and available in sizes 22, 26 and 30 mm diameter. Initial fitting by a doctor or nurse is desirable, but not essential, and there is no expected need for future follow-up visits. FemCap™ must be

used with a spermicidal gel, and may be worm continuously for up to 48 h in all, including 6 h after last intercourse. The manufacturer's stated pregnancy rate of 10.5 per 100 women for 1 year of use in US trials requires independent confirmation. The Oves™ cap, also an over-the-counter product used with spermicide, arrived on the UK market with almost no efficacy data and since 2002 has ceased to be available. The Gynaeseal™ diaphragm–tampon devised by an Australian and mentioned in the last edition of this book, seems to have sunk without trace.

4 *Intracervical devices*: both medicated and non-medicated devices with some kind of flange or protruding arms to anchor them in the lower part of the uterus are possibilities that have been studied.

5 *Vaginal rings*: WHO did some preliminary work on a silicone rubber ring that released nonoxynol-9 at a constant rate for at least 30 days. This seems a very promising approach, but it should use a more advanced spermicide and one day – hopefully – a microbicidal substance to be used in addition to any chosen contraceptive. This would be invaluable worldwide, empowering women who often cannot persuade their partners to use a condom.

 PATIENT QUESTIONS

QUESTIONS ASKED BY USERS ABOUT VAGINAL CONTRACEPTION

4.77   Can I use some kind of cap if my womb tilts backwards?

It is a myth that this makes it impossible to use the method. Some positions of your cervix (entrance to the womb) can make it preferable for you to be given an arcing diaphragm and could result in rejection of a cervical cap but the method is not ruled out if you wish to use it.

4.78   In the US they have inserters for diaphragms – are they available here?

Yes they are, but you need to ask yourself whether your wish to use one might be connected with some reluctance to touch yourself in the genital area. This could be overcome by counselling, or perhaps you should think about using another method.

4.79   How do I know where my cervix is?

It is absolutely essential that you feel confident that you can find your cervix, whatever the kind of occlusive cap you are going to use. It is often helpful to ask your doctor or the nurse to tell you in which direction its opening points. You might also find it easier to feel if you use two fingers rather than one.

4.80   How much cream or jelly should I use with my diaphragm?

A common error is to use too much (*see Q 4.44* for the standard instructions). If you find messiness a particular problem but still want to use the method, ask your doctor or nurse about the possibility of following the US teaching of putting spermicide only on the top when it is first inserted (but continue to follow all the other rules you were taught). Delfen™ foam might be preferable.

4.81   Can the cap fall out when you go to the toilet?

Normally this will not happen. If it does, soon after intercourse, consider postcoital contraception (*see Chapter 10*). Moreover, if your diaphragm or other cap comes out it might be that you have a prolapse, or the wrong size, or are not inserting it correctly. So you should make an early appointment to discuss things with the doctor or nurse.

4.82   Can caps and diaphragms be fitted with strings to help removal? I have difficulty in getting mine out.

There are no longer any marketed with strings. You might have been taught to use just one finger to hook out the diaphragm and the solution to your problem could well be just to use two fingers, one each side of the front rim. FemCap™ has a special removal strap.

4.83   How do I check the diaphragm is in good condition? Its dome has become much softer and floppier and it has lost its new whiteness – do these changes matter?

You should hold your diaphragm up to the light and stretch it, being careful not to damage the rubber with your fingernails. If no holes are seen, and if the rim can readily be restored to a reasonable shape, then all is well. The change in colour and texture of the rubber is quite normal.

4.84   Can I leave the cap in during my periods?

The US Food and Drug Administration (FDA) advises against this because of an unproven extra risk of the rare TSS. It can be used short term to reduce messiness if you fancy lovemaking during any bleeding but a better solution might be Femidom™ (*see Q 4.55*).

4.85   I have heard you can leave the cap in all the time – is this right?

If you follow the rules, yes – almost! It can be in position most of the time if your love life is unpredictable and frequent. The important thing is to remove it at least once in 24 hours, (48 h if you have a FemCap™) always 6 h after the last intercourse, wash it in mild soap and rinse it thoroughly, after which it can be reinserted. Continuous use without giving your vaginal wall an occasional rest seems a bad thing, however (*see Q 4.54*), at least with a diaphragm.

4.86 Can I have a bath or go swimming with the cap in place?

Yes. Although it would be ideal to wait until 6 h after the last intercourse, in case it helps the sperm to escape the action of the spermicide. And if you make love after bathing with the diaphragm in, put some extra spermicide in first.

4.87 I've had a baby – can I go back to using my old diaphragm or cap?

Quite possibly not. It is certainly important to get the fitting rechecked for size, and maybe take the opportunity to rediscuss *all* your contraceptive options. (*See also* Q 4.47).

4.88 How often should I change the diaphragm or cap for a new one?

Only when your inspection (*see* Q 4.83) shows damage, or as recommended by your clinic. Successful regular use of the same one for 2 years is common. Remember too that if you lose your cap you can buy the right size at any pharmacy.

4.89 Is Femidom™ a recommended method?

Yes. Follow the instructions that come with it carefully, every time. As long as you are careful to avoid wrong positioning of the penis (*see* Q 4.57), and the sperm are caught completely within the Femidom™, it is comparable to a male condom both as a contraceptive and for safer sex.

4.90 Can I use a home-made barrier 'in an emergency'?

Improvised barriers can be made. Probably the best is a suitable piece of sponge or plug of cloth, soaked either in vinegar solution diluted 1 in 20 with water or in a lemon juice or soap solution.

4.91 Do you recommend the 'honeycap', which my friend uses?

Definitely not. Available from some doctors in private practice in London, this is really only a size 60 arcing-spring diaphragm that is first soaked in honey for 7 days and then used without spermicide for up to a week at a time. The honey is meant to reduce the risk of vaginal infection or odour, but even this is unproven and its effectiveness has also not been properly tested.

All in all it is highly likely to have the same failure rate as in a 1982 Marie Stopes Centre study of the 'non-spermicide, fit-free diaphragm' (of the same 60 mm size), which amounted to a risk, in the first year, that one in every four users would become pregnant!

The combined oral contraceptive – selection and eligibility

5

STARTING ROUTINES WITH THE COC

CONTRACEPTION AFTER PREGNANCY (SEE QS 11.18–11.32)

MAJOR SYSTEMIC EFFECTS OF THE COC

THE COC AND CIRCULATORY DISEASES

A MORE DETAILED APPRAISAL OF THE CONTROVERSY ABOUT VENOUS THROMBOEMBOLISM (VTE) AND ITS IMPLICATIONS FOR PRESCRIBERS

SELECTION OF USERS AND FORMULATIONS: CHOOSING THE 'SAFER WOMEN', AND THE 'SAFER PILLS'

MORE ABOUT THE AVAILABLE PILL FORMULATIONS

INDICATIONS AND CONTRAINDICATIONS FOR THE COC METHOD, IN DEPTH

MIGRAINE HEADACHES, WITH AND WITHOUT AURA

BACKGROUND: EFFICACY AND MECHANISMS

5.1 What is the definition of oral contraception?

An orally administered substance or combination that prevents pregnancy. Specifically, at the present time such substances are only for use by women. Although steroids and other potential systemic contraceptives can also be given by non-oral routes (see *Qs 6.80–83, Chapters 8 and 11*), in this chapter I will consider only the combined oral contraceptive (COC), which is a combination of oestrogen and progestogen. Unless qualified, the word 'pill' refers to the COC. The progestogen-only pill (POP) is considered in *Chapter 7*.

5.2 What is the history of oral contraception?

This is discussed in more detail elsewhere (see my book *The pill*, details in Further Reading). In brief, it was shown by the early 1900s that the corpus luteum of pregnancy stops further ovulation. In 1921, Haberlandt transplanted ovaries into female rabbits, which rendered them infertile for several months. He suggested that extracts from ovaries might be used as oral contraceptives. In 1941 Marker used diosgenin, from the Mexican yam, as the raw material for sex steroids. This led to the synthesis of norethisterone (known as norethindrone in the US) by Djerassi and his colleagues in 1950. Frank Colton independently produced norethynodrel, which – with mestranol – was the first marketed oral contraceptive. Margaret Sanger, supported by her wealthy friend Catherine McCormack, financed the studies of the biologists Gregory Pincus and M.C. Chang, together with the obstetrician John Rock. After systematic experiments in animals, the first human trials in North America were reported in 1956. In the Puerto Rico field-trial that followed, the intention appears to have been to use progestogen alone, but there was contamination with mestranol. Thus the invention of the 'combined pill' – which was shown later to give much better cycle control than any progestogen-only method – owes a definite debt to chance.

The combined pill became available in the US in June 1960 and in the UK during 1961. In 1963 the Wyeth Company achieved the total synthesis of norgestrel.

The first case report of venous thromboembolism was reported in *The Lancet* in 1961 by an astute British GP. Subsequently, there have been numerous case–control studies and three main prospective (cohort) studies, researching both the adverse and beneficial effects. Much more money has been spent on testing than on originally developing the method.

5.3 What is the usage of the pill, worldwide and in the UK?

Currently around 100 million women rely on the pill. There is enormous variation between countries, and within countries, according to age groups.

The differences have more to do with medical politics, religion and the inertia of institutions than with the acceptability or otherwise of the method to potential consumers. Estimated overall usage varies between less than 10% of married women in Japan through to about 50% in Western Europe. For UK data, *see Table 1.3*, p. 16.

In several surveys over the last 15 years, for the Royal College of General Practitioners (RCGP) and other bodies, up to 95% of sexually active UK women under the age of 30 reported use of oral contraceptives at some time.

5.4 What are the main mechanisms of contraceptive action of the combined pill?

These are summarized in *Table 5.1*. Without exception, all steroidal methods operate by some combination of the mechanisms there described. The COC has a very similar primary action in most women, namely the prevention of ovulation – both by lack of follicular maturation and by abolition of the oestrogen-mediated positive feedback that leads to the luteinizing hormone (LH) surge. The other mechanisms shown in the table – reduction in sperm penetrability of cervical mucus (*see Q 7.16*) and of the receptivity to the blastocyst of the endometrium (*see Q 7.17*) – are primarily back-up mechanisms for the COC. They have greater relevance to the mechanisms of some of the oestrogen-free methods of *Chapters 7 and 8*.

5.5 What are the types of COC?

Current COCs are either fixed-dose or phasic; both types contain oestrogen and progestogen. The ratio of the two is not fixed, however, but changed in a stepwise fashion, either once (biphasic pills) or twice (triphasic pills) in each 21-day course. They are discussed in more detail below (*see Qs 5.179–5.184*). We should note here, however, that – like all COCs – the phasic types remove the menstrual cycle, but these attempt to replace it with cyclical variations, chiefly in the progestogen dose. There is as yet no proof that this has important health benefits (aside, that is, from the giving of a low dose of each hormone).

5.6 What are 'everyday' (ED) varieties of COC? Do they have advantages?

These are regimens that include, usually, 7 days of placebo tablets. They have the advantage of a reduction in the risk that the user will forget to restart her next packet on time – a potent cause of pill failure (*see Q 5.18*). This system is also one way of removing the necessity for numbering, as opposed to putting the day of the week, against the pill blisters in phasic packets (compare Logynon ED™ with Logynon™). A simpler solution, as in Trinovum™, is the use of 7-day phases. 'Sunday start' schemes, with

TABLE 5.1 Various progestogen delivery systems

	COC	EVRA™	POP (old type)	NET-EN	DMPA	Cerazette™	Implanon™
Administration	Oral	Transdermal 7-day patches	Oral	i.m.	i.m.	Oral	Subdermal
Frequency	Daily	Daily	Daily	2-monthly	3-monthly	Daily	3-yearly
Estrogen dose	Low	Low	Nil	Nil	Nil	Nil	Nil
Progestogen dose	Low	Low	Ultra-low	High	High	Low	Ultra-low
Blood levels	Daily peaks & troughs	Steady	Daily peaks & troughs	Initial peak then decline	Initial peak then decline	Daily peaks & troughs	Steady
First pass through liver	Yes	No	Yes	No	No	Yes	No
Major mechanisms							
Ovary: ↓ Ovulation*	+++	+++	+	++	+++	+++	++
Cervical mucus: ↓ sperm penetrability	Yes	Yes	Yes	Yes	Yes	Yes	Yes
Endometrium: ↓ receptivity to blastocyst (a weak effect)	Yes	Yes	Yes	Yes	Yes	Yes	Yes
Consistent use failures/100 WY	0.2–3	0.6–0.9	0.3–4	<2	0–1	0.2–0.9	0–0.07
Menstrual pattern	Regular	Regular	Often irregular	Irregular	Very irregular	Often irregular	Often irregular
Amenorrhoea during use	Rare	Rare	Occasional	Common	Very common	Common	Common
Reversibility							
Immediate termination possible?	Yes	Yes	Yes	No	No	Yes	Yes
By woman herself at anytime?	Yes	Yes	Yes	No	No	Yes	No
Median time to conception from first omitted dose/removal	c. 3 months	c. 3 months	c. 2 months	c. 3 months	c. 6 months	c. 2 months	c. 2 months

*By two mechanisms – no pre-ovulatory follicles formed, plus no LH surges occur.

i.m., intramuscular. 100 WY, 100 woman-years

Note: Cerazette™ contains the same active agent as Implanon™ (desogestrel being a pro-drug for etonogestrel) and shows other similarities.

instructions for extra contraception for the first seven days, are common in the US.

5.7 What are the disadvantages of ED packaging?

This is often (not always) complicated by a starting routine involving a variable number of placebos, so extra contraception has to be advised for up to 14 days. Moreover some women dislike the implication that they are too unintelligent to remember when to stop and restart treatment. It has been suggested that some women think that the dummy lactose (sugar) pills might be bad for them!

For these reasons, ED packaging has never been popular in the UK. However, in other countries well over half of all pill cycles are of this type, which I personally favour as an aid to compliance. There are ways – as with Microgynon ED™ for example – of simplifying the starting routine so as always to start with an active tablet; and perhaps the placebos should be made of bran, as everyone knows that bran is good for you!

5.8 What modified regimens would you like to see marketed?

Given that the pill-free interval (PFI) is 'the Achilles' heel' of the COC's efficacy, there would be particular merit in returning across the board to an earlier scheme of 22 active pills with six placebos. Indeed, even without placebos this might help compliance because the 'finishing day' is then the same day of the week as the 'starting day'.

ED packets of ultra-low-dose monophasic brands with four placebo tablets are coming in at last. Instead of, or as well as, tricycling (*see Q. 5.31*) these regimens with a much shortened pill-free time could be used by women with a history of past conception while taking the COC (*see Q 5.27*). Moreover, with the PFI so shortened, new products for general use can safely offer even lower doses of both hormones than are currently viable. Such products (e.g. Minesse™ or Meliane Light™; other names are on the IPPF website: *www.ippf.org.uk*) are already marketed in some countries. Minesse™ is an effective anovulant despite containing only 15 μg of ethinylestradiol plus 60 μg of gestodene given as 24 tablets followed by just four hormone-free days.

5.9 What about other oestrogen–progestogen agents (especially sequential pills and regimens of HRT)?

High-oestrogen sequential pills were shown to double the risk of endometrial carcinoma and have rightly been consigned to history.

Older women are now frequently given a similar regimen of oestrogen alone, typically for 16 days, followed by oestrogen plus progestogen for 12 days. The oestrogen is, of course, a natural oestrogen, in doses that have a far smaller effect on the endometrium. There is evidence that these regimens do not significantly increase the risk of endometrial cancer, but they are not safely contraceptive.

There is some evidence that the continuous combined HRT regimens reduce cancer risk. Moreover (including tibolone) they are almost certainly contraceptive but are not recommended while there is any residual fertility (only because they might cause irregular bleeding if so used). *See Chapter 11.*

5.10 What link is there between the COC cycle and the menstrual cycle?

Very little, but endless confusion is caused by the fact that women consider their hormone withdrawal bleeds as the same thing as 'periods'. In reality, of course, the normal menstrual cycle is removed during use of the COC. The ovaries show no follicular activity during pill taking (contrast the situation between packets, *see Q 5.15*) and hence produce minimal endogenous oestrogen. Withdrawal bleeding (WTB) is an end-organ response to withdrawal of the artificial hormones and is irrelevant to events elsewhere in the body, and specifically at the pituitary and the ovaries. In physiological terms, everywhere except at the endometrium, the pill causes secondary amenorrhoea for as long as the woman takes it.

Absence of WTB is totally irrelevant to future fertility, although a pregnancy test is indicated after two WTBs have been missed: sooner if there are good reasons to suspect pill-failure. Aside from pregnancy testing, it is pointless to investigate this.

Breakthrough bleeding (BTB) is likewise a purely endometrial response but it might be heavy enough to simulate a 'period' to the woman. This also needs explaining in advance as a reason to continue taking her daily pills with extra diligence (until an early appointment), rather than stopping.

Lack of adequate instruction about WTB and BTB commonly causes avoidable 'iatrogenic' pregnancies (*see Qs 11.12 and 11.17*).

5.11 What is the importance of the pill-free interval (PFI)?

Enormous – yet it is still not fully explained in most pill leaflets or by many prescribers. It influences all the following issues:

1 The efficacy of the COC, in that lengthening the PFI risks ovulation whereas mid-packet pill omissions are unimportant
2 The improved recommendations once pills are omitted or vomited
3 Short- or long-term use of interacting drugs or use of the pill if past 'breakthrough pregnancies' have occurred
4 The minimizing of health-risks (fewer pills per year than continuous use).

All these points will be expanded in the next group of questions.

EFFECTIVENESS OF THE COC – CIRCUMSTANCES IN WHICH IT CAN BE REDUCED

5.12 What is the efficacy of the COC?

There is no simple answer to this question because efficacy is so user-dependent. According to Trussell, during 'perfect use' only 0.1% of women in the US will experience a pregnancy during the first year of use, but in 'typical' use he gives a figure of 5% – a fifty-fold range! In the UK the FPA settles for 'over 99% effectiveness' for consistent users (*see Qs 1.18–1.19*).

The theoretical effectiveness approaches 100% partly because of the adjunctive mechanisms mentioned above (*see Q 5.4*). However it appears that for some women the modern (less than 50 μg oestrogen) pills are only just sufficient for efficacy, particularly if omitted tablets lead to the slightest lengthening of the pill-free week. Minor errors of compliance are extremely common and most pill takers (through provider failure) are uninformed about the importance of the pill-free time.

The slightly higher pregnancy rate with modern pills is thus explained chiefly in terms of 'reduced margin for error'. But, regrettably, this problem is often amplified by insufficient pill teaching by hurried healthcare professionals, who regularly omit any explanation of the implications of the pill-free interval (*see Qs 5.15–5.28*) and fail to back this with the user-friendly FPA leaflet on the combined pill.

5.13 What is the effect of increasing age on efficacy?

The Oxford/FPA study shows the (slight) expected decline in pregnancy rate with increasing age, due mainly to declining fertility and also some reduction in the frequency of intercourse (*see Table 1.2*, columns 3 and 4, and *Q 1.19*). The latter effect does not of course apply to older couples in new relationships, which are becoming more common.

5.14 Are overweight women more likely to conceive while taking modern ultra-low-dose COCs?

No. This has not been demonstrated, although it might be expected pharmacologically because a 80-kg woman receives exactly the same dose in normal pill taking as her 40-kg friend. Moreover, there is a definite weight influence on the efficacy of some never-marketed progestogen-only methods (*see Q 7.14*) and also of the skin patch EVRA (*see Q6.80*).

My own theory is that the combined pill is contraceptively so very strong, along with its back-up actions, that it has sufficient margin to cope with women of any weight. Other factors like compliance will affect efficacy far more (relatively) than body mass, which is perhaps more detectable as a factor if a systemic method has a method-failure rate above 1/100 woman-years.

5.15 As it is the contraceptive-free part of the pill-taking cycle, does the PFI have efficacy implications?

Precisely. When you think about it we have here a bizarre contraceptive: one that we providers actually instruct the users not to use – for 25% of the time. Any systemic contraceptive must be at its lowest ebb when it is longest since it was actually ingested (*Fig. 5.1*). Hardly surprisingly, biochemical and ultrasound data demonstrate varying degrees of return of pituitary and ovarian follicular activity during the PFI.

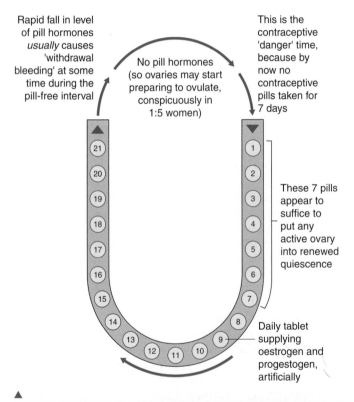

Rapid fall in level of pill hormones *usually* causes 'withdrawal bleeding' at some time during the pill-free interval

No pill hormones (so ovaries may start preparing to ovulate, conspicuously in 1:5 women)

This is the contraceptive 'danger' time, because by now no contraceptive pills taken for 7 days

These 7 pills appear to suffice to put any active ovary into renewed quiescence

Daily tablet supplying oestrogen and progestogen, artificially

Fig. 5.1 The pill cycle displayed as a horseshoe. Q 5.15. *Note*: a horseshoe is a symmetrical object and thus the pill-free interval (PFI) can be lengthened (resulting in the risk of conception) either side of the horseshoe – by forgetting pills at the beginning or at the end of the packet. See also Figure 5.4 (and Qs 5.30 and 5.31) and the issue of patient choice with regard to arranging to have far fewer PFIs and therefore bleeds.

Figure 5.2 shows the findings from a 1979 study based on patients attending the Margaret Pyke Centre. It is the rapid and sustained decline in the artificial hormones at the start of the PFI (top half of *Fig. 5.2*) that leads to the WTB. More importantly in this context, the figure shows the resulting slight average increase in (natural) estradiol, implying regular

The pill-free week

Fig. 5.2 The hormone changes of the pill-free week. Q 5.15. Changes through the pill-taking cycle in the blood levels of both the ingested artificial hormones (oestrogen (O) and progestogen (P)) and in follicular activity as demonstrated by growth of the dominant follicle by ultrasound. Note the rapid return to low ovarian activity during the first 7 days of pill taking. The bottom half of the figure is from a study of patients attending the Margaret Pyke Centre. WTB, withdrawal bleeding.

return of ovarian follicular activity during the pill-free week. Wide standard deviations are also shown, meaning that in a subgroup the levels are high – indeed as high as has been observed well into the follicular phase of spontaneous menstrual cycles.

In a more recent study by the Margaret Pyke Centre, apparently preovulatory-type follicles of diameter 10 mm or more were present on the seventh pill-free day in 23% of 120 pill takers; in three women the follicle was 16–19 mm in diameter (i.e. potentially only 1–2 days from fertile ovulation). In the other women there was no important change, suggesting continuing quiescence of their ovaries.

However, for the purpose of maintaining contraception all we have to be concerned about is the extreme cases. Among them, breakthrough ovulation is most likely to follow any lengthening of the PFI. Most important, such lengthening can result from omissions, malabsorption due to vomiting and drug interaction involving pills either at the start or at the end of a packet. See the legend to *Fig. 5.1*: pill taking is depicted as a horseshoe because a horseshoe is a symmetrical object.

Clearly, the advice that is still sometimes given – to take extra precautions to the end of her packet – is wrong: it fails to allow for ovarian activity returning in the pill-free time.

5.16   So what is the scientific basis of the advice we should give a woman who has missed pills for any reason?

In 1996, a fascinating study of previously regular pill takers by Smith et al found that if only 14, or even as few as seven, pills had been taken since the last PFI, no women ovulated after seven pills were subsequently missed! (Although one woman in the seven-pills-then-seven-missed-pills group got very close, producing progesterone – albeit at non-fertile levels.) This and other work can be summarized by three propositions:

1   Seven consecutive pills are enough to 'put the ovaries to sleep' (thereafter pills 8–21 in a packet, or many more if she tricycles, simply maintain the ovaries in quiescence).
2   Seven pills can be omitted without ovulation, as indeed is regularly the case in the pill-free week.
3   More than seven pills missed in total risks ovulation.

5.17   So what do you now (2004) recommend for missed COCs?

Fig 5.3 answers this question.

Note that the recommendations have changed quite substantially since the last edition. An algorithm was produced following the WHO 'Practice Recommendations' meeting of a WHO Scientific Working Group in London during October 2001. This is gratifyingly similar to what colleagues

Every time you miss one or more active pills (days 1–21)

| 1 Take a pill as soon as you remember | → | 2 Take the next pill at the usual time | → | 3 Keep taking active pills as usual, one each day |

In these special cases, ALSO follow these special rules:

| Started pack more than 1 day late? | Missed any 2 or more pills of first 7 pills? (days 1–7) | | Missed any 2–4 pills of last 7 active pills? (days 15–21) |

- Avoid sex or use an extra method for 7 days
- PLUS immediate use of hormonal emergency contraception (EC) if sexual exposure since end of the preceding pack of active pills
- Return to next active pill within 12 hours of the EC treatment

- Finish all active pills in the pack
- Do not take last 7 (inactive) pills in 28-pill pack
- Do not wait 7 days to start next 21-pill pack
- Start a new pack

If you miss any of the 7 inactive pills (in a 28-pill pack only):

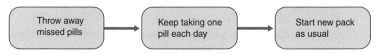

| Throw away missed pills | → | Keep taking one pill each day | → | Start new pack as usual |

▲

Fig. 5.3 What to do if you miss one or more pills. Q 5.17 (adapted from Johns Hopkins University Bloomberg School of Public Health, Population Information Program and WHO's Practice Recommendations. **Note**: For what to do if five or more pills are missed during days 8–21, see Q 5.22.).

and I recommended in 1995 (Korver T, Goorissen E, Guillebaud J. British Journal of Obstetrics and Gynaecology 1995; 102: 601–7). Fig. 5.3 has resulted after further discussion by the UK FPA and the Faculty of Family Planning, and a couple of minor changes to remove some ambiguity. At the time of writing I am hoping that this figure, and the text that follows here, will be in all important ways congruent with what will appear in the new editions of the UK FPA's leaflets – intended for launch in 2004.

The new advice remains firmly based on the above pharmacology but also takes account of further studies which show that the current UK advice is 'contraceptive overkill', in two respects:

1 the recommendations about added contraception if pills are missed later than day 7 in a pack, and

2 the definition of what constitutes 'missed pill(s)' (i.e. as the trigger for the pill-taker – or rather non-taker! – to take a specified action other than getting back to pill-taking). The WHO Scientific Working Group judged from available data that the number of women who might conceive by a less demanding definition – away from the previous 'more than 12 h late' – would be negligible. In *Fig. 5.3* the new definition of the earliest trigger for an appropriate action (which differs according to the weeks of the pill-cycle) therefore is:

■ two missed pills or
■ more than 1 day late in pill-taking.

NB In my interpretation these are actually the same thing: if we talk in whole numbers of hours, both mean taking action if one pill is late by 25 hours (or more) and the next in the sequence by one hour (or more).

Note that in 'late restarters' or those missing any two or more pills in the first week, the 7 days of added contraception are logical in view of point 1 in *Q 5.16*. This is because if there is already some follicular activity – which applies (almost) only at *the start of the packet after the PFI* and then only to just around one-fifth to one-quarter (23%) of a pill-taking population – seven tablets seem to be capable of putting any ovary back into a quiescent state. Moreover, if it has been too late to stop ovulation, this is likely to occur (and after ovulation the egg quickly ceases to be fertilizable) during the same 7 days of condom use.

For added safety, emergency contraception is now recommended additionally if intercourse has occurred during a PFI which has been lengthened

■ to anything beyond 8 days in a late restarter or
■ in an equivalent way through the missing of two or more tablets out of the first seven.

If 28-day packaging is used the woman must be carefully taught which are the dummy 'reminder' tablets, for omission if she misses any of the last seven active pills. All women should be asked to return for the exclusion of pregnancy if they have no bleeding in the *next* PFI.

5.18 It is easy to see from Figures 5.1 and 5.2 that missing pills at the start of a packet, lengthening the contraception-losing time to more than 7 days, could well be 'bad news!' but what about omitted pills in the middle of a packet?

Tablets *omitted following on prior tablet-taking for 7 or more days*, and not followed by a PFI, are very low risk omissions for breakthrough ovulation.

If we allow for the one woman who nearly ovulated and the small numbers in the study just quoted in *Q 5.16*, once seven tablets have been taken, at the very least up to four pills may be missed mid-packet with impunity. (For 5 or more pill-omissions, *see Q 5.22*)

Yet because of a wrong analogy with the normal menstrual cycle, unless we prescribers re-educate them, patients worry most about missed pills when it matters least, in mid-packet. Unless they have been taught (as after more than 40 years of the COC it is surely high time they were so taught! – *see Q 5.21*) they will rarely even seek advice when pill omissions or a stomach upset have led to a lengthening of the pill-free time, or (at the end of a pack) will now be leading to a similar lengthening. These are the most serious situations of all, but are not seen as such by women who think, for example, 'I just started my pack a bit late!'

5.19 What are the implications of late-packet pill omissions?

If a woman omits a number of tablets in the last week of her preceding packet and is allowed to recommence the next packet on her usual starting day (something she is sure to do, unless otherwise instructed), there will be an ovulation risk at the end of the thereby lengthened pill-free time, after what is a falsely reassuring withdrawal bleed. Indeed, if this has already happened by the time she is first seen and she has been sexually active during the extended PFI, this would indicate emergency contraception plus 7 days of an additional method. And, if she is not seen until much later, perhaps in the antenatal clinic, any questioning about missed pills must include asking about tablets she might have missed before the last menstrual period (LMP).

If she is properly taught, however, and follows the scheme in Figure 5.3, going straight on to the next packet, she will actually be more protected than usual due to having a shorter PFI. Hence the removal, now, of any need to advise an added method for 7 days, except when five or more tablets are missed (*Q 5.22*) – and even that is being ultra-cautious.

5.20 Should this advice for late tablet omissions (*Q 5.19*) be different if the woman is on a triphasic pill brand?

No; at the end of the packet she should start immediately with the first (lower dose) phase tablets (*see 5.174–5.179*). She will probably have a 'withdrawal-type' bleed, but contraceptive efficacy will nevertheless still be increased. This is a different situation from postponing 'periods' as described at *Q 5.179*.

5.21 Clearly it would be better if there emerged a new generation of pill-takers who understood this physiology ahead of time!

And it could happen, with our help as providers. In my opinion every new pill-taker has the right to know the basics of the 'contraception-losing' pill-free interval, which are not that complicated to explain in lay terms:

- that it is a time when the ovary is 'let off the hook'
- that she could very well be one of the 23% with extra ovarian activity (*see* Q 5.15)
- that her contraceptive safety in and after the PFI depends crucially, not only on having taken the previous packet well but also on starting her next packet on time – so if she switches methods there are not seven 'safe' carryover days ... (*Q11.17*)
- that missing pills at the end of a packet is like making her pill-free break early by mistake, which is why it would be a bit silly to add on the regular break on top.

In my experience, when this bit of simple explaining is done, current missed pills advice becomes understandable and compliance with it much more probable. It takes a bit of time, but this basic pill-teaching (whether by a nurse or a doctor) is well worth making time for – backed always by the latest version of the UK FPA's leaflet (*Q 5.12*).

5.22 What if the pill-taker has actually or effectively missed five or more pills? (such gross omissions, except for during the first week, being deliberately omitted in *Figure 5.3*)

It might be worth asking her the question (in addition to sorting her immediate problems) whether, after missing that many pills, she considers that she is a suitable person to be a pill-taker! It is logical to offer her one of the more forgettable options in future, such as an implant or IUD/IUS.

The WHO Scientific Working Group states in their Practice Recommendations that given continuing sexual exposure, five or more pills omitted in mid-packet (pill days 8–14) and in the last week (pill days 15–21) do justify:

- emergency contraception (i.e. in the UK Levonelle™) and
- the advice for the next 7 days to use an additional method, such as condoms and
- for such massive omissions in either of these weeks, that after returning to pill-taking through to the end of the current pack the woman should skip her next PFI, going straight to the first pill of her next pack.

5.23 What other now outdated 'rules' for missed pills are there that a pill-taker might have read or been taught?

1 The 'take precautions from now to the end-of-packet' rule is probably commonest and is delightfully *simple*; but sadly (*see* Q 5.19) it is also dangerously *wrong* for missed pills near the end of a pack.
2 The 'take precautions for the next 14 days, whatever happens' advice is acceptable; since the *second* 7 days of the fortnight does cover the time of

ovulation risk at the end of a PFI that has been lengthened by missed pills just before it (i.e. near the end of a pack). But because it is so counter-intuitive, many men as well as women see use of the unpopular sheath method as pointless, especially just after what they (falsely) see as a reassuring 'period'.

We however know that the ovary can be ovulating in synchrony with the endometrium bleeding, since that happens only because of exogenous hormone withdrawal.

5.24 What about emergency contraception for the *very* late pill re-starter who is continuing to be sexually active?

To minimize the chance of disturbing an implanted pregnancy, which in present UK law is only legal if the terms of the Abortion Act are complied with, my view is that (with continuing sexual exposure) any intervention should not be later than day 14 of any such greatly lengthened PFI: i.e. after seven missed pills, which could of course have been either before or after it. This calculation assumes that the very earliest likely ovulation might occur after 9 completed days that are pill-free, to which are added 5 days for the usual expected interval between ovulation/fertilization and implantation. Copper IUD insertion would be the preferred method of emergency contraception in such a case, see Chapter 10.

> But the main message from this section, *Qs 5.12–5.24*, is that for almost all mid-packet and late-packet (days 8–21) pill omissions postcoital treatment would be over-treatment.

5.25 What advice for vomiting and diarrhoea?

If the vomiting started less than 2 h after a pill was swallowed, another active tablet should be taken. If the replacement tablet (e.g. taken in emergency from the end of a pack) and a second one 25–26 h or more later both fail to stay down – i.e. once two or more pills have been effectively missed, as defined in *Q 5.17* – the actions described in *Fig 5.3* should be triggered, depending as usual on the phase of the pill-cycle.

In a long illness with vomiting of consecutive pills sufficient to produce lengthening of the PFI, extra contraceptive precautions should be continued for 7 days after it ends; if a subsequent PFI would be lengthened it should be omitted, once again as indicated by Fig. 5.3. Warn that breakthrough bleeding (BTB) is now likely.

Diarrhoea alone is not a problem, unless it is of cholera-like severity!

5.26 Surely the above discussion of the PFI takes too little account of the adjunctive contraceptive effects (*see Q 5.4*)?

Actually, these do not change the argument about the PFI. The most important extra effect is probably the progestogenic reduction in sperm penetrability of cervical mucus. But this too will be at its lowest ebb at the end of any PFI which has been lengthened: obviously, since it is then as long as is possible since progestogen was last ingested.

Once tablet-taking is resumed, however, the pills in the next pack should be able to operate usefully, both by the mucus effect and by their anti-implantation effect on the endometrium.

5.27 Pending the marketing of packets with a shortened PFI, what is the best regimen for women who have had a previous combined pill failure?

Some of these women claim perfect compliance but most will admit to the complete omission of no more than one pill. Most women admit to missing tablets from time to time (in one NOP survey the modal number missed per year was 8!), yet very few conceive. One can therefore argue that the ability to do so after missing only one tablet selects out those who are likely to have ovaries with above average return to activity in the PFI.

Therefore all women in this group should in my view be advised to take two or more packets in a row, the so-called bicycle or tricycle regimens (*see Q 5.31* and *Fig. 5.4*), followed by a shortened PFI. Often 6 days is a good choice in these cases because it is easy to remember, with each PFI start day now being identical to the finish-day – but the gap can be shortened even further in a 'high-risk' case (*see Q 5.36*).

Tricycling is surely more logical than the reaction of many doctors after a woman conceives on the pill, a summary of which is 'read her the Riot Act about better pill taking and give her the same one as before!' Even giving her a stronger formulation might be of less relevance than eliminating plus shortening the PFIs.

▲

Fig. 5.4 Tricycling a monophasic COC. Q 5.27. *Note:* must be monophasic packs. The pill-free interval (PFI) is usually shortened to 4 days if greater efficacy is required – but this can be 7 days if tricycling is not being done for efficacy reasons. Variants that run two or four or more packets together are also possible. WTB, withdrawal bleeding.

5.28 Aren't there other disadvantages to taking a PFI?

Yes: in summary, the 'cons' of the PFI are:

1 It makes the COC method less effective.
2 The withdrawal bleeds can be heavy or perceived as a nuisance.
3 In some women, migraines or other types of headache occur during the PFI, triggered by hormone withdrawal.
4 On theoretical grounds, compared with the normal cycle, it is 'unphysiological' to have a whole week with almost no oestrogen circulating (in the majority with quiescent ovaries, that is, not the 23% who start producing their own).

5.29 With all these snags, why do we continue to recommend the PFI to anyone?

Because one can list quite a few 'pros' of the PFI as well:

1 Many women like monthly bleeds to reassure 'that all is normal', and that they are not pregnant, more frequently than every 10–13 weeks as in tricycling. Explaining pill physiology can overcome this objection in cases where tricycling is indicated.
2 Avoids the complaint of bloatedness, which some experience through the last weeks of a tricycle.
3 Can avoid the breakthrough spotting that sometimes occurs, especially with low-dose pills during the last packet of a tricycle sequence.
4 Tricycle regimens do entail taking more tablets per year: 15–16 packets rather than the 13 when a regular PFI is taken. This increase in the hormone dose taken runs counter to the general philosophy of giving the lowest dose of both hormones for the desired effect of contraception.
5 One has to remember that all data generated from epidemiological studies about the (great) safety and the (remarkable) reversibility of the COC have been gained from women who were taking regular monthly breaks. So it might be best to stay with that concept for most pill takers. In confirmation of that view:
6 In one study HDL-cholesterol suppression (*see* Q 5.99) by the COC brand in use was restored towards normal by the end of the PFI. In a major randomized, controlled trial now being analysed at the Margaret Pyke Centre, this phenomenon has been confirmed for other important substances, including coagulation factors. Hence the PFI might prove to be good for homeostasis – allowing regularly some degree of recovery from systemic effects of the pill. This concept is entirely theoretical, of course.

5.30 What do you conclude, given the advantages of the PFI?

1 It can be useful to point out to a woman who actually wants to continue with the method but 'someone has suggested' that she ought to 'take a break' from the pill after 10 years' use, that she has already taken 130 breaks. Or, put another way, she has really only taken it for $7\frac{1}{2}$ years!

2 With the above list of 'pros' it would seem wise generally to cut the gap between packets primarily when there are indications – although one of these can certainly be the woman's own choice (*Table 5.2*). In the short term this can be done upon request if the woman wishes to avoid a 'period' on a special occasion like her honeymoon (*see Q 5.184* and *Fig. 5.15* (p. 225) for the procedure if a phasic brand is in use).

There are also longer-term indications for eliminating the PFI, as in *Table 5.2* and *Q 5.31*.

5.31 When is the tricycle pill regimen (or one of its variants) indicated? And what is Seasonale™?

The regimen has nothing to do with triphasic pills. Indeed, it necessitates use of monophasic pills, which are simply run together – three or four

---

TABLE 5.2 Indications for the tricycle regimen using a monophasic pill, or its variants (Q5.31)

1 At the woman's choice

2 Headaches, including migraine with non-focal aura, and other bothersome symptoms occurring regularly in the withdrawal week (*see Q 5.28*)

3 Unacceptable heavy or painful withdrawal bleeds

4 Paradoxically, to help women who are concerned about absent withdrawal bleeds (this concern and the nuisance of pregnancy testing therefore arising less often!)

5 Premenstrual syndrome – tricycling can help if COCs used to treat PMS

6 Endometriosis: a progestogen-dominant monophasic pill can be tricycled, for maintenance treatment after primary therapy

7 Epilepsy: this condition benefits from relatively more sustained levels of the administered hormones (*see Q 5.36*), i.e. and may be treated with an enzyme-inducer see (8)

8 Any enzyme-inducer therapy

9 Suspicion of decreased efficacy (*see Q 5.27*) for any other reason

Notes:

1. In view of the possibility that the monthly pill-free interval (PFI) has health benefits (*see Q 5.29*), and it certainly means less hormone is ingested per year of pill-taking: one of these indications should normally apply. See also Appendix A 'named patient use' because the tricycle regimens are unlicensed.

2. In circumstances (1) to (6) in the table there is no special need to shorten the PFI, when one is taken.

packets in a row – followed by a PFI of the selected length (7 days, or less if the indication is to increase the efficacy of the method) (see *Fig. 5.4*).

Seasonale™ is a brand in the US – apparently due to arrive in the UK before long – that uses dedicated packaging to provide four packets of the equivalent of Microgynon-30™ in a row followed by a 7-day PFI. This will produce four WTBs – one bleed in each season of the year! Many women will welcome this choice, provided they also accept the implications of three extra packets of hormone per year. If the indication is pill-withdrawal headaches, they should get only four bad headaches per year – instead of the usual 13! *Table 5.2* summarizes the indications for tricycling.

5.32 What is the significance of BTB or spotting after the first pack during 'tricycling'?

If it occurs during the second or third packet in a woman who had no BTB problems with 21-day pill taking, and if none of the explanations in *Table 5.15 (see Q 5.168)* applies, then it is most likely to be an 'end-organ' effect. In other words, the current formulation is proving to be incapable of maintaining this woman's endometrium beyond a certain duration of continuous pill taking, i.e. without the 'physiological curettage' of a WTB. Although we lack data, it is my belief that this type of BTB is less likely to be due to low blood levels of the contraceptive steroids than when BTB occurs in the other circumstances (discussed in *Qs 5.161–5.176*).

Therefore the first step, if this is a problem to the woman, is to try a shorter continuous sequence of pills, e.g. by 'bicycling' (two packets in a row) – rather than to use a stronger pill. Another option during annoyingly prolonged BTB is to simply take a pill-free break of 4–7 days and restart. This is always contraceptively safe if at least seven pills have been taken since the last PFI.

DRUG INTERACTIONS AFFECTING THE COC

5.33 What is the enterohepatic cycle?

After pill ingestion, the progestogens are 80–100% bioavailable from the upper small bowel, but ethinylestradiol (EE) is subject to extensive 'first-pass' metabolism, chiefly by being conjugated with sulphate in the gut wall (*Fig. 5.5*). After absorption, the artificial oestrogen and progestogen are carried in the hepatic portal vein to the liver. Liver metabolism then or later (after the steroids have been transported around the body), creates metabolites of both steroids. The liver mostly forms glucuronides. Once these conjugates re-enter the lumen of the bowel, the bowel flora (chiefly *Clostridium* species) remove the sulphate and glucuronide groups. This restores some EE for reabsorption and, in some women, can help to maintain its level in the circulation.

However, in the case of all the artificial progestogens in current use, the progestogenic metabolite that is reabsorbed after the action of the bowel organisms is biologically inactive. This has the important implication that non-enzyme-inducing antibiotics can have no effect on the efficacy of the progestogen-only pill (POP) or indeed any progestogen-only method.

Moreover, according to researchers in Liverpool, both studies in women with an ileostomy and formal studies with relevant antibiotics suggest that, in the vast majority of COC takers, the recycling even of the oestrogen seems to be unimportant for maintaining efficacy. There is some detectable reduction of the area under the curve (AUC) for EE in a few women when relevant antibiotics are coadministered, but ovulation has not been shown.

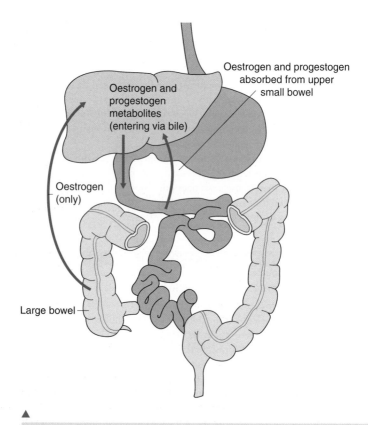

▲

Fig. 5.5 The enterohepatic circulation. Q 5.33. *Note*: the progestogen does not recirculate in a pharmacologically active form.

It is generally agreed, however, that because we do not know which few individuals might be affected by any antibiotics that destroy the relevant bowel flora, it is medicolegally best to play safe, as described in *Q 5.35*.

5.34 What is the effect on pill efficacy of drug interactions linked with the enterohepatic cycle?

These can reduce the pill's efficacy in two main ways, both related to the pharmacology of *Fig. 5.3*:

1   The first and by far the more important mechanism is by induction of liver enzymes, which leads to increased metabolism and thus elimination in the bile of both oestrogen and progestogen. Various drugs are involved, as detailed in *Table 5.3*. The main ones of clinical importance are rifampicin and its relatives, some antiretroviral drugs used in the treatment of HIV, griseofulvin and a number of antiepileptic drugs. Among the latter, note that valproate, clonazepam, clobazam and all other newly marketed antiepileptics except for topiramate (including vigabatrin and lamotrigine) are *not* enzyme inducers.

2   Alternatively, disturbance by certain antibiotics of the gut flora that normally split oestrogen metabolites arriving in the bowel can reduce the reabsorption of reactivated oestrogen in a very small (but unknown) minority of women. The more relevant ones – as much medicolegally as clinically – are also listed in *Table 5.3*. Note the following:

   (a)   This problem does not relate to any of the drugs used to prevent or treat malaria, except one – doxycycline – which has recently acquired that indication; nor (probably) to trimethoprim; nor, certainly, because they somewhat inhibit hepatic metabolism, to co-trimoxazole, sulfonamides and erythromycin (*Table 5.3*).

   (b)   The effect applies only to short-term antibiotic treatment or, in long-term therapy, at the time of change to a new antibiotic. This is because the bowel flora rapidly develop antibiotic resistance, in under 2 weeks.

Antibiotic-related diarrhoea is unlikely to be a problem because diarrhoea has to be 'cholera-like' before absorption is affected.

5.35 What should be advised during short-term use of any interacting drug?

1   *Enzyme inducers*: if, for example, griseofulvin is to be used (up to say 6 weeks – if longer, *see Q 5.40*) in the treatment of a cutaneous fungal infection, extra contraceptive precautions are advised for the duration of the treatment. These should be continued for a further 7 days, with omission of the next PFI if the last potentially ineffective pill was taken in the last 7 days of the current pack. Rifampicin is such a powerful

TABLE 5.3 The more important drug interactions with oral contraceptives

Class of drug	Approved names	Main action	Clinical implications for COC use
Drug that can reduce COC efficacy			
Anticonvulsants	Barbiturates (esp. phenobarbitone) phenytoin, primidone, carbamazepine, oxcarbazepine, topiramate	Induction of liver enzymes, increasing their ability to metabolize *both COC* steroids	Tricycling with shortened PFI preferred, using 50 µg oestrogen COCs, increasing to max. 90 µg if BTB occurs. *Sodium valproate, vigabatrin, lamotrigine and clonazepam* are among anticonvulsants *without* this effect (Q 5.35)
Other drugs			
(a) Antitubercle	Rifamycins (e.g. rifampicin, rifabutin)	Marked induction of liver enzymes	Short term, see text Long term, use of alternative contraception is preferred, e.g. DMPA (*see Q 8.11*)
(b) Antifungal	griseofulvin	Induction of liver enzymes	As for anticonvulsants
(c) Most protease inhibitors and other antiretroviral agents	e.g. ritonavir, nevirapine	Induction of liver enzymes	Do not use COCs – DMPA or LNG-IUS are often good choice (+ continuing use of condoms). For all antiretroviral drugs, details available from www.hiv-druginteractions.org
(d) Miscellaneous	Tacrolimus, modafinil	Induction of liver enzymes	As for anticonvulsants
(e) Other antibiotics	Penicillins, ampicillin and relatives, tetracyclines, cephalosporins	Change in bowel flora, reducing enterohepatic recirculation of ethinyloestradiol (EE) only, after hydrolysis of its conjugates	Short courses – *See Q 5.35* Long-term low-dose tetracycline for acne – no apparent problem, probably because resistant organisms develop, within about 2 weeks. POP is unaffected by this type of interaction NB doxycycline now in use as antimalarial prophylaxis

TABLE 5.3—cont'd

Class of drug	Approved names	Main action	Clinical implications for COC use
Drugs that can increase COC blood levels			
	Paracetamol	Competition in bowel wall for conjugation to sulphate. Therefore, possibly more EE available for absorption	No effect on the progestogen Advise: at least 2 h separation of the analgesic from the time of pill taking
	Co-trimoxazole	Inhibits (weakly) EE metabolism in liver	None, if short course given to low-dose COC-user
	Erythromycin, ketoconazole	Potent inhibitors of EE metabolism	

Notes:

1. St John's Wort, widely used as 'Nature's Prozac', is an enzyme inducer. Because its potency in different batches is marked and can very up to 50-fold, it is unsuitable for use by COC- or POP-takers (CSM warning notice issued). However, it might be being taken by a woman requesting emergency contraception, see Q 11.30.

2. Tretinoin, isotretinoin, miconazole and lansoprazole, despite rumours to the contrary, do not pose a clinical problem.

3. *See Q 5.45* for interactions potentially altering actions of other drugs.

enzyme inducer that even if it is given only for 2 days (as, for instance, to eliminate carriage of meningococcus), increased elimination by the liver must be assumed for 4 weeks thereafter. Extra contraception with elimination of the relevant one or two PFIs should be recommended to cover that time. This advice applies also to a relative of rifampicin, rifabutin.

2 *Other antibiotics*: the large-bowel flora responsible for recycling oestrogens are reconstituted with resistant organisms in about 2 weeks. In practice, therefore, if the COC is commenced in a woman who has been taking a tetracycline long term (e.g. for acne or as malaria prophylaxis), there is no need to advise extra contraceptive precautions. There is a potential problem only – although this is now believed to pose a small risk – when the antibiotic is changed or first introduced in the treatment of a long-term pill taker. Even then, extra precautions need to be sustained only for the first 2 weeks, but plus the usual 7 days (i.e. 3 weeks in all), with elimination of the next PFI, if the first 2 weeks' antibiotic use extended into the last 7 days of a pack.

5.36 Given that no action is required with long-term use of 'ordinary' (non-enzyme-inducing) antibiotics, what should be done if long-term use of an enzyme inducer is required?

1 *Rifampicin/rifabutin*: these are such potent enzyme inducers that in some women a five-fold increase in the rate of metabolism of the COC was seen by the researchers in Liverpool, who recommend alternative methods of contraception for long-term users of rifampicin, i.e. avoiding the COC altogether, even in the higher-dose tricycling regimen described below. Fortunately, the main COC hormone affected is EE, so the injectable progestogen depot medroxyprogesterone acetate (DMPA, *see Qs 8.2ff*, and especially *8.11*) is an option.

2 *Other long-term enzyme inducers*: mainly anticonvulsant therapies. Here too an alternative contraceptive option such as an intrauterine method (IUD or IUS) should be considered seriously; this is a WHO 3 situation (*see Q 5.119*). DMPA might be a good choice (*see Q 8.11*) or the IUS (*Q 9.149*).

However, if the COC is strongly preferred after counselling it is usual to:

■ Prescribe an initial dose of 50–60 μg oestrogen. This normally means starting with two tablets daily of a 30-μg product, commonly Microgynon-30™, or a 20-μg plus a 30-μg combination (*see Q 5.37*) – always on a 'named patient' basis (see Appendix A). The only 50-μg single tablet now marketed in the UK (Norinyl-1™, which contains norethisterone, *see Q 5.130*) is unsuitable in my view because it contains mestranol, which is a prodrug for EE and its conversion in vivo is not more than about 75–80% efficient, so it effectively provides only 37.5–40 μg of EE. More important than the pill(s) used, however.

■ At the Margaret Pyke Centre we also advise that the tricycle regimen described in Q 5.31 is used. This reduces the number of contraceptively 'risky' PFIs. It is particularly appropriate for epileptics because the frequency of attacks is often reduced by the maintenance of steady hormone levels. We strongly recommend that the woman also shortens the PFI at the end of each tricycle to 4 days. A 'diary card' can help her in this; but the main thing is to explain that her 'period' (withdrawal bleed) will tend to continue into the start of the next pack.

5.37 What if it seems more appropriate to use a gestodene-, desogestrel- or norgestimate-containing COC for a pill-taker needing treatment long term with an enzyme inducer?

In selected cases I would prescribe two sub-50 μg pills a day, e.g. one Marvelon™ plus one Mercilon-20™ from the desogestrel 'ladder' (*see Q 5.129* and *Fig. 5.12*). But whenever two or more are prescribed daily, the grounds – as here – must be solid and record-keeping must be meticulous ('named patient use', see Appendix A), because the manufacturer will not accept product liability should a serious problem arise. The same applies if extra pills have to be taken to control BTB (*see Q 5.38*).

5.38 What could signal the need to consider either an important drug interaction or the need for two pills?

Having excluded other causes (*see Q 5.168*), BTB might be the first clue to a drug interaction in the first place. But it could also be used as an indication to consider further increasing the dose or to advise a change of method. If the user of an enzyme-inducing drug develops BTB on the COC, the first step is to try fewer packs in a row. If the problem persists, try two or more tablets a day, if necessary to provide a combined oestrogen content of 80 or 90 μg (suggested maximum; and *see Q 5.39* and Appendix A), titrated against the BTB.

5.39 How can one explain this increased dosage to a woman, i.e. that she is not receiving a 'dangerously' strong pill regimen?

The risk of this policy, given that BTB is not a fully accurate measure of blood levels (*see Qs 5.160–5.168*), must be assessed carefully by the prescriber, especially if the woman has any risk factor for arterial or venous disease. Thereafter it can be explained that, as described more fully in Qs 5.162–5.168, one is only attempting to give the minimum dose of both hormones to finish just above the threshold for bleeding. Reassure her that she is metaphorically 'climbing a down escalator'. In other words, her increased liver metabolism means that her system is still basically receiving a low-dose regimen while she is taking a 50–60-µg dose. She is exposed to more metabolites but this is not believed to be harmful.

5.40 Can a woman go straight back to the normal dose and regimen as soon as the enzyme inducers are stopped?

No: it could be 4 or more weeks before the liver's level of excretory function reverts to normal. Hence if any enzyme inducer has been used for 6 weeks or more (or at all in the case of rifampicin), Professors Michael Orme and David Back of Liverpool recommend a delay of about 4 weeks before the woman returns to the standard low-dose pill regimen. This delay should be increased to 8 weeks after more prolonged use of established enzyme inducers. And logically there should then be no gap between the higher- and the low-dose packets (*see Table 5.4*).

5.41 What are the implications of long-term and possibly changing antibiotic treatments in women suffering from acne or (for example) cystic fibrosis?

- *On long-term antibiotics and when first starting oral contraception*: no problem (*see Qs 5.34 and 5.35*).
- *On oral contraception, when first starting antibiotics, or at each switch to a new broad-spectrum antibiotic*: here the counsel of perfection would be to use an additional method such as the condom for the first 3 weeks, to permit antibiotic resistance to develop (*see Q 5.35*).

In practice, these precautions are frequently not observed, yet breakthrough pregnancies resulting from this mechanism seem extremely uncommon.

5.42 What about anion-exchange resins like cholestyramine, or activated charcoal or guar gum, which is sometimes used to treat postprandial reactive hypoglycaemia? Might they impair pill absorption?

Any such effect appears to be minimal but a potential problem could be eliminated by taking them at least 4 h before or 2 h after the pill – or indeed any other oral drug.

5.43 What drugs can increase the bioavailability of ethinylestradiol? Does a high intake of vitamin C do this?

- New research on the vitamin C interaction shows no increase in circulating levels of EE and no rebound on discontinuation, refuting earlier concerns.
- Any effect of paracetamol – in competing for EE conjugation and therefore raising EE blood levels – is probably clinically unimportant.

However, in the absence of a definitive (negative) study, it is still best to advise separating pill taking from the paracetamol by a couple of hours.

■ Co-trimoxazole, erythromycin, clarithromycin, itraconazole and the interferons inhibit liver CYP 3A4 enzymes and so also tend to increase the bioavailability of the COC.

Dose adjustment of the COC or the other drug does not seem to be clinically necessary for any of the above.

5.44 Is the rumour about an interaction between the pill and grapefruit juice founded on fact?

Yes, this one is, although not the one that it might make the pill fail; it is the other way round. Grapefruit is a rich source of flavonoids, which compete for the enzymes that metabolize EE, so increasing bioavailability (and blood levels). But even in high grapefruit consumers this is unlikely to cause any significant added prothrombotic risk from the pill. If concerned, the simple solution is to ensure grapefruit juice is always quaffed at least 2 h after the time of pill taking.

5.45 Are any of the interactions in which COCs affect the metabolism of other drugs of any clinical significance?

Oral contraceptive (OC) steroids are themselves weak inhibitors of hepatic microsomal enzymes. So they might lower the clearance of diazepam, tricyclic antidepressants, prednisolone, ciclosporin and some other drugs – including, according to some reports (but not others), alcohol. Only the enhanced toxicity of *ciclosporin* is important clinically; the others are unlikely to be noticed.

COCs (and progestogens alone) inhibit the metabolism of warfarin to a variable extent, potentially raising the International Normalized Ratio (INR). Also, independently, it can itself alter clotting factors. Thus the interaction is unpredictable and the combination needs very careful monitoring by more frequent INRs, at least initially.

However, in specific individuals the combination is sometimes appropriate on a WHO 3 basis. The contraindication to the COC after a venous thrombosis, for example, is only WHO 4 (absolute) after anticoagulation ceases. COCs are also, sometimes, the only acceptable method for women on long-term warfarin, due to structural heart disease and atrial fibrillation risk (*see Q 5.139*).

As COCs tend to impair glucose tolerance, sometimes cause depression and can raise blood pressure, they naturally tend to oppose (pharmaco-dynamically) the actions of antidiabetic, antidepressant and antihypertensive treatments, respectively. With respect to hypertension, see the important point in *Q 6.9*; but otherwise this type of effect is fairly easily compensated for clinically by monitoring the dose/response of the other drug.

5.46 What else, apart from treating my patient, should I do if I suspect a drug interaction of any type?

Practitioners who do detect possible drug interactions are asked to continue the practice of completing a yellow card for the Committee on Safety of Medicines.

5.47 Should women with an ileostomy or colostomy avoid hormonal contraception for fear of absorption problems, or be given a stronger brand than usual?

Despite the interference in the enterohepatic cycle after an ileostomy, the bioavailability of EE, as well as levonorgestrel was not detectably altered (Grimmer et al. Contraception 1986; 33:51–59). Efficacy would not be expected to be impaired unless there was associated significant small bowel disease and malabsorption.

Yet, because of anecdotes of unexpected conceptions, due presumably to reduced reabsorption of EE from the large bowel (*see Qs 5.33 and 5.34*) in apparently compliant women with an ileostomy, I would now recommend added precautions or a regimen with fewer and shorter PFIs in such women (*see Q 5.31*). But I would not advise increasing the COC dose solely on these grounds.

Colostomy, however, does not (and would not be expected to) have any effect on the enterohepatic circulation of oestrogen.

5.48 Does coeliac disease impair absorption of the COC?

No. Paradoxically, while this disease is active the diminished function of the gut wall leads to less conjugation of absorbed EE. So more bioactive EE is absorbed than usual! Once coeliac disease is successfully treated, absorption is normal.

STARTING ROUTINES WITH THE COC

5.49 What factors need consideration in devising starting routines for the COC?

1 First and foremost, women with short cycles can ovulate very early in the second week of the menstrual cycle. Hence the value of the day 1 (or 2) start, to ensure seven tablets are taken in time (*see Q 5.16*) and with no need for additional contraception from the outset (see *Table 5.4*).

2 First-timers can usefully be warned that their first 'period' might come on after only about 23 days. Also that each new pack should start after

no more than 7 days and this will always be on the same day of the week (*see Qs 5.50 and 5.51*).

3   There are studies, especially from Israel, showing that the older routine of a day 5 start has one advantage: less BTB and spotting in the first cycle. This is well worth considering, and the 1998 Tel Aviv study showed a higher rate of early discontinuations for bleeding in the group that started on day 1. If this is preferred, or with 'Quick starts' that are even later in the cycle (as is perfectly acceptable if any earlier intercourse is judged to have been adequately protected, or in selected cases immediately after emergency contraception), extra precautions for 7 days are advisable. It is my practice also to advise this whenever the first tablet of the first pack is taken on day 3 or later (see *Table 5.4*).

4   After a first-trimester pregnancy has ended, the earliest fertile ovulation seems to occur no earlier than about day 10.

5   After a full-term pregnancy (in the absence of breastfeeding) the earliest possible fertile ovulation has been shown biochemically at around day 28. However, starting too early has to be avoided because of evidence that the oestrogen in the combined pill can increase the risk of puerperal thromboembolism. The coagulation factor changes of pregnancy are largely reversed by 2 weeks. So for most a start date of day 21 is appropriate. Starting the COC should be further delayed in those at highest risk of any form of thrombosis, including the obese, and after severe pregnancy-related hypertension or the HELLP syndrome (hypertension, elevated liver enzymes, low platelets) with persistent biochemical abnormalities, with alternative contraception for 7 days if the pill is therefore started beyond day 21.

6   The COC can be started immediately after injectables such as DMPA. But of more interest is the fact that the COC can also (and often very usefully) be given concurrently with DMPA. For example, on restarting after major or leg surgery that has been covered by DMPA (*see Q 6.17*) or to control bleeding problems (*see Q 8.48*). See Q 8.53 for relevant advice if the prospective pill taker is already overdue her most recent injection.

These and my other recommendations for the COC are summarized in *Table 5.4*. See Q 7.56 for the progestogen-only pill, which is more suitable than the COC during lactation.

CONTRACEPTION AFTER PREGNANCY

This important subject is discussed in much more detail in *Qs 11.18–11.32*, including when there is amenorrhoea, how not to commence use of a new medical method (IUD, injectable or pill) when an implantation has (or might have) already occurred (*see Q 11.22*).

TABLE 5.4 Starting routines for combined oral contraceptives (as recommended by J Guillebaud – WHO Practice Recommendations differ slightly)

	Start when?	Extra precautions for 7 days?
1 Menstruating	Day 1	No*
	Day 2	No†
	Day 3 or later	Yes†
	Any time in cycle ('Quick start')	Yes†
2 Postpartum		
(a) No lactation	Day 21 (low risk of thrombosis by then‡, first ovulations reported day 28+)	No
(b) Lactation	Not normally recommended at all (POP/injectable preferred)	
3 Post-induced early abortion/miscarriage	Same day or next day to avoid postoperative vomiting risk	No
4 Post-trophoblastic tumour	1 month after no hCG detected	As 1
5 Post-higher dose COC	Instant switch§	No
6 Post-lower or same dose COC	After usual 7-day break	No
7 Post-POP	First day of period	No
8 Post-POP with secondary amenorrhoea, not pregnant	Any day (Sunday? see Q 5.51)	No
9 Post-DMPA (risk of pregnancy excluded see Q 11.22)	Any day (see text, may overlap the methods)	No‖
10 Other secondary amenorrhoea (risk of pregnancy excluded, see Q 11.22)	Any day (Sunday? see Q 5.51)	Yes

TABLE 5.4—cont'd

	Start when?	Extra precautions for 7 days?
11 First cycle after postcoital contraception (see Q 10.41)	1st day/or no later than day 2 'Quick start', i.e. immediately, as Q 10.42	No Yes

*Extra precautions if packet advises starting with a number of placebos before the active pills.

†Delay into day 2 can sometimes help, to be sure a period is normal. WHO's Practice Recommendations (2002) are less cautious and only after day 5 advise extra precautions for the 7 days that seemingly make any ovary quiescent (Q 5.16). Starts beyond day 5 (i.e. not waiting for that elusive next period) are entirely acceptable if the prescriber is sure there has been no risk of conception up to the starting day.

‡Puerperal thrombosis risk lasts longer after severe pregnancy-related hypertension or the related HELLP syndrome, so delay COC use until the return of normal BP and biochemistry (Q 5.49). But a history of HELLP in an earlier pregnancy is irrelevant (WHO).

§This advice is because of anecdotes of rebound ovulation occurring at the time of transfer.

‖Unless overdue most recent injection – if so, see Q 8.53.

Note: in presence of amenorrhoea, exclusion of there being either a blastocyst or sperm in the upper genital tract can be done by obtaining a negative sensitive pregnancy test after minimum 14 days of abstinence or 'very safe' contraception, *see Q 11.22*

A point to mention here is that, after excluding pregnancy during amenorrhoea, the COC can often best be started on the next Sunday (plus additional precautions for 7 days); this avoids future bleeds at weekends (*see* Q 5.51).

5.50 What single question screens for accurate pill taking?

Simply: 'What day of the week do you start each new pack?' If a pill taker states the day with confidence, all is well. If she hums and haws or says 'It all depends', there's a problem!

5.51 Can I help my patients to avoid the withdrawal bleed (WTB) at weekends?

Yes, but only if you think to discuss the point! With most starting routines, depending on the weekday their first period happens to start and the length of their WTB, perhaps one-third of all pill takers will bleed during part of one weekend in every four. This is completely unnecessary.

Starting the pill on the first Sunday of the next period is one option. This is popular in the US but must be combined with extra precautions for 7 days. Otherwise, during follow-up at any time, you can simply advise shortening any PFI with a start on, say, Sunday or Monday, thereby ensuring that future bleeds will occur only on weekdays.

MAJOR SYSTEMIC EFFECTS OF THE COC

5.52 Which studies have provided our present information about the wanted and unwanted effects of the COC?

 There have been many case–control studies but much of the most useful data has been generated by cohort studies. Wherever possible, statements made in this book are based on congruence of the findings of all the studies, by different investigators in different populations. Three of the most important are:

1 *The Royal College of General Practitioners' (RCGP) study*: in brief, 23 000 married pill users were recruited from 1400 GP practices and matched (only for age) with a similar number of married control women not using the COC. The GPs informed the study coordinators of all subsequent medical effects, based on every surgery attendance or hospital referral for in- or outpatient care (including for pregnancy). Ex-users have been similarly followed up.

2 *The Oxford/FPA study*: launched in the same year (1968), this study has similarly followed a total of over 17 000 clinic attenders since its start. In this study, users of different reversible methods of contraception act as controls for each other; 56% used oral contraceptives at the outset,

compared with 25% who were diaphragm users and 19% who were fitted with an IUD.

3 *The Nurses' Health study*: In 1976, 121 700 female registered nurses in the US completed a mailed questionnaire including items relevant primarily to risk of cancer and circulatory disease. Follow-up questionnaires are sent every 2 years to update the risk factor data and to ascertain any major medical events.

The completeness of the follow-up in all the above studies is exemplary, for example, for fatal outcomes, ascertainment in the Nurses' study runs at about 98%. There is also much useful information now becoming available through the Fertility Regulation Group of the Cochrane Collaboration.

5.53 What are the strengths and deficiencies of the main cohort studies?

They have the strengths of similar prospective epidemiological studies, particularly with regard to the completeness of data collection over the years, and the possibility of assessment of non-comparability between the groups compared, and of biases. However, they share obvious weaknesses:

1 Random allocation was impossible, so pill users are different from non-users in many important ways: in the Walnut Creek Study, for example, COC users tended to be on average taller, more physically active, more likely to smoke or drink in moderation (although not more likely to be heavy smokers or heavy drinkers), to sunbathe more frequently, to have initiated sex earlier and to have had more partners than non-users.

2 All the studies tended to include fewer teenagers than are now normally found amongst a pill-using population, partly because the unmarried are so difficult to follow in long-term prospective studies.

3 In the UK studies, a large number of initially recruited women were lost to follow-up just because they moved house. However, checks on the characteristics of a sample of the latter have not shown them to differ in such a way as to significantly bias the results.

4 By the time the cohort studies report, they are invariably providing information about yesterday's contraceptives. Much of the above data generated by the studies relates to brands containing at least 50 µg of oestrogen and the recently marketed progestogens are under-represented.

5.54 What are case–control studies and what can we learn about the COC from them?

Case–control studies are retrospective: cases are recruited with a condition of interest (e.g. venous thromboembolism, VTE) and attempts are made to match the women with 'controls' (admitted to the same hospital or from the same community) who are free of the condition but otherwise as similar as possible. The basic idea is that if the frequency of pill use is greater in cases (relative risk more than 1) the pill might be causing the condition, if it is less (relative risk less than 1) the pill might be protective. Useful studies of this kind are quoted repeatedly in this book, many organized through WHO. Case-control studies never provide absolute rates (attributable cases per 100 000 of population) although these can be roughly calculated if the background prevalence of the condition is known. These studies have a number of problems we cannot discuss in detail here, but here are some:

1. They are obligatory for very rare events like thrombosis and diseases that take many years of exposure for any causation to become apparent, like arterial wall disease or cancer. But they are notorious for the problems of bias and confounding. Epidemiologists try very hard to correct for these but certain confounders (predisposing factors for which pill use or use of particular brands of pill might be a marker, leading to an association that is coincidental, not causative) might be unknown. In interpreting the observed association of VTE with pills containing desogestrel (DSG) and gestodene (GSD), the confounding effect of duration of use (meaning that use of older brands became associated with being a lower-risk woman through the 'attrition of susceptibles') has been a major bone of contention since that unfortunate CSM letter of October 1995.

2. Epidemiology is particularly weak when it comes to assessing odds ratios (or relative risks) that are not much above or below unity (in the ranges 1–2 and 0.5–1). Yet for common conditions these could mean an important attributable risk or benefit.

3. Because of the low prevalence of use, we are unlikely ever to have useful epidemiological data on the side-effects of the POP.

4. It is more difficult to study beneficial than adverse relationships; the death that does not take place as a result of some protective effect is far more difficult to recognize than the one that is linked to COC use. However, good data are available for most of the benefits in Q 5.56.

5.55 Can we identify the 'best buy' among the different pills, for benefits versus risks?

In summary, no. We have to say that thus far all the methods of epidemiology, even when backed by 'biological plausibility', have proved too insensitive as research tools for this to be done with any specificity. Preoccupation with metabolic minutiae (common among rival drug firms in the 1980s and early 1990s) can also be misleading. (*See also Qs 5.107–117.*)

But there are good data to show that we should give formulations with the lowest acceptable dose of both the oestrogen and progestogen. It is also clear that it is essential to have a range of different products for prescribers and users to exercise effective choice – in relation both to the initial prescription, and subsequently, when minor side-effects occur.

ADVANTAGES AND BENEFICIAL EFFECTS

5.56 What are the beneficial effects of the COC?

These can be listed as follows:

CONTRACEPTIVE

1 Highly effective – and the regular withdrawal bleeds give regular reassurance of that fact.
2 Highly convenient, especially sexually (non-intercourse-related).
3 Reversible (*see Qs 5.61 and 5.62*).

NON-CONTRACEPTIVE – MAINLY GYNAECOLOGICAL

4 A reduction in the rate of most disorders of the menstrual cycle:
   (a) less heavy bleeding, therefore
   (b) less anaemia
   (c) less dysmenorrhoea
   (d) regular bleeding, and timing can be controlled (*see Qs 6.85*) with no bleeding at weekends (*see Q 5.51, 6.86*) or even arranged to occur only about four times a year through tricycling as an option (*see Q 5.31*)
   (e) fewer symptoms of premenstrual tension overall (*see Q 5.133*), especially if tricycling is tried, although some women do experience similar symptoms on the COC itself
   (f) no ovulation pain, which can be severe in some cycles.
5 Less pelvic inflammatory disease (PID) (*see Q 5.59*).
6 Fewer extrauterine pregnancies – because ovulation is inhibited, and as a long-term result of (5).
7 Less benign breast disease (*see Q 5.96*).
8 Fewer functional ovarian cysts (*see Q 5.60*).
9 Less need for hospital treatment due to bleeding from or size of fibroids (*see Q 5.96*).
10 A beneficial effect on some cancers, notably carcinoma of the endometrium and epithelial cancers of the ovary (*see Qs 5.75 and 5.76*). Also, very probably, a reduced risk of colorectal cancer (*see Q 5.74*).

MISCELLANEOUS

11 Fewer sebaceous disorders especially acne (only with selected oestrogen-dominant COCs) (*see Q 6.60*).

12 No acute toxicity if overdose is taken: only vomiting, and in prepubertal girls the likelihood of WTB a week or so later.

13 Protection from osteoporosis and control of climacteric symptoms in older women up to age 50 (as a valid alternative to natural oestrogen replacement therapy, in risk-factor-free women needing contraception whose ovaries are beginning to function less well, *see Q 11.38*). The same can apply to younger women with premature ovarian failure or oligomenorrhoea (*see Qs 5.65–5.67*). But the COC has been found not to improve bone density when the comparison is with normal cycling women receiving oestrogen from their own ovaries.

14 Beneficial social effects (e.g. postponing childbirth until after tertiary education, as an option). Other possible benefits have been identified in some studies but have yet to be fully confirmed:

15 Reduction in the rate of endometriosis (*see Q 6.51*).

16 Less trichomonal vaginitis (*see Q 6.52*).

17 Maybe less TSS (*see Q 6.53*).

18 Less thyroid disease (both overactive and underactive syndromes according to the RCGP study).

19 Maybe less rheumatoid arthritis (*see Q 6.59*).

20 Fewer duodenal ulcers. This apparent effect could well be a good example of confounding (*see Q 5.54*): anxious women prone to ulcers might also be more influenced by the media to avoid COCs.

5.57 What is thought to be the unifying mechanism of the benefits, especially the gynaecological benefits? How can this be useful in counselling prospective pill takers?

The removal of the normal menstrual cycle and its replacement by a situation that more closely resembles the physiological state of pregnancy. Women who, due to frequent pregnancies and prolonged lactation, have few menstrual cycles during their reproductive lives (say 50 rather than the 450 plus that would now be typical in developed countries) are less likely to get all the symptoms and conditions listed at items (4), (7), (8), (9), (10), (15) and (19) in *Q 5.56*. The similarity of the protection that the COC gives against ovarian and endometrial cancers, for example, is probably because there is much less chromosomal activity in the endometrium and ovaries than in cycling women. Less chromosomal activity means less chance of harmful mutations during frequent epithelial cell divisions.

So taking the pill is in some ways more 'normal' than using a barrier contraceptive and having numerous menstrual cycles because the latter are in reality 'abnormal' and tend to promote gynaecological pathology, i.e. all the conditions at items (4), (7) to (10) and (15) in *Q 5.56*. In a real sense, any woman who has been on the pill for 10 years has had iatrogenic amenorrhoea for 10 years, but of a benign, pregnancy-mimicking kind because oestrogen and progestogen are still available to the relevant tissues.

Some women find this story reassuring, that in summary the pill can be truly said to tend to 'restore normality'. It reduces the dangers of too many menstrual cycles among those many who now do the 'unnatural' thing, by not having huge families (*see also* Q *5.133*).

5.58 Does lowering doses to reduce the risks also reduce the benefits of gynaecological or non-gynaecological pathology, in comparison with the older high-dose formulations?

There has to be some real doubt about this and it will take years to resolve. The protection against functional cysts (*see* Q *5.60*) is definitely reduced by such pills, although there is certainly no proof that it no longer exists. The modern more oestrogenic pills might well also be less protective against benign breast disease, fibroids and endometriosis, which are benefited by relatively more progestogen. My own (entirely theoretical) concern is particularly about the triphasics (*see* Q *5.179*), which imitate (albeit imperfectly) the normal cycle. This might not be such a good idea because eliminating the normal cycle seems, as we have just seen, to be relevant to the mechanism of the gynaecological benefits.

There is usually no such thing as a 'free lunch'! But we can be sure of one good thing: any oral contraceptive that regularly blocks ovulation ought to retain the protective effect against ovarian cancer.

5.59 By how much does the COC protect against PID, and what is the mechanism?

The protective effect against symptomatic PID appears large, a 50% or more reduction in the risk of hospitalization for the disease. This is such a major cause of subfertility (*see* Q *9.49*), that in many parts of the world it is probably a significant non-contraceptive benefit of the pill.

Although suggestions that the COC might facilitate transmission of HIV have been largely discounted (*see* Q *6.70*), there is nothing to suggest protection against any of the sexually transmitted viruses (except there are data that all STIs are important in promoting the sexual transmission of HIV, hence the COC might reduce the risk of HIV infection indirectly through the reduced risk of PID).

MECHANISM

It seems likely that progestogens reduce not only the sperm penetrability of cervical mucus (*see* Q *5.4*), but also its 'germ penetrability'. Indeed, the two might even be connected, in that spermatozoa can act as 'bio-vectors': there is some evidence that sexually transmitted organisms such as *Chlamydia* and the gonococcus actually 'hitch a lift', using the sperm as their means of transport to the upper genital tract!

Chlamydia carriage is actually more frequent in COC takers than controls (not easy to interpret, as controls might use more condoms). So infection and sexual transmission of organisms are probably not impeded at the level of the cervix/vagina: the beneficial effect of the progestogen is likely to be one of protection of the upper genital tract.

However, silent or less severe infection that can still occlude the tubes is not uncommon in pill takers. There is some evidence that the COC attenuates the symptoms of *Chlamydia*, and this could be an adverse effect if it led to the condition being underdiagnosed and undertreated. Yet the overall effect of the COC on this cause of infertility must still be positive, given the Farrow study (*see Q 5.61*).

However, safer sex requires condom use as well ('Double Dutch').

5.60 By how much does the COC protect against functional ovarian cysts, and what is the mechanism?

The reduction has been shown in practically all studies. In a study in Boston, pill users were one-fourteenth as likely to develop such cysts as non-users. Although benign, such cysts often result in surgery.

Functional cysts are caused by abnormalities of ovulation. Most of the time, the COC abolishes all kinds of ovulation (both normal and abnormal). However, the POP increases the risk of cyst formation (*see Q 7.34 and also Q 5.58* regarding the lowest-dose combined pills).

REVERSIBILITY OF THE COC

5.61 Are COCs fully reversible as just stated (*see Q 5.56*)? Do they impair future fertility?

The short answers to these questions are 'yes' to the first and 'no' to the second. In the Oxford/FPA study, for example, among previously fertile women who gave up contraception, by about 30 months over 90% of the ex-pill-users had delivered: a proportion that was indistinguishable from that for ex-users of the diaphragm and IUD. There was a definite delay of 2–3 months in the meantime taken to conceive, probably due in part to the advice pill takers are often given (*see Q 6.48*).

More recently, a study by Farrow et al (published in 2002 in *Human Reproduction* 17:2754–2761) of 12 106 pregnant women showed that prolonged use (> 5 years) of the COC before the 8497 planned conceptions was associated with a decreased risk of delay in conceiving – even for nulliparous women. Quite the opposite finding to what, since the very first day the COC was marketed, has been a prime concern. Indeed, I find in my visits to Africa that fear of infertility continues to put people off the pill unnecessarily (*see Q 5.69*).

It is also interesting that, when this study was done (it began in the early 1990s), so many (3545 or 29%) of the conceptions were still 'accidental'.

5.62 What, then, is 'post-pill amenorrhoea'?

This term should be abolished (*see Q 5.63*). It is commonly used to mean secondary amenorrhoea of more than 6 months' duration following discontinuation of the COC. Most authorities now believe that the association is casual rather than causal. Of 1862 inhabitants of Uppsala county, Sweden, 3.3% reported a history of amenorrhoea of longer than 3 months. Amenorrhoea of more than 6 months' duration occurred in 1.8% of the population, most frequently in women under the age of 24. So this is quite a common condition. If a woman is predisposed but instead takes the COC for many years, any episodes that would otherwise have been recognized will be masked by the regular withdrawal bleeds induced by her contraceptive. In such a woman, the pill could easily be unfairly blamed for her 'after pill' secondary amenorrhoea when it could in fact be revealed only 'after pill'.

Moreover, studies show that the probability is not associated with formulation, nor – in most studies – with duration of use. Professor Jacobs of University College London has shown that the distribution of diagnoses was the same in cases of secondary amenorrhoea after the pill as in non-post-pill cases; and in the two groups the types of treatment needed, the frequency with which they were employed and the excellent outcome in terms of cumulative conception rates were all the same. All this argues very strongly against a specific pill-induced syndrome causing secondary amenorrhoea.

5.63 What are the bad effects of continuing to use the term 'post-pill amenorrhoea' at all?

1 It leads to a tendency on the part of many doctors to defer investigation of patients with amenorrhoea that develops after the pill, thereby delaying the diagnosis and treatment of potentially serious conditions. Instead, as there is no specific syndrome, after 6 months without a period all cases of secondary amenorrhoea should be referred for investigation and appropriate treatment – whether they are 'post-pill' or 'post-condom'!

2 A second unfortunate result of accepting amenorrhoea after the pill as a real condition is that it deters doctors from prescribing oral contraceptives to women for whom they otherwise might be suitable. A past history of secondary amenorrhoea is good example (*see Q 5.67*). In some conditions, as we shall see, the COC can be positively beneficial and it is still frequently being needlessly withheld.

3   Amenorrhoeic women often develop feelings of guilt that treatment with the pill has caused their amenorrhoea and has wrecked their chances of ever having a baby. In the first place, it is most unlikely that the pill had anything to do with their problem and, secondly, even if it did, modern therapy of amenorrhoea is so effective that cumulative pregnancy rates approaching 100% can be confidently expected.

5.64 How are such cases of secondary amenorrhoea investigated?

The Royal College of Obstetricians and Gynaecologists (RCOG) in association with NICE has issued (2003) evidence-based guidelines on the management of the infertile couple in primary and secondary care.

It is important for all concerned to be clear whether the woman currently desires a pregnancy. It is crazy but not unheard of for high technology to be used to induce ovulation in a woman who promptly requests a termination when the resulting ovum is fertilized (*see* Q 11.17)!

It is beyond the scope of this book to go into details of hospital investigations for secondary amenorrhoea but three of the most helpful tests are simple and non-invasive, and can be arranged by an interested GP.

1   *Weight and height*: from which can be calculated the body mass index (BMI):

$$\frac{\text{weight (kg)}}{\text{height (in m}^2)}$$

This is easily derived on a pocket calculator in the surgery, or from charts, and should normally be in the range 19–26.

2   *The progestogen challenge test*: this is usually performed by giving medroxyprogesterone acetate (MPA) 5 mg daily for 5 days. If this is followed by a WTB it means that the woman's oestrogen status is either normal or high. Absence of the WTB means subnormal oestrogen (see below).

3   *Ultrasound scan of the ovaries*: the third of this trio of valuable and uninvasive tests.

Other important tests in oligo- or amenorrhoeic women are: plasma prolactin, thyroid function, FSH and LH.

5.65 What are the risks of prolonged amenorrhoea? How should women be treated subsequently if they do not want a pregnancy?

The management depends very much on the diagnosis and particularly on oestrogen status, as well as whether the woman is actually ready yet for fertility enhancement.

Prolonged amenorrhoea and oligomenorrhoea (say, less than four periods a year) are not by any means always innocuous conditions, according to Professor Jacobs. They should always be investigated, and management then depends on the diagnosis.

POLYCYSTIC OVARY SYNDROME (PCOS) VERSUS 'POLYCYSTIC OVARIES'

This is not the same as the finding of polycystic ovaries on ultrasound scan, which is a very common finding seen in more than 20% of normal women, studied both on the pill and off it. So far as we know it is only clinically of importance if the ultrasound finding is linked with symptoms: irregular or absent menses with, usually, evidence of excessive androgen (acne or hirsutes). Those symptoms, with the scan findings, do then add up to the 'syndrome'. These women, even if amenorrhoeic, have high levels of both oestrogen and androgens, and with the latter goes a low level of sex hormone binding globulin (SHBG). Oddly enough, their problem seems to be mediated through insulin-like growth factors, linked with carbohydrate and lipid metabolism (syndrome X), and putting on weight sets up a number of vicious metabolic circles – and risks, especially of arterial damage.

The most important therapeutic point therefore is to help a non-overweight PCOS woman to stay slim and, if her BMI is above 30, she will benefit greatly by losing weight by increasing her unrefined carbohydrate intake and taking regular exercise. If hirsutes is a problem she might require a consultant-led high-dose cyproterone acetate and oestrogen regimen, followed by Dianette™ (*see Q 6.64*) or Yasmin™ or Marvelon™ for maintenance.

If acne alone is the problem, perhaps with some irregular menstrual cycling, there is no need to refer. Dianette™ (*Q 6.64*) can be prescribed, usually followed (once the symptoms are controlled) by the pill – this is an indication in my view for one of the modern 20–35-µg oestrogen varieties with DSG or GSD. Yasmin™ could also be used: it is the same price as Dianette™, although more expensive than other COCs. The intention of the combined treatment is to increase SHBG, so binding androgens, and also to protect the endometrium from overstimulation.

Be very cautious, however, if the BMI is above 30, and all ethinylestradiol-containing products should normally be avoided above a BMI of 39.

SECONDARY AMENORRHOEA IN LOW NORMAL OR UNDERWEIGHT WOMEN

This is often weight-related amenorrhoea and common in track athletes. The concern here is that they have no follicular oestrogen, little extraglandular oestrogen from peripheral conversion of androgen in fat depots and, moreover, have enhanced metabolism along the pathway that degrades oestrogens to antioestrogens. All these mechanisms lead to low oestrogen levels and a serious risk of osteoporosis. If the amenorrhoea has continued for more than 6 months, a progestogen challenge test (*see Q 5.64*) or an estradiol measurement should be arranged, with ideally also a bone scan if it is low (less than 100 pmol/L).

These women are theoretically also at risk of heart disease, like women with a premature menopause, if the hypoestrogenic state were to continue for a very long time. They should certainly stop smoking, which also lowers plasma oestrogen, and be encouraged to put on weight. They are usually very opposed to taking hormones but they might be better off healthwise on an oestrogen-dominant and 'lipid-friendly' pill than using barrier contraception alone. Opposed natural HRT oestrogens could be used if preferred – they would be as good for prevention of osteoporosis, but it is a myth that HRT would be any better than the COC for this indication.

HYPERPROLACTINAEMIA

This requires specialist treatment, e.g. with bromocriptine or another dopamine agonist drug. Hypo-oestrogenism is not a problem in treated cases, if they are cycling and have normal libido. The COC is usable simultaneously with a dopamine agonist but it is relatively contraindicated. Used alone there is the risk of enlarging a macroadenoma, potentially endangering eyesight, and the advice of the specialist in charge should be sought.

AMENORRHOEA WITH NORMAL OESTROGENIZATION YET NO PCOS (POSITIVE PROGESTOGEN CHALLENGE, OVARIES SHOW NO OVULATION BUT EVIDENCE OF FOLLICULAR ACTIVITY)

Here there is the contraceptive problem that at any time the woman might ovulate. There are no special grounds for using the COC, but neither is it contraindicated. The cap or even just Delfen™ foam or a sponge (*see* Q 4.64) would be fine, if acceptable, until the first spontaneous period occurs. Because this suggests the return of ovulation, the woman would then be advised to consider transferring to a more effective method – not excluding the COC as an option.

5.66 In summary, what is the place of the COC for women with amenorrhoea?

It is positively beneficial to use the COC in a number of these cases. Its oestrogen content definitely helps where the oestrogen status is low, especially to prevent long-term problems such as heart disease and osteoporosis. And the progestogen content of the COC can also be of value in PCOS women with oestrogen excess and no endogenous progesterone, to protect their uterus from carcinoma of the endometrium.

5.67 What advice should be given to a healthy woman who gives a past history of secondary amenorrhoea but is currently seeing normal periods?

All the evidence suggests that there is no reason to refuse the COC to such women, although they must understand that with or without the pill they might at some future time have difficulty in conceiving. Future fertility can never be proved in advance of becoming pregnant. Another important point is to investigate such a woman first if her current menses are in fact still erratic, for example, if she is experiencing less than four periods per year. She might well have the polycystic ovary syndrome (*see Qs 5.65 and 5.66*).

5.68 To preserve future fertility, should pill users take regular breaks of say 6 months, every 2 or every 5 years?

The answer here is an unusually confident 'no'. This follows from *Q 5.61*: the pill is a reversible means of birth control, whose reversibility is not dependent on duration of use. Too often breaks demonstrate very well to the woman that her fertility is unimpaired – by an unplanned pregnancy! See also *Qs 5.29, 5.30 and 6.72*, which add a health-related (rather than a fertility-related) perspective to this same issue of duration of use/taking breaks.

5.69 Contrary to the common myth about its reversibility, doesn't the COC in fact much reduce the likelihood of infertility?

Yes (see the Farrow paper quoted in *Q 5.61*). Many of the benefits of the pill (*see Q 5.56*) relate to conditions that can readily impair fertility and childbearing, specifically:

1 less pelvic infection
2 fewer ectopic pregnancies
3 less endometriosis
4 less growth of fibroids, a cause of miscarriage
5 fewer functional ovarian cysts, a cause of unnecessary surgery
6 less surgery altogether, for all the conditions listed here, a frequent cause of pelvic adhesions and consequent infertility
7 fewer unwanted pregnancies: which can lead in various ways to secondary infertility (e.g. by infected abortions of all kinds, or by puerperal infection).

For the same reasons, there is no logic in pill takers being specially earmarked for a regular annual bimanual examination (*see Q 6.3*)!

MAIN DISADVANTAGES AND PROBLEMS

5.70 What are the major established unwanted effects of COCs?

 These are summarized here before more detailed consideration. They fall under four main headings:

1 Circulatory diseases (*see Qs 5.97–5.117*).
2 Liver disease:

(a) liver adenoma (*see Q 5.96*), or carcinoma (*see Q 5.95*)

(b) cholestatic jaundice (*see Q 6.35*)

(c) gallstones (*see Q 6.37*).

3 Adverse effects on some cancers (*see Qs 5.71–5.95*).

4 Unwanted social effects.

The latter are hotly debated. Discussion ranges over whether removal of the fear of pregnancy has in some societies tended to promote intercourse with multiple partners, with its consequences on marital and emotional stability, STIs and so on, or whether other simultaneous changes, such as the decline in religious belief, have been more important factors.

> There are, of course, numerous other possible but fortunately less 'major' unwanted side-effects. 'Minor' side-effects are never to be seen as 'unimportant' – practically all that have been described will be considered in later sections of this chapter.

THE COC AND NEOPLASIA (BENIGN AND MALIGNANT)

5.71 Does the COC influence the rates of benign and malignant neoplasms?

It should not be surprising that artificial hormones can influence neoplasia but recent research has confirmed the expectation that the effect of hormones would not be all in one direction. Some benign neoplastic conditions are benefited by OC use (e.g. benign breast disease), some are promoted (e.g. liver adenomas). Similarly, two cancers are now clearly shown to be less frequent in pill users (carcinoma of the ovary and endometrium); whereas the COC might possibly act as a co-carcinogen in the case of two other common cancers (cervix and breast). The literature is complex and the jury is still out.

5.72 Why has it taken so long to begin to show associations between the pill and neoplasia?

The main reason is summarized in the word 'latency'. There can be up to 30 years between first exposure to an agent and its manifestation in the incidence of tumours. Even the largest prospective studies tend to have too few numbers and take too long to give an answer. Hence data have been obtained mainly from case–control studies, which are notoriously subject to bias. Other problems relate to the following:

1 The specificity of any co-carcinogen to the species, to the tissue and to tumour histology.

2   Time of life is relevant – in animal models chemicals can have contrary actions, promoting or inhibiting tumours according to when in the life of the individual exposure takes place.

3   Formulation: not only differing ratios of progestogen to oestrogen, but also different progestogenic chemicals, are used around the world. It is particularly unfortunate that most studies cannot disentangle the effects of specific formulations (apart from generally showing that low-oestrogen pills usually have a lesser effect).

5.73 What is the benefit/risk balance sheet for neoplasia and the pill, so far as is currently known?

The situation can best be explained to a patient in terms of 'swings and roundabouts' (*Fig. 5.6*). Some cancers are definitely less frequent in pill users (endometrium and ovary); others might be more frequent (but in none of those shown is a causative link proven beyond all doubt). For all remaining common malignancies (e.g. of the respiratory, gastrointestinal or renal tracts), there seems no association, or certainly no adverse association, at all. A similar balance sheet can be struck for benign neoplasia (*Fig. 5.7*).

The bottom line in counselling is: Populations using the pill might develop different benign or malignant neoplasms from non-users but computer models using the best currently accepted data and assumptions do not so far indicate that the overall risk of tumours is increased. (There is no proof of an overall reduction of risk either.) Now let us consider some of the details.

5.74 What is the influence of the COC on colorectal cancer?

Several studies, both cohort and case–control, now find that COC use reduces this risk. The largest of the latter (Fernandez et al 1998 *Epidemiology*

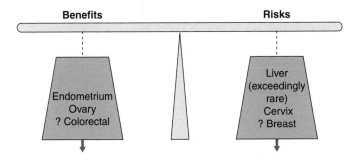

Fig. 5.6 Cancer and the pill. Q 5.73.

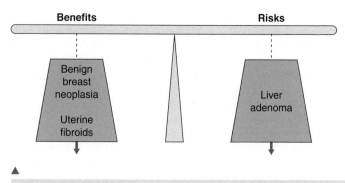

Fig. 5.7 Benign neoplasia and the pill. Qs 5.73 and see also Q 5.96.

9:295–300), found a 60% risk reduction among ever-users. However, this protective effect was not shown in other studies, so this benefit (unlike the cancer benefits in the next two questions!) is not fully established.

5.75 What is the influence of the COC on carcinoma of the ovary?

Good news! Many studies have yielded results pointing in the same direction, namely that epithelial ovarian tumours are less frequent in COC users. Overall, the risk is reduced by about half. There is increasing protection with increased duration of use amounting to a two-thirds reduction after more than 5 years, and the largest study shows that the protective effect lasts for at least 15 years after pill taking ceases. This is good news indeed, because ovarian cancer carries a high mortality.

5.76 What is the influence of COC use on carcinoma of the endometrium?

More good news, the risk of this cancer in ever-users is again reduced by about 50%. Four studies show increasing protection with increasing duration of use and three studies show some degree of persistence of the effect after stopping the method, lasting – according to one of them – for at least 15 years.

The similarity of the beneficial effects of the COC on these two cancers is striking, but not surprising (*see* Q 5.57).

5.77 What is the influence of the COC on trophoblastic disease (hydatidiform mole)?

There is no evidence that the incidence of any form of this tumour of pregnancy is increased by past pill use.

However, workers at Charing Cross Hospital in London have shown that usage of the combined pill after this diagnosis, and before human chorionic gonadotrophin (hCG) has reached undetectable blood levels, doubles the likelihood that the patient will require chemotherapy for incipient choricarcinoma. Other researchers, notably from America, have completely failed to show this association, but their chemotherapy policy is far more aggressive. See RCOG guidelines on trophoblastic pregnancies (2003).

The London team remains convinced of a causative link. Because it is not clear if the effect is due more to the progestogen than to oestrogen, they continue to recommend that all hormonal methods are avoided, if possible (WHO 3, *see Q 5.119*), until the hCG levels are undetectable, in urine at first, then confirmed in the blood. Emergency contraception is however WHO 2, using POEC (*Q 10.29*).

Thereafter, most importantly, this history is definitely WHO 1. IUDs are WHO 3 or even 4 when hCG levels are high (a scan should first exclude invasive cancer involving the uterine wall). Fortunately, in the vast majority of cases the hCG levels do become undetectable within 2 months of evacuation of the mole. The prohibition against hormonal methods, which is only precautionary (and not advised by WHO itself, or in the US at all) is therefore usually short-lived and not as long as until the next conception – usually advised after there have been at least 6 months with no hCG detectable.

5.78 What is the influence of the COC on carcinoma of the cervix?

Evidence exists of a modest increased risk of both squamous cell and the much rarer adenocarcinoma of the cervix. Studies on cervical cancer are complicated by confounding with the sexual variables, i.e. by the problem of getting accurate information about different patterns of sexual activity, both for women and their partners. The prime carcinogen is clearly sexually transmitted, probably a virus or combination of viruses (specific strains of the human papillomavirus (HPV) being the prime candidates). Cofactor(s) are important: cigarette smoking currently stands most accused in that role (at least doubling the risk in developed country studies).

Yet most studies, do show an association between incidence of, and now also in mortality from, this cancer, plus its premalignant forms (CIN), and use of the COC. But is the association causative or casual? The Oxford/FPA cohort study supports the former view by demonstrating an effect of duration of pill use among nearly 7000 parous women. No effect of duration of IUD use was found among over 3000 users of that method with whom they were compared. The incidence of all forms of cervical neoplasia combined rose from 0.9/1000 woman-years in those with up to 2 years' pill use to 2.2/1000 woman-years after 8 years. In the first report of this study, all 13 cases of invasive cancer occurred in women in the oral contraceptive group. The frequency of taking cervical smears for cytology was similar. In their most recent report (Vesey et al. 2003 *Lancet* 362:185–191) only 1 of 17 deaths from this cancer was in a newer user of the pill.

The International Agency for Research on Cancer (IARC) pooled multicentre case–control study published in 2002 (Moreno et al 2002 *Lancet* 359:1085–1092) found that if high-risk human papillomavirus (HPV) had already been found, implying exposure to the prime carcinogen, there was an increased risk of invasive cancer of the cervix with increasing exposure to the COC. A systematic review (Smith et al. 2003 *Lancet* 361: 1159–67) of 80% of the world's data found for HPV-positive women that the odds ratios for use of COCs for cases versus controls increased significantly with greater durations of use (1.3 for 5–9 years and 2.5 for 10 or more years' use). The relative risk was not detectably increased among COC-users for <5 years.

5.79 What is your overall assessment of the association with neoplasia of the cervix?

The COC does not increase the likelihood of acquiring HPV. But once a high-risk strain is present in the cervix, the 2002 Moreno study (along with other data) suggests that the COC is a cofactor, increasing the rate at which CIN progresses through the preinvasive stages to invasion. It is probably weaker in this respect than cigarette smoking. Even if the two cofactors are combined, it is believed that routine 3-yearly screening by cervical cytology will suffice, ensuring that, barring human errors, almost all preinvasive lesions can be diagnosed in time and treated pre-emptively. And past treatment for such lesions is no more than WHO 2 for pill continuation (with ongoing cytological surveillance).

The influence of the COC is clearly many times less than the influence of sexual lifestyle of the woman or her partner(s). COC users should have regular cytological and, as necessary, colposcopic surveillance (*see also Q 5.80*).

5.80 Should women discontinue COC use once an abnormal cervical smear has been detected?

It is currently entirely acceptable to continue COC use during the monitoring of a mildly abnormal cervical smear, during definitive treatment of cervical intraepithelial neoplasia (CIN) and subsequently. These are weak, relative contraindications (WHO 2, *see Q 5.119*): although the recurrence risk for the problem would of course be minimized if the couple were prepared to use a barrier method instead or as well (*see Qs 3.26 and 4.17*).

THE COC AND BREAST CANCER

5.81 What is the association between breast cancer and COC use?

The incidence of this disease is high and therefore it must inevitably be expected to develop in women whether they take COCs or not. As the recognized risk factors include early menarche and late age of first birth, use by young women was rightly bound to receive scientific scrutiny. However, if there is a real causative link with pill use, use by older women will obviously result in more attributable cases, because the incidence rises steeply with age above 35 years (*Fig. 5.8*).

The literature to date is copious, complex, confusing and contradictory! Research is complicated by the problems related to latency, changes in formulation, time of exposure and high-risk groups.

5.82 What is the main risk factor for breast cancer?

Age, because it affects everyone (unlike family history, or possession of the rare but hazardous risk factor of carrying a *BRCA* gene). It seems that cumulative duration of exposure of breast tissue to ovarian hormones – or to substitutes to them (notably those in the combined pill or HRT) – means a cumulative increased risk of cancer, starting in the mid-thirties, as shown in *Fig. 5.8*.

Is the risk from those substitutes the same as or greater than from a woman's exposure (over the same duration) to the hormones from her own ovaries? For the usual combined HRT (oestrogen plus progestogen), rather

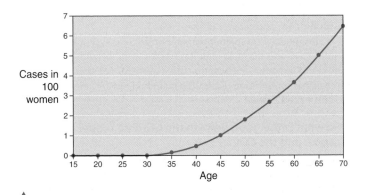

▲

Fig. 5.8 Background risk: cumulative number of breast cancers per 100 women, by age. Q 5.81, 5.82.

than oestrogen alone, the answer for current users now appears to be 'greater' – but with no detectable added risk in ex-users after 5 years (see the Million Women Study (2003) *Lancet* 362:419–427 for full details).

A COC study (Marchbanks et al 2002, *see Q 5.86*) was essentially negative for added breast cancer risk, in a population aged 35 to 64 at diagnosis, for any duration of previous use. Since all pill-takers are effectively 'menopausal' (i.e. their inactivated ovaries produce virtually no oestrogen nor progesterone), this reassuringly means that replacement of ovarian hormones by ethinylestradiol plus progestogen for all those years had not affected their breasts more than functioning ovaries would have done – with respect to breast cancer risk later in life.

However, as now to be discussed, earlier work still clearly suggests that the COC source of hormones increases breast cancer risk compared with the ovarian source in two categories: current users and recent ex-users.

5.83 So what was the model proposed in the 1996 paper by the Collaborative Group on Hormonal Factors in Breast Cancer? (CGHFBC)

The group reanalysed original data from 90% of all the available epidemiological data worldwide. This relates to over 53 000 women with breast cancer and over 100 000 controls from 54 studies in 25 countries. In its publication (Collaborative Group 1996 *Lancet* 347:1713–1727), the group proposed a widely accepted model (*see Qs 5.87–5.90*) – of an increase in risk through pill usage of 24%, but with diminution in ex-users and complete disappearance of added risk by 10 years. The strongest risk factor was confirmed as age of the woman: this is believed to be linked, as just mentioned, to cumulative exposure of the breast to oestrogen/progestogen hormones. They found that the most important predictor of added risk with the COC was recency of use.

This model showed disappearance of risk in ex-users, but recency of use of the COC was the most important factor: with the odds ratio unaffected by age of initiation or discontinuation, use before or after first full term pregnancy, or duration of use. The main findings are summarized in *Table 5.5* and below.

5.84 So what is the good news in the CGHFBC model of breast cancer and the COC?

Combined oral contraceptive (COC) pill users can be reassured that:

■ Although the small increase in breast cancer risk for women on the pill noted in previous studies is confirmed, the odds ratio of 1.24 signifies an increase of 24% only while women are taking the COC and for a few years thereafter, diminishing to zero after 10 years.

TABLE 5.5 The increased risk of developing breast cancer while taking the pill and in the 10 years after stopping	
User status	**Increased risk**
Current user	24%
1–4 years after stopping	16%
5–9 years after stopping	7%
10 plus years an ex-user	No significant excess

(Collaborative Group on Hormonal Factors in Breast Cancer, 1996)

■ Beyond 10 years, after stopping there is no detectable increase in breast cancer risk for former pill users.

■ The cancers diagnosed in women who use or have ever used COCs are clinically less advanced than those who have never used the pill; and are less likely to have spread beyond the breast.

This reanalysis shows that these risks are not associated with duration of use, the dose or type of hormone in the COC, and there is no synergism with other risk factors for breast cancer (e.g. family history – see below).

The risks for progestogen-only contraceptives (POPs and injectables) failed to reach statistical significance. However, this does not exclude a real effect, which in that case would be very similar for those methods to the model for the COC. See *Qs 7.52* and *8.38* for the practical implications.

5.85 What is the not-so-good news?

Mainly, this affects use by those with pre-existing risk factors; and by older women, who are now permitted to use the COC to age 50 if they choose to do so, provided they are fully healthy non-smokers (*see Q 6.75*). If the background risk for the individual is greater, whether because of increased age or a family history, the applicable percentage increase in *Table 5.5* necessarily means more attributable cases (than in women without any breast cancer risk factor).

As *Fig. 5.8* shows, irrespective of the use of hormonal contraception the cumulative risk of breast cancer in young women is very small, being 1 in 500 in women up to age 35. But the cumulative risk increases with age thereafter, to 1 in 100 at age 45 and 1 in 12 by age 75. The increase in COC-attributable cases as age of last use increases has been calculated, and is shown in *Table 5.6*. Most importantly, for a given age at last use the excess risk is little affected by a women's prior duration of oral contraceptive use. Everything seems to depend on recency of use (i.e. current or within 10 years) at the given age.

TABLE 5.6 Cumulative risk of breast cancer by recency of use. Showing usage in different age groups, the cumulative numbers of breast cancer cases per 10 000 women in never-users of oral contraception and the cumulative number per 10 000 women who had used oral contraception for 5 years and who were followed up for 10 years after stopping

Pill use for 5 years or any duration*	To age 20	To age 25	To age 30	To age 35	To age 40	To age 45
Breast Cancers diagnosed by:	Age 30	Age 35	Age 40	Age 45	Age 50	Age 55
Never-users:	4	16	44	100	160	230
Users who stopped 10 years earlier	4.5	17.5	49	110	180	260
Excess number of cases of breast cancer per 10 000 women	0.5	1.5	5	10	20	30

*Because the CGHFBC researchers state that for a given age at last use the excess risk is little affected by a women's prior duration of oral contraceptive use.

5.86 In 2002, what was the good news about breast cancer and the pill (the CDC study)?

A large, well-conducted study by the US Centers for Disease Control (CDC) (Marchbanks et al 2002 *New England Journal of Medicine* 346:2025–2032) of 4575 women aged 35–64 with breast cancer, and matched controls, reported no increased COC-related risk – odds ratio of 1 or less. This applied across the board and for all the following: current users, past users, long-term users, users with a family history and users starting COCs at young age. The latter was particularly reassuring, negating the so-called 'time-bomb' for ex-users in this older age group with a high incidence for breast cancer – even for those exposed before a first full-term pregnancy. This study is very reassuring, given that COC-exposure in the population was > 70 %, although it is not the last word by any means.

5.87 Why do we not now simply go with anyone's first impression from the CDC study that it is no worse for the breast if sex hormones come from the COC instead of the ovaries?

First, 'one swallow does not make a summer', and the CGHFBC study does have the virtues of size, plus the data coming from numerous different centres. Moreover, technically:

■ The upper confidence interval of the overall odds ratio was 1.3. This places the 24% increase shown in the 1996 pooled analysis within the bounds, i.e. they might still be corresponding to reality.

■ Crucially, most of the cancers in the CDC study would have been diagnosed more than 10 years after stopping the COC and hence would be non-pill-caused ones on the CGHFBC model anyway (*see Q 5.84* and last line of *Table 5.5*).

■ The CDC study unfortunately tells us nothing about those few women (often with genetic predispositions) who are diagnosed with cancer under age 35 (this important group was not recruited).

■ The CDC study also has very little data about women who carry on taking the COC until the menopause. Very few of the latter were in the studied population, although such long-term use has been permitted as a choice in more recent years.

So the CGHFBC model should certainly continue to be applied to the last two important groups (*see Qs 5.91 and 5.92*).

5.88 Can the adverse CGHFBC findings be explained by surveillance bias?

If reality is as the CDC study suggests – that there is truly no increase in risk when the breasts are exposed to the pill's hormones as opposed to those produced by the ovary, at least for cancer diagnosis at age 35–64 and when exposure to the COC has been mainly before age 35 – what explains the earlier findings?

The collaborative group conceded from the outset that their findings, of less advanced cases being identified in current or recent takers of the pill but more of them being found at each given age, could actually be explained wholly or in part by surveillance bias. This would imply that pill takers, both during and after the years of use of the method, were relatively more 'breast aware' than non-takers, and so would have more excision biopsies. One would then have to postulate that this did not apply to the US women of the CDC study, perhaps because in that country there is a more universal anxiety about this condition, affecting all categories of women.

But as already stated, the CDC study amplifies the reassurances of the earlier analysis rather than refuting it: because most of the cancers studied would have been diagnosed more than 10 years after stopping the COC and hence on the CGHFBC model would be background-risk cancers, not caused by the pill, anyway (see *Table 5.5*).

5.89 So what are the clinical implications for routine pill counselling?

The Faculty of Family Planning in the UK states that pill users should be informed of/counselled about the uncertainties with regard to breast cancer and the COC, but reiterates the advice given by the CSM that there need be no fundamental change in prescribing practice.

One effect of the essentially negative CDC study of 2002 is to remove pressure to raise this issue proactively at the first visit with young pill users. However, any questions they have should be answered with complete transparency and, even if they are not asked, at an appropriate time the topic should always be addressed. Women should be encouraged to practise breast awareness and report any unusual changes promptly.

In summary, women using COCs can be reassured that:

■ There might be little or no added breast cancer risk for women through using the pill. If it exists, the highest likely estimate is 24% and then it applies only while women are taking the COC and for a few years thereafter; it reduces to zero after 10 years.

■ Beyond 10 years after stopping there is no detectable increase in breast cancer risk for former pill users.

■ No excess COC-related *mortality* from this has been shown (Beral et al 1999 *British Medical Journal* 318:96–100).

■ The cancers diagnosed in women who use or have ever used COCs are clinically less advanced than those who have never used the pill and are less likely to have spread beyond the breast.

■ The risks, even if existing, are not associated with duration of use or the dose or type of hormone in the COC and there is no synergism with other risk factors for breast cancer (e.g. family history).

■ Women who do have a strong family history (breast cancer under age 40 in a sister or mother) do indeed have a pre-existing problem: but the percentage extra risk is the same for them as for girl-friends without the family history. They might certainly use the COC (WHO 2) if they so wish. But they should be advised to request reassessment whenever new data are obtained, and every 5 years.

■ The balancing protective effects of COCs against malignancy of the ovary and endometrium and possibly large bowel are always worth mentioning.

The known contraceptive and non-contraceptive benefits of COCs might seem so great to many (but not to all) as to compensate for almost any likely lifetime excess risk of breast cancer.

5.90 How do you explain the worst-case scenario to a pill taker if the CGHFBC model continues to be the one we fundamentally accept?

I use the fourth column of *Table 5.6*, divide the numbers by 10, and ask her to visualize two concert halls each holding 1000 women (*Fig. 5.9*). Imagine that the first hall is filled with 1000 pill takers, all now aged 45 but all having

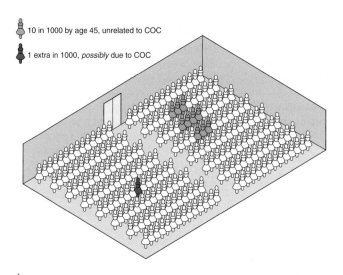

10 in 1000 by age 45, unrelated to COC

1 extra in 1000, *possibly* due to COC

Fig. 5.9 Cumulative incidence of breast cancer during and after use of COC until age 35. Q 5.90 (from Guillebaud 1998 *Contraception today*, 3rd edn, p 10. London, Martin Dunitz. With permission. Based on data from the Collaborative Group on Hormonal Factors in Breast Cancer 1996). See also Table 5.6.

used the COC for varying durations of time then stopping when they reached age 35 (a common situation). The (cumulative) number of cases of breast cancer would be 11 in concert hall 1. However, in hall 2, which is filled with never-takers of the pill also all currently aged 45, there would be 10 cases, i.e. there is only one extra pill-attributable case/1000 in hall 1. Moreover, if the pill is acting only as a cofactor then it is very possible that this woman would have developed the disease without the pill at a later age anyway.

The remaining 989 women in hall 1 will, from this time on, have only the same risk of breast cancer as the women in hall 2, i.e. no ongoing added risk because it is over 10 years since their last pill. This is a very important point to explain, with the overall risk rising so much with age.

Finally, the cancers diagnosed among the pill takers in hall 1, already and in future, will tend to be less advanced than those in hall 2.

5.91 What about pill use by an older woman?

As *Table 5.6* shows, without a change in relative risk there is an increased attributable risk with age. For example, there are 30 extra cases per 10 000 for ex-users now aged 55 who stopped the COC 10 years before, rather than the 10 extra cases of column 4 (which, with 1000 as the denominator, was the basis for *Fig. 5.9*). This must be explained and might be acceptable to many with the balancing from the established protection against cancer of the ovary and endometrium. But to my mind these new data will increasingly lead to more older women choosing from other options that are now available (especially IUDs and the IUS).

5.92 What about COC use in high-risk groups for breast cancer, specifically (A) those with a family history of a young (under 40) first-degree relative with breast cancer or with a predisposing BRCA gene? And (B) women with benign breast disease (BBD)?

Here we see the effect of having a larger background risk than the generality of women: rather as just discussed for older women. The 24% increment is not believed to be greater but when applied to a bigger background risk means more attributable cases. Therefore both these are relative contraindications (WHO 2, *see Qs 5.119, 5.136*). However, if a past breast biopsy showed epithelial atypia this in my view is at least WHO 3, and warrants obtaining the advice of the patient's oncologist/histologist.

Different women will react differently to the same information, given as it should always be in a balanced way. Some will ask for a method where no possible increase in breast cancer risk has been suggested, above that she has to live with. If however the woman chooses the COC as she is entitled to do, given its benefits, it should be a low oestrogen formulation for a limited duration, with specific counselling and reassessed every 5 years or so.

5.93 What is the prognosis if a woman develops breast cancer while on the COC? Should women with this history ever use hormonal methods in future?

The prognosis is better than for a prior condom user (see above). Nevertheless, most authorities advise that the pill should be discontinued and women with a history of this cancer should normally avoid combined OCs thereafter. Progestogen-only methods are acceptable during remission, defined by WHO as after 5 years, following discussion with the oncologist and with continued surveillance.

5.94 Has the last word been spoken on this issue?

No way! Research continues. The above (*Qs 5.81–5.93*) seems the best that we can make of available data at present.

5.95 What is the influence of the COC on other cancers?

PRIMARY HEPATOCELLULAR CARCINOMA

Case reports and three case–control studies have suggested that COC use might promote this rare cancer. The annual attributable risk is estimated as less than 4 per million users. It might very well be much less, especially given that liver cancer is usually fatal within 1 year of diagnosis, yet there has been no increase in deaths in the US or Sweden where the COC has been widely used since the 1960s. Instead, there has been a gradual increase in incidence and mortality in Japan, where the COC is seldom used.

Moreover, the pill association is not established in hepatitis-B-infected livers – fortunately, as that is the main risk factor.

Once again, smoking rears its ugly head: increasing the relative risk of this cancer by a factor of four even without the COC. A past history of liver tumours (benign as well as malignant) absolutely contraindicates the COC thereafter (*see also Q 6.65 re* cyproterone acetate).

MALIGNANT MELANOMA OF THE SKIN

An increased risk, particularly of the superficial spreading type of this cancer, was suggested among COC users; most other studies show no link. It is becoming increasingly probable that the association is not causal – related to the pill itself – but to the confounding variable of exposure to ultraviolet light.

Women in long-term remission after melanoma, and also after apparent cure following conservative treatment for cancer of the ovary and cervix, can use COCs – provided their oncologist agrees.

No association has been shown with malignancy involving any other organ or tissue.

5.96 What is the influence of the COC on benign neoplasms?

See *Fig. 5.7*, page 150.

1   *Benign breast disease (BBD)*: a definite protective effect has been shown, which increases with duration of use and is probably attributable to the progestogen component of the pill. The protection in some studies seems to be restricted to the most common but less serious forms of the disease without epithelial atypia, the latter being considered the premalignant variety (*see Q 5.92*). This might explain the paradox that COCs protect against BBD developing in the first place but have no demonstrable protective effect against breast cancer.

2   *Hepatocellular adenoma*: this tumour occurs about ten times more frequently in users of COCs than in other women, but the background prevalence is so low that the incidence among COC users is still tiny (around 1/100 000 users per year). The risk is greatest in older women using relatively high-dose pills for a long period of time (*see Q 6.39*).

3   *Focal nodular hyperplasia (FNH) of the liver*: this has also been linked, and can regress with COC withdrawal (*see Q 5.134* for prescribing implications).

4 *Other benign tumours showing no association*: these include benign trophoblastic disease (but *see Q 5.77*) and prolactinoma of the pituitary gland. For some years it was widely held that COC use increased the risk of the latter but two good case–control studies have provided strong evidence against the association (*see also Q 5.136*).

5 *Fibroids*: while older high-oestrogen OCs were believed to cause fibroids to increase in size, current more progestogen-dominant brands have been shown to reduce the risk of hospital referral for fibroids. However, this benefit has not been confirmed for the most recently marketed COCs.

THE COC AND CIRCULATORY DISEASES

5.97 Which circulatory diseases have been shown to be more common in COC users?

To expand from *Q 5.70*:

1 *Systemic hypertension*: this is not so much a disease in its own right as it predisposes to and does its damage through the arterial circulatory diseases below. Detection of this is crucial, in determining eligibility for the COC and for ongoing safety in use of the method.

2 *Venous disease*:
   (a) deep venous thrombosis
   (b) pulmonary embolism
   (c) rarely thrombosis in important single veins, e.g. mesenteric, hepatic or retinal.

3 *Arterial diseases*: these include:
   (a) myocardial infarction
   (b) thrombotic strokes
   (c) haemorrhagic strokes
   (d) other arterial events affecting solitary but vital vessels, such as mesenteric or retinal arteries.

5.98 Can any of these risks be explained by known metabolic changes induced by the artificial hormones of the COC? In particular, what is the influence of the oestrogen content?

Over the years, biochemistry has been of only very limited help. Very many studies have been done but the true meaning of many of the findings has been difficult to interpret – particularly those thought to relate to arterial disease (*see Q 5.99* and *Table 5.7*).

Alterations in clotting factor levels induced by oestrogen might be thrombogenic. More important changes include reduced levels of antithrombin III and protein S but there are also increased levels of fibrinogen and several of the vitamin K-dependent coagulation factors. These changes help to explain the increased risk of venous thrombosis, particularly if the woman already has a congenital or acquired predisposition such as factor V Leiden and antiphospholipid antibodies (*see Qs 5.112 and 5.114*).

However, it is likely that if there is already significant arterial wall disease, oestrogen might also promote superimposed arterial thrombosis. There is evidence of a compensatory increased fibrinolytic activity, also an oestrogen effect. This might in part explain the rarity of overt disease, especially arterial disease, in non-smoking pill users.

Hepatic secretion of many different proteins is stimulated by oestrogens. These proteins are involved in: the transport of hormones, vitamins and minerals, the control of blood pressure and immunological processes. When oestrogen is given, the stimulatory effect can sometimes be suppressed by concomitant administration of a progestogen. But the interactions are complex: there might also be synergism or independence of the effects, and differences between progestogens (see *Table 5.7*).

Finally, synthetic oestrogens have been shown to raise arterial blood pressure both in short-term challenge experiments and in longer-term studies.

The protective increase in fibrinolysis is impaired by heavy smoking.

5.99 What is the influence of the progestogen content on metabolism and risk?

1 The risk of venous thromboembolism, which still seems to be primarily caused by oestrogen, might be modified by progestogens in some way as yet to be fully explained (*see Qs 5.107–5.111*).

2 Provided oestrogen is also given, increasing the dose of progestogen leads to an increased rate of diagnosis of clinical hypertension. (However, when given without oestrogen, as in the POP or DMPA, progestogens have not been shown to have an important adverse effect on blood pressure.)

3 When oestrogen was kept constant, the incidence of arterial diseases – both as a group and individually – was correlated with the progestogen dose in some early epidemiological studies. This has only been shown for norethisterone (NET)–levonorgestrel (LNG) group progestogens, often unhelpfully referred to as the 'second generation'.

4 Many studies, including a randomized, controlled trial (RCT) at the Margaret Pyke Centre, have shown that if a constant dose of oestrogen is given then the oestrogen-induced high-density

TABLE 5.7 Some metabolic effects of combined oral contraceptives

	Blood level	Remarks
Liver		
Liver functioning	Altered	These many changes cause no
(a) generally	in all users	apparent long-term damage to the
(b) specifically		liver itself. The liver is involved,
Albumen	↓	however, in the production of most
Transaminases	↑	of the changes in blood levels of
Amino acids	Altered	substances shown elsewhere in
Homocysteine	↑	this table, including the important
		changes in carbohydrate and lipid
		metabolism, and coagulation factors
Blood glucose after		These change, barely detectable
carbohydrate ingestion	↑	with the latest pills, can partly
Blood lipids	Altered, mostly ↑	explain the increased risk of
HDL-cholesterol – in low		arterial disease with earlier
oestrogen/progestogen-		preparations
dominant COCs	↓	
Clotting factors		
(a) generally	Mostly ↑	Both the pill and smoking affect
(b) specifically		these interrelated systems.
Antithrombin III, Protein S		Fibrinolysis is enhanced by COC
(anticlotting factors)	↓	in the blood, but reduced in the
Fibrinolysis	↑	vessel walls.
Tendency for platelet	↑	Protein S is lowered less by EE-
aggregation		containing pills combined with
		LNG than with DSG
		(*see Q 5.111*)
Hormones		
Insulin	↑	These hormone changes are
Growth hormone	↑	related to those affecting blood
Adrenal steroids	↑	sugar and blood lipids (above)
Thyroid hormones	↑	
Prolactin	↑	
LH	↓	These effects are integral to
FSH	↓	contraceptive actions. However, the
Endogenous oestrogen	↓	first three tend to rise in some
Endogenous progesterone	↓	women during the pill-free week.
		Hence any effective lengthening of
		the pill-free time can lead to an
		LH surge and ovulation
Minerals and vitamins		
Iron ↑		This is a good effect for women
		prone to iron deficiency

TABLE 5.7—cont'd

	Blood level	Remarks
Copper	↑	
Zinc	↓	Effects unknown, but not believed
Vitamins A, K	↑	to cause any health risk for most
Riboflavine, folic acid	↓	pill-users. Pyridoxine is discussed
Vitamin B$_6$ (pyridoxine)	↓	in Q 6.23
Vitamin B$_{12}$ (cyanocobalamin)	↓	
Vitamin C (ascorbic acid)	↓	
Binding globulins (including SHBG)	↑	These globulins carry hormones and minerals in the blood. Because their levels increase in parallel with the latter, the effective blood levels of the hormones or minerals are usually not much altered
Blood viscosity	↑	
Body water	↑	This retention of fluid explains some of the weight gain blamed on the pill
Factors affecting blood pressure	Altered	Drospirenone in Yasmin™ might lower associated ↑ aldosterone secretion and sodium retention, Qs 6.33, 6.62
Renin substrate	↑	Changes do not correlate as well
Renin activity	↑	as expected with the rare
Angiotensin II	↑	incidence of frank pill-related hypertension
Immunity/allergy		
Number of leucocytes	↑	See Qs 6.69–6.71
Immunoglobulins	Altered	
Function of lymphocytes	Altered	

Notes:

1. In the table ↑ means the level usually goes up, ↓ down.
2. 'Altered' means that the changes are known to be more complex, with both increases and decreases occurring within the system.
3. The changes are generally (a) within the normal range, (b) similar to those of normal pregnancy.
4. These effects are obviously highly relevant to the interpretation of many laboratory tests. See Q 6.79.

lipoprotein (HDL)-cholesterol increase is reversed by LNG- and NET-containing pills, whereas it is permitted by DSG or GSD if present (*see Q 5.110*). Prior to the CSM's letter of October 1995 and the subsequent 'pill-scare', it was widely thought and promoted by the relevant manufacturers that lack of reduction of HDL-cholesterol would be beneficial (to the arterial walls). This view is now less confidently held – at least for women without risk factors – because there is increasing evidence that no formulation of COC is atherogenic (or in particular promotes heart attacks) unless there is first an arterial risk factor such as smoking.

5 When such arterial risk factors are present, however, it remains a tenable hypothesis that these apparently 'lipid-friendly' products might reduce arterial disease risk, relative to other products (*see Q 5.115*).

5.100 Given the importance of blood pressure in arterial disease, what effects does the COC have?

In the majority of combined pill users there is a slight, measurable increase in both systolic and diastolic blood pressure within the normotensive range. Early large studies showed a 1.5–3 times higher relative risk of clinical hypertension. Modern varieties with reduced biological impact of the oestrogen and progestogen (both are relevant because there is synergism once oestrogen is being taken) have reduced but not eliminated this risk. However, the new progestogen drospirenone in combination with EE as Yasmin™ led in one premarketing study to a very small but significant fall in mean blood pressure. Whether this will translate into greater safety of that formulation for arterial disease, especially when there are risk factors, remains for further study and reports.

Predisposing factors include strong family history, and a tendency to water retention and obesity. Past pregnancy-associated hypertension (toxaemia) does not predispose to hypertension during OC use, in controlled studies. But the RCGP study showed that past toxaemia history (which might be a 'marker' for essential hypertension, not diagnosed before the pregnancy) does predispose to myocardial infarction, especially in smokers (*see Q 5.136*).

Hypertension is an important risk factor for the arterial diseases to be considered in detail below, especially heart disease and both types of stroke.

5.101 As of 2003, what do we really know about how the COC affects the various cardiovascular diseases?

A most useful summary of the worldwide epidemiological findings was published by the WHO in 1998 in their periodical Progress in Human

Reproduction Research (which also contains all the most important references). In view of the amount of heat that has been generated on this subject since October 1995, I reproduced much of this (with permission, slightly rearranged and with a few comments of my own) in the last edition (1999). But for this new edition a shortened form (still making a longer than usual answer!) will suffice.

CARDIOVASCULAR DISEASE AND STEROID HORMONE CONTRACEPTIVES
On 3–7 November 1997, WHO convened in Geneva a Scientific Group Meeting on Cardiovascular Disease and Steroid Hormone Contraception. Acknowledging the major changes that have taken place in the hormonal content of combined oral contraceptives and prescribing patterns, the Scientific Group paid particular attention to studies that included data collected after 1980.

The Scientific Group concluded that the incidence and mortality rates of all cardiovascular diseases (stroke, myocardial infarction and venous thromboembolism) in women of reproductive age are very low. Any additional cardiovascular disease incidence or mortality attributable to oral contraceptives is very small if the users do not smoke and do not have other cardiovascular risk factors. The background papers prepared for the meeting have been published in the journal *Contraception* (March 1998, vol. 57). The final report of the Scientific Group Meeting was published in 1998 by WHO (Technical Report Series, No. 877).

Venous thromboembolism (VTE)
The Scientific Group concluded that:

■ Current users of COCs have a low absolute risk of VTE, which is none the less 3–6 times that in non-users. The risk is probably highest in the first year of use and declines thereafter, but persists until discontinuation.
■ After use of COCs is discontinued, the risk of venous thromboembolism drops rapidly to that in non-users.
■ Among users of COC preparations containing less than 50 μg of ethinylestradiol, the risk of venous thromboembolism is not related to the dose of oestrogen. [**JG: Rather, this expected link has as yet neither been shown, nor disproved.**]
■ COCs containing desogestrel or gestodene probably carry a small risk of VTE beyond that attributable to COCs containing levonorgestrel.
■ There are insufficient data to draw conclusions with regard to COCs containing norgestimate.
■ The absolute risks of VTE attributable to use of oral contraceptives rise with increasing age, obesity, recent surgery, and some forms of thrombophilia.

■ Cigarette smoking and raised blood pressure, which are important risk factors for arterial disease, do not appear to elevate the risk of venous thromboembolic disease. [**JG: This is a valid working summary, although some data still suggest a link with smoking.**]

■ There are insufficient data to conclude whether there is a relation between VTE and the use of progestogen-only contraceptives. [**JG: Yet in WHO's own *Eligibility Criteria* book (2000) a past history of VTE is seen as no more than WHO 2 (see Q 5.119) for all the progestogen-only contraceptives! UK practice is similar, in the absence of any established causative link; see Vasilakis et al 1999 Lancet 354:1610–1611.**]

■ The relative risks of venous thromboembolic disease observed in users of combined oral contraceptives in developed countries appear to be applicable to developing countries.

Acute myocardial infarction (AMI)

Data are available which show that increasing age, cigarette smoking, diabetes, hypertension and raised total blood cholesterol are important risk factors for AMI in young women. The Scientific Group concluded that:

■ The incidence of fatal and non-fatal AMI is very low in women of reproductive age. Women who do not smoke, who have their blood pressure checked and who do not have hypertension or diabetes are at no increased risk of AMI if they use COCs when compared with never-users of the same age. [**JG: Indeed, in every study, including the four main cohort studies and the 1999 MICA case–control study, this disease has effectively not been reported in a pill taker unless she also smoked or had another arterial risk factor, and is regardless of pill-formulation.**]

■ There is no increase in the risk of AMI with increasing duration of use of COCs. There is no increase in the relative risk of AMI in past users of COCs. [**JG: This is not the pattern to be expected if the COC, alone, in the absence of arterial risk factors, were atherogenic.**]

■ Women with hypertension have an increased absolute risk of AMI. The relative risk of AMI in current users of COCs with hypertension is at least three times that in current users without hypertension.

■ The increased absolute risk of AMI in women who smoke is greatly elevated by use of COCs, especially in heavy smokers. The relative risk of AMI in heavy smokers who use COCs might be as high as 10 times that in non-smokers who do not use COCs. [**JG: See *Table 5.8.***]

■ Although the incidence of AMI increases exponentially with age, the relative risk of AMI in current users of COCs does not change with increasing age.

TABLE 5.8 Estimated number of cardiovascular events at different ages among non-users and users of combined oral contraceptives in developed countries by smoking habits

Number of events	Age (years)		
(per million woman-years)	20–24	30–34	40–44
Non-smokers – Non-users			
Acute myocardial infarction	0.13	1.69	21.28
Ischaemic stroke	6.03	9.84	16.05
Haemorrhagic stroke	12.73	24.28	46.30
Venous thromboembolism	32.23	45.75	59.28
Total	51.12	81.56	142.9
Non-smokers – Users*			
Acute myocardial infarction	0.20	2.55	31.92
Ischaemic stroke	9.04	14.75	24.07
Haemorrhagic stroke	12.73	24.28	92.60
Venous thromboembolism	96.68	137.30	177.80
Total	118.70	178.90	326.40
Smokers – Non-users			
Acute myocardial infarction	1.08	13.58	170.20
Ischaemic stroke	12.06	19.67	32.09
Haemorrhagic stroke	25.46	48.55	138.90
Venous thromboembolism	32.23	45.75	59.28
Total	70.83	127.60	400.50
Smokers – Users*			
Acute myocardial infarction	1.62	20.36	255.30
Ischaemic stroke	18.09	29.51	48.14
Haemorrhagic stroke	38.19	72.83	231.50
Venous thromboembolism	96.68	137.30	177.80
Total	154.60	260.00	712.70

*Blood pressure was checked in users.
Source: Farley TMM, Collins J, Schlesselman JJ. 1998 Hormonal contraception and risk of cardiovascular disease: an international perspective. *Contraception* 57:211–230.

- The available data do not allow the effect of the dose of oestrogen on the relative risk of AMI to be evaluated independently of the type and dose of progestogen.
- There are insufficient data to assess whether the risk of AMI in users of low-dose COCs is modified by the type of progestogen. The suggestion that users of low-dose COCs containing gestodene or desogestrel might have a lower risk of AMI than users of low-dose formulations containing levonorgestrel remains to be substantiated. [**JG: Since then,**

both the Transnational Study and Tanis et al 2002 (*New England Journal of Medicine* 345:1787–1793) have shown this, with relevant statistical significance, among smokers (*see* Q 5.115).]

■ The above conclusions appear to apply equally to women in developed and developing countries.

Ischaemic stroke

The Scientific Group concluded that:

■ The incidence of fatal and non-fatal ischaemic stroke is very low in women of reproductive age, but increases with increasing age.

■ The reported estimates of relative risk of ischaemic stroke associated with use of combined oral contraceptives have decreased since the earliest epidemiological studies linking use of oral contraceptives with stroke.

■ In women who do not smoke, who have their blood pressure checked, and who do not have hypertension, the risk of ischaemic stroke is increased about 1.5-fold in current users of low-dose combined oral contraceptives compared with non-users. There is no further increase in the risk of ischaemic stroke with increasing duration of use of COCs. Women who have stopped taking COCs are at no greater risk of ischaemic stroke than women who have never used oral contraceptives.

■ Women with hypertension have an increased absolute risk of ischaemic stroke. The relative risk of ischaemic stroke in current users of COCs with hypertension appears to be at least three times that in current users without hypertension.

■ The absolute risk of ischaemic stroke in women who smoke is about 1.5–2 times that in non-smokers; this risk is multiplied by a factor of 2–3 if such women are current users of COCs.

■ The risk of ischaemic stroke in users of COCs containing high doses of oestrogen is higher than that in users of COCs containing low doses of oestrogen.

■ There are insufficient data to allow any conclusion to be drawn about whether the risk of ischaemic stroke is related to the type or dose of progestogen contained in low-dose COCs.

These conclusions appear to apply equally in developed and developing countries. [JG: Careful prescribing in relation to headaches especially migraine with focal neurological aura (*see* Qs 5.151–5.159) should further reduce the risk of this catastrophic complication, but we need more data.]

Haemorrhagic stroke

The Scientific Group concluded that:

- The incidence of fatal and non-fatal haemorrhagic stroke is very low in women of reproductive age in both developed and developing countries. In women aged less than 35 years, who do not smoke and who do not have hypertension, the relative risk of haemorrhagic stroke associated with use of COCs is not increased. There is no increase in the risk of haemorrhagic stroke with increasing duration of use of oral contraceptives. Women who have previously used oral contraceptives are at no greater risk of haemorrhagic stroke than women who have never used them.
- Women with hypertension have an increased absolute risk of haemorrhagic stroke. The relative risk of haemorrhagic stroke in current users of COCs with hypertension might be 10 times that in current users without hypertension.
- The risk of haemorrhagic stroke in women who smoke is up to twice that in non-smokers; in women who are current users of COCs and who smoke, the relative risk is about 3.
- The incidence of haemorrhagic stroke increases with age, and current use of COCs appears to magnify this effect of ageing.
- There is no evidence that either the oestrogen or the progestogen constituent of COCs is related to the risk of haemorrhagic stroke.

These conclusions appear to apply equally in developed and developing countries (see *Table 5.8*).

Possible biological mechanisms for cardiovascular effects

The complexity of the mechanisms underlying cardiovascular disease has been increasingly recognized over recent years. COCs affect lipoprotein and carbohydrate metabolism, haemostasis, and mechanisms regulating blood pressure. An influence on the functioning of the endothelium of blood vessels and arterial tone also seems likely. The Scientific Group suggested that the potential significance of these changes should be investigated and interpreted using new models of vascular pathophysiology. The Scientific Group concluded that:

- Epidemiological observations are more likely to be accepted if they are biologically plausible, although the absence of such an explanation does not exclude a causal relationship.
- The biological mechanisms underlying cardiovascular disease involve a complex interplay between lipoprotein metabolism, humoral regulators such as insulin, coagulation and fibrinolysis, the renin–angiotensin–aldosterone system, and the functioning of the endothelium of blood vessels.
- COCs do not increase the risk of developing diabetes mellitus. They have little effect on fasting plasma concentrations of glucose and insulin

but cause modest elevations in the plasma levels of glucose and insulin after an oral glucose challenge and might increase insulin resistance. The clinical significance of such changes in otherwise healthy young women is unknown, especially in relation to arterial disease.

■ The changes in metabolism of lipoproteins in plasma induced by use of COCs have been extensively studied. Low-dose COCs increase fasting plasma levels of triglycerides but have only minor effects on low-density lipoproteins (LDL), lipoprotein or total cholesterol. The effect on HDL depends on the balance of oestrogen and progestogen. The clinical significance of such changes is uncertain in the context of current low-dose formulations.

■ COCs alter the plasma concentrations of many components (including their activation markers) of both the coagulation and fibrinolytic systems. These changes are less marked with COCs containing low doses of ethinylestradiol and even less so with progestogen-only contraceptives. Hereditary conditions such as antithrombin III defect and factor V Leiden mutation predispose women to venous thromboembolism. These disorders might underlie a large proportion of idiopathic venous thromboembolic events, perhaps one-third of those seen in Caucasian women. This effect is increased in women using COCs.

■ The prevalence of hereditary conditions such as antithrombin III defect and factor V Leiden mutation is about 5% in Caucasian women but is lower in other populations. The positive predictive value of screening for these disorders is very low. [**JG: See** *Qs 5.112 and 5.113.*]

■ Even low-dose COCs cause modest elevations in blood pressure that might increase the risk of arterial disease. In healthy young women with a low background risk of arterial disease, small increases in blood pressure attributable to use of COC are likely to have minimal effects on the absolute risk of arterial disease.

■ Comparative studies of users of low-dose COCs suggest that the dose and type of the progestogen component influence the effect of these preparations on lipid and lipoprotein metabolism and haemostasis. The clinical significance of these differences is uncertain.

Recommendations for further research

The Scientific Group made a number of recommendations regarding areas of future research related to the risk of cardiovascular disease and the use of steroid contraception – interested readers are referred to the last edition of this book or to WHO Technical Report 857.

Making informed choices about COCs

Any assessment of the risk of cardiovascular disease associated with COCs is complex. Nevertheless, it is clear that mortality rates from cardiovascular disease are extremely low among women of reproductive age, and that the added risk of using steroid contraceptives is also very low. Within the context of the everyday risks of modern life, steroid contraceptives are safe. Factors that need to be taken into account when determining a woman's risk of cardiovascular disease while using COCs include:

■ the age-specific incidence of each cardiovascular condition
■ the strength of the association between use of COCs and each cardiovascular outcome
■ the woman's age and presence of other risk factors for cardiovascular disease, such as smoking and a history of hypertension
■ whether there are important differences in risk between particular formulations of COC and, if so, the choice of formulation.

The number of cardiovascular events attributable to the use of COCs is very small, especially among users of all ages who do not smoke and among younger users who smoke. [JG: **This is shown very clearly in *Table 5.8*, which comes from the same WHO publication, especially as the numbers shown are per million women per year.**] The number of associated deaths is even smaller and, again, is highly dependent on whether the user is a smoker. Any small increase in risk of cardiovascular disease must be considered against the very high contraceptive efficacy of COCs and the rapid reversibility of this effect after they are stopped. The use of less reliable alternative methods of contraception (or the avoidance of any contraception) exposes women to an increased risk of pregnancy, a condition that is associated with a higher incidence of venous thromboembolic disease than that associated with the use of any of the currently available low-dose COCs. In addition, COCs are associated with many non-contraceptive benefits, including a reduced risk of endometrial and ovarian cancer. By any standards, all of the currently available low-dose COCs can be regarded as safe.

The Study Group concluded that:

■ Any increase in incidence of, or mortality from, cardiovascular disease attributable to use of COC is very small if users do not smoke and do not have other risk factors for cardiovascular disease (*Table 5.8*). For example, among users of COCs who do not have risk factors for cardiovascular disease, the annual risk of death attributable to use of oral contraceptives is approximately 2 deaths per million users at 20–24 years of age, 2–5 per million users at 30–34 years of age and approximately 20–25 per million users at 40–44 years of age. [JG: **In *Fig. 5.11* I use a summary risk of 10 per million (= 1:100 000) for the total all-age and all-cause mortality risk of the COC.**]
■ The risk of mortality from cardiovascular disease attributable to use of oral contraception is much greater (up to 10-fold) among women aged

40–44 years than among women aged 20–24 years. [**JG: A very relevant point this, now we have several new highly effective choices for the older woman, despite the convenience for her of the COC** (*see Q 11.39*).]

■ At any given age a woman who smokes but who does not use oral contraceptives is at greater risk of death from arterial disease than a user of oral contraceptives who does not smoke. [**JG: Worth saying this to some women – and men!**]

■ The benefits of blood-pressure measurement in reducing the risk of cardiovascular disease attributable to use of oral contraception increase with the age of the user. [**JG: And WHO found that not having BP taken at all is a good surrogate for poor healthcare of pill takers!**]

■ Venous thromboembolic disease is the most common cardiovascular event among users of oral contraceptives. However, it contributes very little to any increase in the number of deaths since the associated mortality (maximum 2%) is relatively low compared with that associated with arterial diseases. Long-term disability from non-fatal venous thromboembolic disease is also low.

5.102 What is the difference between relative risk and absolute or attributable risk?

This is a most important distinction, which is not often understood by either patients or journalists, notably in relation to venous thromboembolism (VTE). Twice almost nothing out of a million is still almost nothing! Pill-takers can relate to the analogy that being given a second lottery ticket does not make you hugely more likely to win even though doubling your chances:

A small relative risk might easily cause more attributable cases than a large one, if the background prevalence is high – and vice versa.

In *Table 5.9* the first set of figures (A) actually apply to the frequency of hepatocellular adenoma in controls as compared with COC users using older 50-μg-plus pills. The second set (B) come from *Table 5.8* (*see Q 5.101*), which itself is from the 1998 report of the WHO's special Scientific Group. They apply to smokers aged 40–44, who would have an increase in relative risk of acute myocardial infarction (AMI) of only 1.5 if they additionally took the modern low-dose pills at that age; but the attributable number of extra cases (absolute risk) is 85 per million. Contrast only 19 extra cases of hepatoma in the first set of figures (A), despite a 20-fold greater relative risk.

Neither statistic is good news (both are dangerous conditions). But the difference in the excess number of cases caused explains why it was reasonable to accept, for 50-μg-plus pills, a 20-fold increase in the risk of benign liver tumours. However, a mere 50% increase in AMI through more modern pills is widely considered unacceptable for smokers above age 40.

TABLE 5.9 Attributable risk

Background prevalence	Relative risk	No. of cases	No. of cases attributable
(A) 1 in 10^6	$\times 20$	20	19
(B) 170 in 10^6	$\times 1.5$	255	85

Note: This many times an infinitesimal risk can still be infinitesimal. See Q 5.102

5.103 Patients are naturally anxious about the known adverse effects of the combined pill on cancer and circulatory disease. Assuming they otherwise wish to use the method, how can this anxiety be reduced?

See Q 5.101, the section on 'making informed choices', and *Figs 5.10 and 5.11*. The media do the general public a disservice by tending to exaggerate the bad systemic effects and by not pointing out the counterbalancing non-contraceptive benefits, aside from the advantages of efficacy, reversibility and convenience. Another form of counterbalancing is shown on the right-hand side of *Fig. 5.10*, namely the comparison with the risks of pregnancy (so effectively avoided by the COC) and the avoidance of the risk and inconvenience of the alternative methods.

Potential users can be reminded that there are many other risks in life. However intelligent and educated, most of us are amazingly 'risk-illiterate'.

Note: All to be viewed in the context of risks of life generally

Fig. 5.10 The risks versus the benefits of hormonal contraception (see Fig. 5.11 for the risks of life generally). Q 5.103.

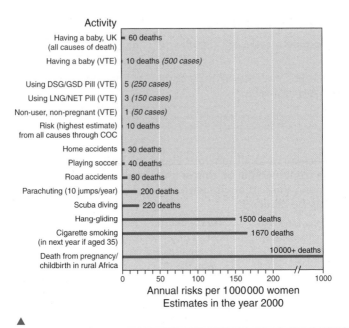

Fig. 5.11 The risks of various activities (annual number of deaths per 1 000 000 exposed). Q 5.103. With regard to cancer, in this figure excess cancer mortality is assumed to be zero (see Q 5.73 and Fig. 5.6) (sources: Dinman 1980 *Journal of the American Medical Association* 244:1226–1228; Mills et al 1996 *British Medical Journal* 312:121; Anonymous 1991 *British Medical Journal* 302:743; Strom 1994 *Pharmacoepidemiology*, 2nd edn, pp. 57–65. Chichester, John Wiley; Guillebaud 1998 *Contraception today*, 3rd edn, p 20. London, Martin Dunitz). COC, combined oral contraceptive; DSG, desogestrel; GSD, gestodene; LNG, levonorgestrel; NET, norethisterone; VTE, venous thromboembolism.

Many risks are far greater than pill taking, yet cause minimal concern: for example having babies or travelling by car (*Fig. 5.11*) – let alone smoking!

For those who are not very numerate, risks are best expressed in relative terms: 'The risk of dying through pill taking is less than one-hundredth of the risk of death through smoking 20 cigarettes a day', for example.

Life is pretty risky: believe it or not, each year one has a 1:1000 chance of having to visit a Casualty Department through a home injury from a bottle or a can. At least three deaths have been reported at the Brompton hospital through allergy to hamsters.

Among one million men, the risk of dying (from all natural causes) is one in a million:

- in the next 7.5 h if aged 40
- in the next 5 min if aged over 65!

Finally, prospective pill takers can be reminded that the tiny risks of the COC can be further reduced: by careful prescribing of lower-dose preparations, with good subsequent monitoring (*see Qs 5.118, 5.136 and 6.1*).

5.104 What effect does smoking have on the mortality of arterial disease in pill users?

Given the relevance of smoking as a serious risk people take for granted, it is salutary to note that the 1983 report of the RCGP showed (and later data are congruent) that the pill user who also smoked was not only more likely to suffer a heart attack but was also much more likely to die as a consequence – a higher case-fatality rate was noted in smokers.

5.105 How can a busy doctor ever convey enough information about COCs to enable worried women to make a fully informed decision?

So much is now known about the method that this is becoming ever more difficult to do. The advice of the Medical Defence Societies is:

A doctor has the duty to give such warnings and carry out such checks as are considered by his/her peers to be necessary having regard to the relevant circumstances of the case. There is no obligation to explain every risk but there is the need to be forthright in explaining risks.

In other words, you should be frank about what is known and honest about what is not yet known; communicate the main pros and cons of the method as in *Qs 5.56, 5.70–5.103*; explain the practicalities, rules for missed pills, minor side-effects – most especially breakthrough bleeding; and allow time for questions. Full records should be kept. A pretty tall order!

For most busy practitioners who wish to maintain high standards 'allow time' means more accurately 'make time', plus delegate. In the real world, how do women present? In the middle of a busy surgery, as like as not needing postcoital contraception (see Chapter 10, a whole chapter to take account of there!) first, and then to start the COC before their follow-up visit. Can all this ever be done well without the availability of counselling by a (family planning-trained) nurse, supplemented by you perhaps at the end of your surgery or during the next dedicated family planning session (*see Q 11.16*)?

5.106 What else is important as an adjunct to good counselling?

The written word! In my view, counselling should always be supplemented by a leaflet and I think the best is still the FPA's leaflet on the combined pill. Among other things, this has advice for missed pills and a medicolegally important list of those side-effects that should lead the woman to seek urgent medical advice (*see Q 6.13*). But new pill-takers must *always* also receive the PIL (licensed patient information leaflet) that relates to the specific product.

Finally, much medical time can be saved if those women who desire the impossible, a 2-h consultation about oral contraception are referred to my comprehensive paperback entitled *The Pill* (see Further Reading)!

A MORE DETAILED APPRAISAL OF THE CONTROVERSY ABOUT VENOUS THROMBOEMBOLISM (VTE) AND ITS IMPLICATIONS FOR PRESCRIBERS

5.107 Now that the dust has settled, what is your take on that letter from the UK Committee on the Safety of Medicines (CSM) on 18 October 1995 regarding VTE?

There is still a range of expert views about the four publications on COCs and VTE published in December 1995 and January 1996, mentioned above in the long WHO extract. They were carefully performed and reasonably congruent with each other. They reported a doubling of the odds ratio for users of desogestrel/gestodene-containing products (DSG/GSD-containing or so-called 'third generation' progestogens) in comparison with the 'second generation' levonorgestrel or norethisterone-containing ones (here called 'LNG/NET pills').

The 'generation' terminology is ambiguous and best avoided. I now much prefer to refer to the *relative oestrogen dominance* of each formulation (*see* Q 5.110).

5.108 Yet has not the accuracy of this finding been queried?

Indeed: by many authorities in the US and in continental Europe – including those involved in the Transnational study, one of the pivotal studies just mentioned. They believe that the whole of the apparent association can be explained not by cause-and-effect but by:

- Prescriber bias (prescribers being selectively more likely, prior to October 1995, to use DSG/GSD products for first-timers and women thought to be at risk of VTE).
- The 'attrition of susceptibles' or 'healthy user effect' (LNG/NET pills being more commonly used by longer-term users and parous women who would be less likely as a population to suffer a VTE, because those who had had this disease would no longer be using the method).
- Diagnostic bias resulting from prescriber bias, in that women put on DSG/GSD pills because of a perceived higher risk might then also be more likely to be referred for accurate investigations leading to this easily-overlooked diagnosis being made more often than among LNG/NET pill users.

Evidence for these alternative explanations for the finding comes from:

■ In 1996, Lewis and co-workers on the Transnational study showed a significant trend of increasing risk of VTE for the progestogens in COCs, related solely to the recency of their introduction to the market.

■ There is also the very odd WHO finding that Mercilon™ with 20 μg of EE, the artificial oestrogen well-recognized as creating prothrombotic coagulation changes, was significantly associated with more cases of VTE than Marvelon™ with 30 μg.

Neither of the above are biologically plausible, yet they might be readily linked to prescriber bias and the healthy user effect.

But for honest seekers after the truth (you – the reader – and I!) the question remains whether there could be some real difference between DSG and GSD versus LNG or NET combined products in allowing EE to cause VTE events despite the non-causative explanations – although clearly these must apply in part (see below).

5.109 In your opinion, where does that leave us as prescribers?

At the time of writing (July 2003), personally, I am sure the apparent doubling is a worst-case scenario, because of the exaggerating effects of the above biases and confounders. But even allowing for these, I am prepared to accept some difference of VTE risk when comparing the DSG/GSD pills with the LNG and NET ones (*see Q 5.110*).

5.110 Is it biologically plausible that the same 30-μg dose of ethinylestradiol (EE) would have different effects when combined with the two different types of progestogens?

There is a degree of biological plausibility, yes, because we have known for years that NET (somewhat) and LNG (more so) behave in some respects as antioestrogenic progestogens:

1 A dose of 30 μg EE raises SHBG, raises HDL-cholesterol and tends to improve acne.

2 In a randomized controlled trial at the Margaret Pyke Centre we have found that if LNG 150 μg is combined with the same 30-μg dose of EE, as in Microgynon™/Ovranette™, then SHBG goes up less than with EE alone and HDL-cholesterol is actually slightly lowered (i.e. the EE effect is reversed). Moreover, clinically, acne may be worsened. Therefore LNG (and, in high enough dose, NET) is clearly capable of opposing the oestrogenicity of EE in its biochemical effects (e.g. SHBG) and in some of its somatic effects (e.g. acne).

3 However, combined with desogestrel 150 μg, as in Marvelon™, the same dose of EE raises SHBG more, raises HDL-cholesterol and tends to improve acne – all very like EE would do on its own.

Thus, on those three criteria (among others) DSG/GSD pills allow EE to have more of its oestrogenic effects than LNG ones do. As prothrombotic coagulation changes are also primarily oestrogen-related, a similar difference in VTE potential has always been possible.

5.111 But surely no-one has been able to show a consistent difference in the effects of the two types of progestogen upon the coagulation factors that are altered by oestrogen?

On the contrary, such differences are now emerging in relation to so-called acquired activated protein C resistance (the work of Rosing and others in the Netherlands) and to the lowering of protein S, which are both oestrogenic effects. In a further study on volunteers, we showed (Mackie et al 2001 *British Journal of Haematology* 113:898–904) that protein S was reduced more in users of DSG than LNG formulations ($P < 0.0001$). Protein S decreased significantly when switching from LNG to DSG pills, mirrored by a similar and significant increase with switching from DSG to LNG formulations. Yet both products (Marvelon™ and Microgynon™) contain the same 30 μg dose of EE.

This fits well with my hypothesis that LNG 'opposes the oestrogenicity' of EE in the COC. For actual thrombosis to occur we suggested a further triggering factor was a likely prerequisite. But pill takers whose levels of protein S were in the lowest percentiles (of whom there would be more in non-LNG-containing products) might be expected to be at greatest risk.

5.112 What are the main hereditary predispositions to VTE? And what action should be taken if one is suspected?

Women with possible hereditary thrombophilia, or who give a clear family history of idiopathic thrombosis in a parent or sibling under 45 (see *Table 5.10*, p. 188), should ideally not be prescribed any COC until thrombophilia has been excluded. The main abnormalities are factor V Leiden (the genetic cause of activated protein C resistance), which is the most prevalent; and deficiencies of protein C, protein S and antithrombin III. Any of these, once known about, absolutely contraindicate all EE-containing pills (although actually, given the background rarity of VTE, the attributable risk from having any of them is not great, *see Qs 5.102 and 5.113*). On the other hand even if they are not found the woman cannot be totally reassured.

The haemostatic system is immensely complicated. Almost half of truly idiopathic cases of VTE are not explainable by modern coagulation testing since by no means all the predisposing abnormalities of the haemostatic system have yet been characterized. Therefore, as shown in *Table 5.10* (p. 188), the COC is still WHO 2 if a woman with a positive family history has negative test results. She might indeed use the pill method but should be specifically advised about the early symptoms of thromboembolism. Like all with a single relative contraindication for VTE she should normally receive a LNG/NET pill.

5.113 If resources are available, why do we not simply screen everyone who asks to go on the pill for a predisposing factor to VTE?

Because it is neither cost-effective nor good practice to screen for the hereditary thrombophilias in cases without well-defined family history criteria (i.e. thrombophilia in the family or idiopathic thrombosis in a parent or sibling under 45). Given that each year there are only three extra cases of VTE among 1000 pill takers, with the most common thrombophilia, factor V Leiden, compared with pill users without this predisposition, 997 of 1000 never actually get a thrombosis. They prove, in a real sense, to be 'false positives'; and then there are other predispositions that are not yet measurable (leading to many 'false negatives'). Given the cost of comprehensive testing, it would cost £100 000s to save one life by untargeted screening. More harm than good would result.

5.114 What are the acquired thrombophilias, and when should they be looked for/screened for?

Antiphospholipid antibodies (such as the unhelpfully named lupus anticoagulant) can appear in various connective tissue disorders, especially systemic lupus erythematosus (SLE). They should be looked for whenever such a disorder is suspected but screening for these in *healthy* women is not cost-effective because, once again, of the number of false positives (women with a detectable abnormality who never get a thrombosis, even during years of pill taking) and false negatives (women who suffer an idiopathic thrombotic event with or without the COC yet have no congenital or acquired abnormality which modern technology can detect).

Antiphospholipid antibodies increase the risk of both VTE and arterial disease and therefore if present they absolutely contraindicate the COC – but not any of the progestogen-only methods.

5.115 Which progestogens might be best for the least arterial wall disease risk? (chiefly AMI and strokes)

There still remains the possibility of a relative benefit to the arterial walls and hence arterial disease from what appear to be the 'good' effects of DSG/GSD and other more oestrogen-dominant brands of lipids: they do not lower HDL-cholesterol as some of the higher dose LNG and NET brands do.

Some epidemiological data on AMI are now available, but not enough to be conclusive. Both the Transnational study and the Tanis study (Tanis et al 2002 *New England Journal of Medicine* 345:1787–1793) have shown – among smokers – that users of low-dose formulations containing levonorgestrel had a statistically significant increased risk of AMI, but no such increase if they used DSG/GSD products. The 1999 MICA study was not confirmatory of this, but a later report from the same group's data did show a lower mortality in myocardial infarction if the smokers who became AMI patients had been using GSD or DSG formulations. More studies are needed to confirm these findings.

5.116 How would you put the VTE risks in perspective?

See *Table 5.8* (p. 169) and *Fig. 5.11* (p. 176). The new studies confirm that all low-dose COCs carry an extremely low risk for healthy women. The UK Department of Health (DoH) issued a helpful statement in April 1999 as follows:

An increased risk of venous thromboembolic disease (VTE) associated with the use of oral contraceptives is well established but is smaller than that associated with pregnancy; which has been estimated at 60 cases per 100 000 pregnancies. Some epidemiological studies have reported a greater risk of VTE for women using combined oral contraceptives containing desogestrel or gestodene (the so-called third generation pills) than for women using pills containing levonorgestrel (LNG) – the so-called second generation pills. *[sic: this category also includes norethisterone (NET) pills].* The spontaneous incidence of VTE in healthy non-pregnant women (not taking any oral contraceptive) is about 5 cases per 100 000 women per year. The incidence in users of second generation pills is about 15 per 100 000 women per year of use. The incidence in users of third generation pills is about 25 cases per 100 000 women per year of use: this excess incidence has not been satisfactorily explained by bias or confounding. The level of all of these risks of VTE increases with age and is likely to be increased in women with other known risk factors for VTE such as obesity.

Women must be fully informed of these very small risks. ... Provided they are, the type of pill is for the woman together with her doctor or other family planning professionals jointly to decide in the light of her individual medical history. [my emphasis]

Note in the above DoH quotation that even though the DoH accepts a real difference between the two 'generations' of COCs – and this is still hotly disputed by some authorities – the estimated annual 'spontaneous' VTE risk per 100 000 users for DSG/GSD pills has been reduced to 25 cases versus 15 for LNG/NET pills. Multiplying by 10, therefore, the difference – being the annual attributable number of cases through using DSG/GSD brands rather than one of less oestrogen-dominant ones – is small, 100 per million. Using these estimates and taking the upper estimate of the 1–2% mortality for VTE, there is only a 2 per million difference in annual VTE mortality between DSG/GSD products and LNG/NET products.

Now, it has been estimated that there is a one in a million risk in each hour of travel by car (Minerva 1988 *British Medical Journal*). Even if the whole of the above difference is accepted as real, therefore, it is small enough, in comparison with other risks (see *Fig. 5.11*) that are taken in everyday life, for a well-informed woman to take if she so chooses. If, for example, she wishes to use or to switch to a DSG/GSD brand on the grounds of 'quality of life', to control so-called minor side-effects such as acne, headaches, depression, weight gain or breast symptoms: if her previous COC was Microgynon™ she can be told that if she simply avoids 2 h of driving in the whole of the next year, in risk terms she is still on Microgynon™ – it is as though she never left off taking it!

5.117 Is intolerance of the LNG/NET pill brands through non-life-endangering but nevertheless 'annoying' side-effects acceptable as sufficient grounds for a woman to use a DSG/GSD brand?

Yes, this is clear in the above DoH quote, indeed it was accepted from the outset, in the original letter circulated by the CSM – provided the woman understood and accepted the tiny excess risk of VTE. In my experience as a counsellor of pill takers, the difference in risk compared with an LNG/NET brand is easily seen by many women as unimportant compared with the risks of life generally.

SELECTION OF USERS AND FORMULATIONS: CHOOSING THE 'SAFER WOMEN', AND THE 'SAFER PILLS'

5.118 What is your recommended framework for good pill management?

We want safer pills for what I call the 'safer women', maximum safety as well as efficacy. But what the safer pills actually are will vary somewhat, depending on research data as it is received, and on characteristics of the woman herself. We need a framework for choice of users as well as choice of pills:

1   Who should never take the pill? (i.e. what are the absolute contraindications, WHO 4?)
2   Who should usually or often not take the pill? Maybe – but then with special advice and monitoring (the relative contraindications now classified by WHO as either WHO 3 or 2, as described in *Q 5.119*.) All these contraindications are described in detail later (*see Qs 5.134–5.138*) because they take so much space that they would hamper this discussion.
3   Which is the appropriate pill?
4   Which second choice of pill? This means taking account of:
    (a) biological variation in the pharmacokinetics of contraceptive steroids (*see Qs 5.160–5.161*)

(b) endometrial bleeding as a possible biological measure of their blood levels (*see Qs 5.162–5.168*)

(c) what is known about their side-effect profile (*see Qs 6.21–6.22*).

5 What is necessary for monitoring during follow-up? Including:

(a) the implications of the PFI (*see Qs 5.15–5.32*)

(b) blood pressure (*see Qs 6.5–6.8*)

(c) headaches, especially migraines (*see Qs 5.151–5.159*)

(d) management of important new risk factors or diseases (*see Qs 6.1–6.18, 6.23–6.71*)

(e) management of minor side-effects (*see Qs 6.19 and 6.20, 6.21 and 6.22*).

The answers to the next questions *re* prescribing are based primarily on my leading article (1995 *British Medical Journal* 311:1111–1112), the statement from the Clinical and Scientific Committee of the Faculty of Family Planning, UK (1996 *British Medical Journal* 312:121) and the above DoH statement in *Q 5.116*. See also *Q 5.101* and the article on evidence-guided prescribing of COCs by Hannaford and Webb (1996 *Contraception* 54:125–129). In my view, none of the later literature substantially challenges this pragmatic framework for prescribing.

5.119 What is the WHO system for classifying contraindications?

This system, which I was able to help to devise at a small WHO working group in Atlanta early in 1994, is described in a WHO document WHO/FRH/FPP96.9. There are four categories, as shown in *Box 5.1*. Numbers 1 and 4 are unchanged when compared to what we are used to (i.e. when the method is always or never usable). The useful new feature of the classification is separation into two categories of relative contraindication.

One of the main purposes of this scheme is to 'loosen up' with respect to contraindications, destroying pill myths that WHO 3 or 4 applies when whatever it is might actually be an indication for the method, WHO 1 (best example being a woman's concern about her future fertility!). The intention is to remove 'medical barriers' to contraceptive use, i.e. wrong or misclassified contraindications, which end by depriving people of what would be the best method for them and so may well result in avoidable pregnancies…

5.120 What should happen at the first visit?

1 Prescribers should first take a comprehensive personal and family history to exclude the established absolute and relative contraindications to the use of COCs. A personal history of definite VTE remains an absolute contraindication to any COC containing EE combined with any progestogen. For others, *see Q 5.134*.

BOX 5.1   WHO classification of contraindications [with amplifications by J. Guillebaud]

WHO 1

A condition for which there is no restriction for the use of the contraceptive method, indeed the condition might even be an indication for it.

'A' is for ALWAYS USABLE [**e.g. COC with history of candidiasis; uncomplicated varicose veins**]

WHO 2

A condition where the advantages of the method generally outweigh the theoretical or proven risks.

'B' is for BROADLY USABLE [**e.g. COC in smoker age 20; history of pregnancy related hypertension**]

WHO 3

A condition where the theoretical or proven risks usually outweigh the advantages, so the prospective user should be advised that another method would be preferable. But – respecting her autonomy – if she accepts the risks and relevant alternatives are contra-indicated or rejected, given the risks of pregnancy as an alternative, the method can be used with caution/additional care and monitoring.

'C' is for CAUTION/COUNSELLING, if used [**e.g. COC in diabetes without known tissue damage; long-term treatment with enzyme inducer drugs**]

WHO 4

A condition that represents an unacceptable health risk

'D' is for DO NOT USE, at all [**e.g. COC with personal history of thrombosis; migraine with aura**]

Notes:

1   Although the A–B–C–D scheme is a helpful aide-memoire to what each category signifies, I will stick with the WHO's 1–2–3–4 classification in this book to avoid any confusion. So, wherever WHO 3 is mentioned, 'Caution, extra counselling' is intended.

2   Clinical judgement is required in consultation with the contraceptive user, especially:

   (a)   in all category 3 conditions – since another method would usually be an even better choice?

   (b)   if more than one condition applies. As a working rule, two category 2 conditions moves the situation to category 3; and if any category 3 condition applies the addition of either a 2 or a 3 condition normally amounts to category 4 (DO NOT USE).

> **BOX 5.1—cont'd**
>
> 3 This scheme is extremely valuable and is used extensively in the rest of this book. However, it is important for the reader to appreciate that the WHO's own classification may differ for some conditions, either from UK practice, or my personal considered judgement of what would be optimal for clients in the UK. Moreover, numerous conditions have not as yet been considered at all by the relevant WHO committee. It should not therefore be assumed that my judgement that a condition is (say) WHO 3 for the POP is necessarily the same as WHO's view, if WHO has a view.

2 The risk factors for VTE and arterial wall disease must be assessed, separately and most carefully. *Tables 5.10* and *5.11* and their footnotes are crucial in this process. Note that in either table, any one risk is WHO 2 or 3 (second or third column of each table) unless it is severe enough on its own to warrant the category WHO 4.

3 Multiple risk factors: as a working rule, two category 2 conditions moves the situation to category WHO 3; and if any category 3 condition applies the addition of either a 2 or a 3 condition normally amounts to category 4. BMI being above 30 is important because it features in both tables. So the patients should be weighed at this visit (but *not* obsessionally at follow-up visits, *Q 6.1*).

4 The blood pressure should be properly measured, to obtain a good baseline reading. Beware if it is already above 140/90. This is WHO 3 (*Table 5.11*) for COCs, meaning another method would be preferable – and is obligatory if any other risk factors are identified.

5.121 Which pill for ordinary first-time users of combined oral contraceptives?

A listing of all the actual pill formulations available and related issues comes later (*see Qs 5.127–5.131*).

1 All marketed pills can now be considered 'first line'. See the section in bold of the DoH statement (*see Q 5.116*). Given the tiny, not yet finally established difference in VTE mortality between the two 'generations', the woman's own choice of a DSG or GSD product or other oestrogen-dominant product (see below), must be respected – and the discussion fully documented:
The informed user should be the chooser.

2 Young first-time users: despite what has just been said, an LNG or NET product should in my view remain the usual first choice. As a rule, one should initially prescribe a low-dose LNG/NET pill, containing no more

than 35 μg EE and no more than 150 μg LNG or 1000 μg NET. Reasons: first-timers include an unknown subgroup who are VTE-predisposed; also, VTE is a more relevant consideration than arterial disease at this age plus the pills are cheaper.

3 Single risk factor for venous thrombosis *or* for arterial disease, including age above 35: *see Q 5.122 and 5.123*.

5.122 Which pill for a woman with a single risk factor for venous thrombosis (e.g. BMI above 30).

A LNG or NET product would be preferred, if COC used at all. This is a WHO 3 situation (*Table 5.10*). Beware also that she is at increasing risk with age.

The choice of type of COC is more difficult if she has a BMI above 30 but also has PCOS (*see Q 5.65*), because oestrogen dominance is important in this condition to raise SHBG and control acne. In such cases the fact that the COC chosen (such as Marvelon™ or Yasmin™) might increase VTE risk more than a LNG-containing brand can often be justified by the medical indication, i.e. the extra therapeutic benefits – beyond just contraception – would be held to justify the anticipated small extra risks.

5.123 Which pill for a woman with a single definite arterial risk factor (from *Table 5.11*) or who is healthy and risk-factor-free but above age 35?

All the studies, including the RCGP study, the Oxford/FPA study, the American Nurses study, WHO (1998), MICA (1999) and the more recent studies have been unable to detect any increased risk of AMI in non-smokers, whether they were current or past pill takers. This means the arterial event risk of using all the modern low-oestrogen brands must be very small, if not absent, for women free of arterial risk factors. But it is high when they are present (the RCGP's relative risk estimate is 20.8 for smoking pill takers), the risk increases with age (see *Table 5.8*, p. 169) and the case-fatality rate for AMI is also much higher (*see Q 5.104*).

There are suggestive data (*see Q 5.115*) that DSG/GSD pills might have relative advantages for arterial wall disease in higher risk women. Therefore switching to a low-oestrogen 20 μg DSG or GSD pill should logically be at least mooted with smokers (and others with a single arterial risk factor) as they get older (say beyond age 35) – for the two reasons:

1 That it is only in the older age group that arterial disease becomes common enough to be relevant to prescribing policy.

2 If she has already been on any COC (EE combined with any progestogen) for some years without a VTE she is relatively unlikely to be one of the individuals with a hereditary (or acquired) predisposition

TABLE 5.10 Risk factors for venous thromboembolism (VTE)

Risk factor	Absolute contraindication	Relative contraindication		Remarks
	WHO 4	WHO 3	WHO 2	
Family history (FH) of thrombophilia or of venous thrombosis in sibling or parent	Identified clotting abnormality of any kind (including acquired type) FH of a defined thrombophilia or idiopathic thrombotic event in parent or sibling < 45 and thrombophilia screen not (yet) available	FH of thrombosis in parent or sibling < 45 with recognized precipitating factor, e.g. major surgery, postpartum, and thrombophilia screen not available	FH of thrombotic event in parent or sibling < 45 with or without a recognized precipitating factor and *normal* thrombophilia screen FH in parent or sibling ≥ 45 or FH in second-degree relative [classified WHO 2 but tests not indicated]	Idiopathic VTE in a parent or sibling < 45 is an indication for a thrombophilia screen if available. The decision to undertake screening in other situations (including where there was a recognized precipitating factor), will be unusual because it is not cost effective – might be done on clinical grounds, in discussion with the woman Even a normal thrombophilia screen cannot be entirely reassuring
Overweight (high BMI)	BMI > 39	BMI 30–39	BMI 25–29	
Immobility	Bed-bound or leg fractured and immobilized	Wheelchair life	Reduced mobility for other reason	

TABLE 5.10—cont'd

Risk factor	Absolute contraindication	Relative contraindication		Remarks
	WHO 4	WHO 3	WHO 2	
Varicose veins (VVs)	Current superficial vein thrombosis in the upper thigh

Current sclerotherapy for VVS (or imminent VV surgery, Q 6.16) | History of superficial vein thrombosis (SVT) in the lower limbs, no deep vein thrombosis | – | SVT does not result in pulmonary embolism, although this past history means caution (WHO 3) in case it is a marker of future VTE risk (not confirmed). Exceptionally, thrombosis of the greater saphenous vein reaching to the saphenofemoral vein junction, can extend into the deep system – such a history is WHO 4 for the COC. |
| Age > 35 | Age > 51 | | Age 35–51 | |

Notes

1. A single risk factor in the relative contraindication columns indicates use of LNG/NET pill if any COC used (see *BNF*).
2. Beware of synergism: more than one factor in either relative contraindication column. As a working rule, two WHO 2 conditions makes WHO 3; and if WHO 3 applies, addition of either a WHO 2 or WHO 3 condition normally means WHO 4 (do not use).
3. The literature on the association of smoking with venous thromboembolic disease offers no consensus (compare arterial disease).
4. Acquired predispositions also exist through disease, especially antiphospholipid syndrome (see text in the list of Absolute Contraindications).
5. There are also important acute VTE risk factors, which need to be considered in individual cases: notably long-haul flights and dehydration through any cause.
6. This is author's classification. WHO categorises FH of VTE in parent or sibling (without further investigation), BMI >30 (no upper limit) and past SVT all as WHO 2.

BMI, body mass index; COC, combined oral contraception; FH, family history; LNG, levonorgestrel; NET, norethisterone; VTE, venous thromboembolism; VV, varicose veins.

TABLE 5.11 Risk factors for arterial disease

Risk factor	Absolute contraindication	Relative contraindication		Remarks
	WHO 4	WHO 3	WHO 2	
Family history (FH) of atherogenic lipid disorder or of arterial CVS event in sibling or parent	Identified atherogenic lipid profile	FH of known lipid disorder or idiopathic arterial event in parent or sibling < 45 and client's lipid profile 'borderline' atherogenic	FH of arterial event with risk factor (e.g. smoking) in parent or sibling < 45 and lipid screen not available	Arterial CVS disease without other risk factors, or a known atherogenic lipid disorder in a parent or sibling < 45 indicate fasting lipid screen, if available.
	FH of a known atherogenic lipid disorder or idiopathic arterial event in sibling or parent < 45 and lipid screening not (yet) available		FH of idiopathic event in parent or sibling ≥ 45 or FH in second-degree relative [classified WHO 2 but tests not indicated]	Despite any FH, normal lipid screen *is* reassuring, means WHO 1 (contrasts with thrombophilia screens, see Table 5.10)
Cigarette smoking	≥ 40 cigarettes/day	15–39 cigarettes/day	< 15 cigarettes/day	Cut-offs are a bit arbitrary
Diabetes mellitus	Severe or diabetic complications present (e.g. retinopathy, renal damage)	Not severe/labile and no complications, young patient with short duration of DM		DM is always at least WHO 3 (safer options available)
Hypertension	BP ≥ 160/100 mmHg on repeated testing	BP 140–159/ 90–99 mmHg	BP < 140/90 mmHg	These levels are in accordance with the British Hypertension Society and WHO
		On treatment for essential hypertension	Past toxaemia (WHO 3 if smoker)	See Qs 5.100 and 5.136 *re* pregnancy toxaemia as a risk factor

TABLE 5.11 Risk factors for arterial disease—cont'd

Risk factor	Absolute contraindication	Relative contraindication		Remarks
	WHO 4	WHO 3	WHO 2	
Overweight	BMI > 39	BMI 30–39	BMI 25–29	
Migraine	Migraine with aura Migraine without aura if severe prolonged attacks (> 72 h) or ergotamine-treated	Migraine without aura plus single WHO 2 arterial risk factor (*Fig. 5.13*)	Migraine without aura	Relates to stroke risk, see text Triptan treatment does not affect the category
Age > 35	Age > 51 (safer options available)	Age > 40 in ex-heavy-smokers to age 35	Age 35–51 in non-smokers (In smokers age > 35 is WHO 4)	In ex-heavy-smokers, category WHO 3 is because earlier arterial wall damage may persist

Notes

1. Beware of synergism: more than one factor in either relative contraindication column. As a working rule, two WHO 2 conditions makes WHO 3; and if WHO 3 applies, addition of either a WHO 2 or WHO 3 condition normally means WHO 4 (do not use).

2. The pill seems to give no added adverse effect in arterial disease unless there is a risk factor. In continuing smokers, COC is generally stopped at age 35, in the UK. But WHO's eligibility criteria surprisingly permit the category WHO 3 above age 35 for smokers if < 15/day.

3. Note overweight appears in both Tables 5.10 and 5.11 – if it is the sole risk factor it indicates use of a LNG/NET pill (i.e. Table 5.10 takes precedence).

4. Some of the numbers selected are arbitrary and perhaps too strict if they are the sole problem (e.g. the COC might actually be allowed, reluctantly, to an otherwise currently healthy 25-year-old admitting to 40 cigarettes a day). However extra caution is wise concerning WHO 3 levels of BP.

5. Numbers also relate to use for contraception: use of COCs for medical indications often entails a different risk/benefit analysis, i.e. the extra therapeutic benefits might outweigh expected extra risks. Once again this is the author's classification: some differences from WHO.

6. Check with local laboratory as to clinical significance of results from fasting lipids.

to venous thrombosis. Those women would be likely to suffer a VTE event relatively early during pill use (or during any full-term pregnancy) and so leave the population of long-term users. (Yet this previous uncomplicated use does not entirely exclude the risk of VTE in future, especially as, like arterial disease, VTE risk goes up with age, see *Table 5.8*, p. 169.)

In the UK, the 20-μg products Femodette™ or Mercilon-20™ are often the most logical choice for these arterial risk women (no later than age 35 though!); and also for completely risk-factor-free women from 35 to 51 years of age. (Loestrin-20™ being less oestrogenic would currently seem a better product if there were any additional concern about VTE risk, although it does have a reputation for poor cycle control.)

5.124 Which pill for a woman who finds she does not tolerate a LNG/NET COC because of persistent breakthrough bleeding or androgenic/other 'minor' side-effects – or who just wants a change?

As already stated, the differential risk between pill types is very small. If a woman does not tolerate an LNG or NET COC because of persistent BTB or 'minor' side-effects such as acne, headaches, depression, weight gain or breast symptoms, or if she wants a change for personal reasons, use of a DSG or GSD product is medicolegally very secure. Once again, the informed user should be the chooser.

5.125 Presumably the verbal consent of women not using the pill brands recommended by the CSM must be well recorded?

Yes: if DSG/GSD pills are chosen (whether for this arterial risk factor indication or just because the woman prefers one of them on quality of life grounds), given the fact that they were singled out by the CSM in 1995 and that advice has not been revoked, there must, for medicolegal security, always be a full contemporaneous record:

■ of the risk factor history
■ that the woman accepts a possibly increased risk of VTE (conveyed in a non-scary way, e.g. as equalling 2 h of driving in a whole year, *see Q 5.116*).

This counselling should always be backed by a user-friendly leaflet, such as the COC leaflet produced by the UK FPA, and it is prudent to note down the date of issue of the leaflet that was given (along with the PIL).

5.126 What about norgestimate, the progestogen in Cilest™?

There remains considerable uncertainty here, through lack of epidemiological data. Intriguingly, one of the main metabolites of norgestimate (NGM) is biologically active (levo)norgestrel (22% by weight, equivalent to about 55 µg of the 250 µg in each tablet). As we saw above, this is a relatively antioestrogenic progestogen so one might expect some counteraction of the oestrogenicity, and maybe therefore the VTE thrombogenicity, of the 35 µg of EE that Cilest™ contains.

We need more data. In practice, we can continue to use Cilest™ without the specific medicolegal anxieties raised by the CSM letter of 18 October 1995. Cilest™ seems to be working out as a useful choice for many women, more oestrogen-dominant than say Microgynon 30™ but not markedly so.

The same considerations with regard to VTE apply to EVRA™, the new contraceptive skin patch (see Q 6.80).

Another progestogenic substance used in UK combination pills is cyproterone acetate, which is an antiandrogen used in the formulation Dianette™ and considered later (see Q 6.64). It is marketed primarily for the treatment of moderately severe acne and hirsutes. Recent work confirms that it is clearly an oestrogen-dominant product, with a statistically increased risk of VTE compared to LNG-containing products. See also Qs 6.60–6.61 with regard to the other antiandrogenic progestogen drospirenone, and its use in Yasmin™ – which (unlike Dianette™) is marketed as a COC.

MORE ABOUT THE AVAILABLE PILL FORMULATIONS

5.127 Which are now considered the 'safer pills'?

It is much easier to say what they are not! The doses in the first brands marketed in the 1960s, on which indeed much of the early epidemiology was based, were clearly too high. On the market then was a brand that gave more of the same oestrogen in a day than is now given in a week; and virtually the same daily dose of a progestogen as now covers a complete cycle (see *Table 5.12*)!

In short, safer pills seem generally to be 'smaller pills'. Both the constituent hormones are capable of unwanted metabolic effects and their epidemiological consequences. After saying that the question is still, after all these years, impossible to answer more specifically. And it will depend on whether one is considering arterial or venous disease.

Above all, we must retain a range of formulations so as to have flexibility in prescribing when 'minor' side-effects occur (see Qs 6.19, 6.20, 6.21, 6.22).

A policy based on preferring 'smaller' pills should reduce the risk of major side-effects. Clinical experience with the lowest doses also shows that, with one exception, minor side-effects are less frequent and less severe.

What is the exception? The obvious one is cycle control: but that can be handled, as part of the follow-up prescribing scheme to be described (see Q 5.160–5.177).

TABLE 5.12 Reduction in doses since combined pills were first introduced

	Dose of sex steroid per tablet in 1962	Minimum of same as used in 2002	Compared with 1962 same dose in 2002 from
Ethinylestradiol (EE)	150 μg in Enovid-10™	20 μg in Femodette™ Mercilon-20™, Loestrin-20™	One week of tablets
Norethisterone (NET)	10 000 μg in Ortho-Novum-10™	500 μg in Ovysmen™/ Brevinor™	One month of tablets

Note: 15 μg EE pills are now marketed in continental Europe.

5.128 What are the fundamental problems in applying a 'safer pills' policy?

1 Almost no RCTs, and too few cohort studies comparing formulations, have large enough numbers and relevant epidemiological end-points. And now that the VTE story that led to the 'pill scare' of October 1995 is largely accepted, it is clear that we all had our hands burnt by relying on (the more easily obtainable) metabolic surrogate markers like HDL-cholesterol.

2 Then there is individual variation. A medium-dose pill for one woman could be in its biological effect a low-dose pill for another, or a high-dose pill for a third.

It is thus a false expectation that any single pill will suit all women. We return to this point below (see *Fig. 5.14* (p. 219) and *Qs 5.160–5.177*).

5.129 What are the pill brands available, and how can they be classified?

The practitioner is faced with a variety of formulations (*Table 5.13*, *Fig. 5.12*). All contain the same oestrogen, EE (or, in the case of Norinyl-1™, a prodrug for it called mestranol, *see Q5.36*). As first proposed by Dr Barbara Law, former Chairman of the Joint Committee on Contraception, they can therefore be grouped in ladders according to the particular progestogen they contain, each lower rung representing a lower hormone content than those above (*Fig. 5.12*). The philosophy behind this display is that the lower down a ladder one is, the less likely is injury if one falls off! Although it is complicated now by the concept of oestrogen-dominance

TABLE 5.13 Formulations of currently marketed combined oral contraceptives

Pill type	Preparation	Oestrogen (µg)	Progestogen (µg)
Monophasic			
Ethinylestradiol/ norethisterone type	Loestrin-20	20	1000 Norethisterone acetate*
	Loestrin-30	30	1500 Norethisterone acetate*
	Brevinor	35	500 Norethisterone
	Ovysmen	35	500 Norethisterone
	Norimin	35	1000 Norethisterone
Ethinylestradiol/ levonorgestrel	Microgynon-30 (also ED)	30	150
	Ovranette	30	150
	Eugynon-30	30	250
Ethinylestradiol/ desogestrel	Mercilon	20	150
	Marvelon	30	150
Ethinylestradiol/ gestodene	Femodene (also ED)	30	75
	Minulet	30	75
	Femodette	20	75
Ethinylestradiol/ norgestimate	Cilest	35	250
Ethinylestradiol/ drospirenone	Yasmin	30	3000
Mestranol/ norethisterone[†]	Norinyl-1	50	1000
Bi/triphasic			
Ethinylestradiol/ norethisterone	BiNovum	35	500 ⎤ 833[‡] (7 tabs)
		35	1000 ⎦ (14 tabs)
	Synphase	35	500 ⎤ (7 tabs)
		35	1000 ⎬ 714 (9 tabs)
		35	500 ⎦ (5 tabs)
	TriNovum	35	500 ⎤ (7 tabs)
		35	750 ⎬ 750 (7 tabs)
		35	1000 ⎦ (7 tabs)
Ethinylestradiol/ levonorgestrel	Logynon (also ED)	30 ⎤	50 ⎤ (6 tabs)
		40 ⎬ 32[‡]	75 ⎬ 92[‡] (5 tabs)
		30 ⎦	125 ⎦ (10 tabs)
	Trinordiol	30 ⎤	50 ⎤ (6 tabs)
		40 ⎬ 32	75 ⎬ 92 (5 tabs)
		30 ⎦	125 ⎦ (10 tabs)

TABLE 5.13—cont'd

Pill type	Preparation	Oestrogen (µg)			Progestogen (µg)		
Ethinylestradiol/ gestodene	Tri-Minulet	30 40 30	}	32	50 70 100	} 79[‡]	(6 tabs) (5 tabs) (10 tabs)
	Triadene	30 40 30	}	32	50 70 100	} 79	(6 tabs) (5 tabs) (10 tabs)
Also: Ethinylestradiol/ cyproterone acetate (marketed primarily as acne therapy not as a standard COC, see Qs 6.22–6.23)	Dianette	35			2000		

*Converted to norethisterone as the active metabolite.
[†]Has to be converted to ethinylestradiol, approx. 35 µg, as active oestrogen so Norinyl-1 ≡ Norimin (Q 5.36).
[‡]Equivalent daily doses for comparison with monophasic brands.

(*Qs 5.130, 5.107–5.111*). The POPs are still definitely the least likely to cause side-effects – on ground level.

5.130 How do the ladders in *Fig. 5.12* differ from each other?

Because norethisterone acetate is converted in vivo (with more than 90% efficiency) to norethisterone, all formulations using it are part of the norethisterone group.

Levonorgestrel and, to a lesser extent, norethisterone appear to reduce the effective oestrogenicity of a given dose of EE, with a probable beneficial effect on prothrombotic blood changes and thrombosis risk. Hence all the other ladders have, in general, more oestrogen-dominant pills, although obviously a change in the oestrogen dominance can also be produced by changing the dose of EE itself. In the UK the lowest dose available is 20 µg, but elsewhere 15 µg doses are now also available.

5.131 Why is D-norgestrel called levonorgestrel? Please explain.

Norgestrel is a racemic mixture of a D-isomer and L-isomer. It is given the prefix 'D' because it shares the same special orientation as other molecules that, by the conventions of stereochemistry, are all called the D-forms. However, when in solution it deviates light in the opposite direction (i.e. to the left) and is therefore known as levonorgestrel.

The opposite applies to L-norgestrel, which rotates light to the right. It is also biologically inactive but it has to be metabolized. Hence, where there is

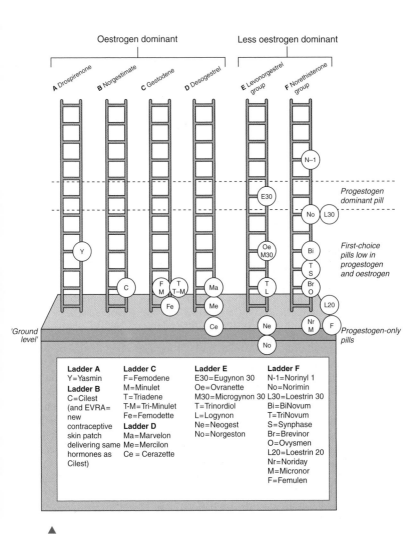

▲

Fig. 5.12 Pill ladders – arranged by progestogen. Q5.129.

Notes 1. Positioning on rungs is somewhat arbitrary: attempts to allow for both dose and potency of constituents.

2. Major distinction between less oestrogen-dominant ladders E and F versus the remainder.

3. Dianette is not shown as it is licensed for short term use for androgenic symptoms, not solely as a COC (*see* Qs 6.64–65).

a choice it is preferable to use the nearest equivalent brand that uses pure levonorgestrel.

INDICATIONS AND CONTRAINDICATIONS FOR THE COC METHOD, IN DEPTH

5.132 For whom is the COC method particularly indicated?

The woman who decides that maximum protection from pregnancy and independence from intercourse are the most important features in her own view. But she can also use it without currently needing contraception (*see* Q 5.133).

It is particularly valuable for the healthy young sexually active non-smoking woman who is sufficiently motivated to be a reliable pill taker. If and when she is at risk of STIs she should be advised to use condoms as well.

5.133 For what (primarily gynaecological) disorders and diseases is the combined pill prescribed?

Because the extra requirement for treatment increases the benefit side of the benefit–risk equation, it might sometimes be acceptable to prescribe higher-dose pills or to give the COC to women with one or more relative contraindications. A specialist's advice should be sought where appropriate.

The COC can be invaluable therapy to:

1 Relieve spasmodic dysmenorrhoea.
2 'Regulate' menstrual cycles. In cases of prolonged bleeding with no demonstrable pathology, but also for true secondary amenorrhoea once characterized. Indeed, the reason for any cycle irregularity or secondary amenorrhoea should always be determined first but then the pill might well be the most appropriate treatment, especially for hypoestrogenic states (*see* Qs 5.65–5.67). Tricycling (*see* Q 5.31) should be offered as a choice.
3 Relieve premenstrual syndrome (PMS). This is not always successful, indeed some women develop similar symptoms when taking the COC. Uncontrolled reports suggest that Yasmin™ (*see* Qs 6.61–6.63) might be better for PMS than other COCs. It is certainly the case that ablating the normal menstrual cycle is well-recognized therapy for PMS. In my experience, using a monophasic COC for that purpose but replacing with a 10–13-week pill cycle through tricycling (as described in Q 5.31) can help to minimize the likelihood of reports back that the replacement reproduced the symptoms. Sufferers usually say that at least they now get the PMS symptoms only towards the end of each tricycle (i.e. only 4–5 times per year) – and sometimes that the episodes are milder as well as less frequent. I have no experience of Yasmin™ used this way, something asking for a proper study!

4   Control menorrhagia. If fibroids are present and surgery not indicated a relatively progestogen-dominant pill should be chosen, with continued monitoring by the same observer.

5   Control endometriosis as maintenance therapy after first-line treatment: use a progestogen-dominant brand – it is perhaps best to start with Microgynon-30™, then perhaps Eugynon-30™ using the tricycle regimen (see *Qs 5.31 and 6.51*).

6   Control functional ovarian cysts (*see Q 5.60*) and ovulation pain if severe.

7   Relieve oestrogen deficiency:
    (a)   in athletes or anorexics with amenorrhoea (*see Q 5.65*)
    (b)   to control gynaecological/menstrual cyclical symptoms in selected healthy non-smoking perimenopausal women under age 51 and still requiring contraception, although becoming oestrogen ± progesterone deficient.

8   Control acne and other manifestations of the polycystic ovarian syndrome (PCOS), despite this not being a condition of oestrogen deficiency but rather of androgen excess (*see Q 5.65*). Oestrogen-dominant pill brands are also useful for acne treatment without PCOS.

9   As prophylaxis against ovarian cancer, for women at high risk (*see Q 5.57*).

Nowadays, other means to control many of the gynaecological conditions above – notably the LNG-IUS (*see Q 9.145ff*) and Cerazette™ (*see Q 7.11*) might be chosen instead.

> Triphasic pills are usually not appropriate for these indications because the intention is often to abolish the normal cycle, and they might too closely simulate it.

5.134 What are the absolute contraindications to (all formulations of) COCs, i.e. WHO 4 in the WHO classification of *Q5.119* ?

Any compilation of contraindications reflects the judgement of the compiler, as much as the available science at the relevant date. The answers to this and the next two questions are as assessed by me in 2003! They are largely congruent with WHO's classification but very many of these conditions have yet to be assessed by WHO.

Many important diseases are considered in considerably more detail elsewhere – please see the Index.

Very few of the contraindications to the COC (whether absolute or relative) apply to the LNG-IUS (*see Qs 9.145 and 9.146*) or to Cerazette™/Implanon™, which can be most useful alternative options providing comparable or greater efficacy for most ordinary users.

PAST OR PRESENT CIRCULATORY DISEASE

- Any past proven arterial or venous thrombosis.
- Ischaemic heart disease or angina.
- Severe or combined risk factors for venous or arterial disease (see *Tables 5.10*, and *5.11*, pp. 188 and 190). Check carefully.
- Known atherogenic lipid disorders (see *Table 5.11*). COC usually avoided unless total cholesterol can be brought below 8 mmol/L. Essential to check with woman's physician: this might become WHO 3 situation.
- Specific prothrombotic abnormalities of coagulation/fibrinolysis, including the congenital thrombophilias with abnormal levels of individual factors and the presence of any acquired thrombophilia, especially the antiphospholipid syndrome.
- Other conditions known to predispose to thrombosis, including severe primary or secondary polycythaemia, Klippel–Trenaunay syndrome, Sturge-Weber syndrome (risk of cerebral/retinal artery thrombosis) blood dyscrasias; some autoimmune and rheumatoid disorders with this risk, including polyarteritis nodosa, scleroderma and severe SLE; and postsplenectomy for any indication if the platelet count is above $500 \pm 109/L$ (WHO 3 if lower platelet count).
- Elective major or leg surgery: from 2 but preferably 4 weeks before, until 2 weeks after full mobilization (do not demand that the COC be stopped for minor surgery such as laparoscopy); during leg immobilization (e.g. after a fracture) or varicose vein treatments; and when going to high altitude if there are risk factors – otherwise WHO 3 (*see Qs 5.140–5.141*).
- Severe inflammatory bowel disease, including Crohn's disease, comes into this category during attacks, or WHO 3 in remissions.
- Migraine with focal aura, and severe migraine ('status migrainosus'); migraine requiring ergotamine treatment.
- Transient ischaemic attacks even without headache.
- Past cerebral haemorrhage, especially if secondary to cerebral venous thrombosis. But this can otherwise be WHO 3 following successful surgery to an aneurysm.
- Pulmonary hypertension/pulmonary vascular disease.
- Structural, including valvular, heart disease wherever there is an added arterial or venous thrombo-embolic risk (discuss with cardiologist, could be WHO 3 especially if on warfarin); atrial fibrillation or flutter (with or without structural heart disease) both sustained and paroxysmal, as high risk of emboli – unless on warfarin with good INR control (WHO 3). See *Table 5.14* and Q 5.139 for more details.

DISEASE OF THE LIVER

- Active liver disease (whenever liver function tests currently abnormal, including infiltrations and cirrhosis).

- Cholestatic jaundice, if pill-related usually WHO 4, but history of cholestatic jaundice in pregnancy is WHO 3; Dubin-Johnson and Rotor syndromes, which are congenital deficiencies of hepatic excretion (but Gilbert's disease is WHO 1–2).
- Liver adenoma, carcinoma. Focal nodular hyperplasia (FNH) (*see Q 5.96*) is WHO 4, but could be WHO 3 with careful imaging during follow-up.
- The acute porphyrias (other porphyrias are in WHO 2 or 3 (*see Qs 6.42 and 6.43*).

> After any viral hepatitis, severe infectious mononucleosis or other reversible hepatocellular damage: COC taking may be resumed 3 months after liver function tests have returned to normal.

HISTORY OF SERIOUS CONDITION AFFECTED BY SEX STEROIDS OR RELATED TO PREVIOUS COC USE

- Acute porphyrias, SLE, cholestatic jaundice, already mentioned.
- Chorea.
- COC-induced hypertension.
- Pancreatitis due to hypertriglyceridaemia.
- Pemphigoid gestationis (formerly called herpes gestationis).
- Stevens–Johnson syndrome (erythema multiforme), if COC-associated.
- Trophoblastic disease but only until hCG levels are undetectable. (In the US this is considered a relative contraindication even when hCG present, partly because chemotherapy is given to almost all cases of trophoblastic disease anyway.)

This is not necessarily a complete list of relevant diseases – see *Q 5.137* for how to assess any new condition affecting your patient.

EXISTING OR POSSIBLE PREGNANCY

UNDIAGNOSED GENITAL TRACT BLEEDING

OESTROGEN-DEPENDENT NEOPLASMS

- Current breast cancer (oncologists rarely may permit COCs in selected cases in prolonged remission defined by WHO as after > 5 years – but always WHO 3).
- All other cancers are normally relative contraindications (WHO 2, rarely 3), supervised use being permitted.

TABLE 5.14 Eligibility for COC-use in some varieties of heart disease

Absolute contraindication	Relative contraindication		
WHO 4	**WHO 3 (must lack features in first column)**	**WHO 2**	
Atrial fibrillation or flutter, sustained or paroxysmal, as high risk of emboli – unless well-controlled on warfarin (WHO 3)	Heart disease or past thrombosis well controlled on warfarin with very careful supervision of INR, which may alter with hormones. [Three exceptions, in first column – plus in all cases reverts to WHO 4 if warfarin stopped]	Dysrhythmias other than atrial fibrillation or flutter	
Pulmonary hypertension or pulmonary vascular disease	Bi-leaflet mechanical valve in mitral or aortic position on warfarin	Valve lesions not yet surgically corrected but uncomplicated including mitral valve prolapse and bicuspid aortic valve; lacking any of the WHO 3 or 4 features of first & second columns	
Pulmonary arterio-venous malformation	All known inter-atrial communications (ASD, PFO) – as always risk of paradoxical embolism e.g. with Valsalva manoeuvre	Any prosthetic or tissue heart valves lacking any WHO 3 or 4 features	
Poor left ventricular function (LV ejection fraction < 30%)	Repaired coarctation with aneurysm and/or hypertension	Fully surgically corrected congenital heart disease lacking any of the WHO 3 or 4 features	
Dilated cardiomyopathy or previous cardiomyopathy with residual LV dysfunction	Marfan's syndrome with aortic dilatation, unoperated	Non reversible trivial L to R shunt e.g. small VSD; trivial patent ductus arteriosus	
Dilated left atrium (> 4cm)		Repaired coarctation without aneurysm or hypertension	
Cyanotic heart disease even taking warfarin		Uncomplicated Marfan's syndrome	

TABLE 5.14—cont'd

Absolute contraindication	Relative contraindication	
WHO 4	WHO 3 (must lack features in first column)	WHO 2
The (post-surgery) Fontan heart, even taking warfarin		Uncomplicated pulmonary stenosis
Bjork Shiley or Starr Edwards valves even taking warfarin		Hypertrophic obstructive cardiomyopathy (HOCM))
Any past venous or arterial thrombo-embolic event with the heart disease – not on warfarin (see second column)		Past pregnancy-related or other cardiomyopathy, fully recovered and with now normal heart on echo-cardiography

Notes

1 **There is a paucity of published information, a very small evidence-base, about contraception in women with heart disease. Hence this Table (which in any event cannot deal with all possible cases) is based on best evidence and opinions available at the time of writing (2003) as here interpreted by the committee mentioned in Q 5.139. This may change as new evidence is obtained.**

2 The prime consideration in decisions about using the COC is *whether or not the condition itself increases the risk of venous or arterial thrombo-embolic events.*

3 If a patient can be classified in more than one WHO category, the more severe category should be applied.

4 The risk of pregnancy should always be balanced against the thrombotic risk of taking the combined oral contraceptive. Thus a high risk in pregnancy due to the heart condition may make COC risks justifiable if alternative effective methods are unacceptable, on the usual WHO 3 basis.

5 Most patients will require discussion with the cardiologist, and periodic reassessment of the suitability or otherwise of the COC in their individual circumstances – because cardiac status is not static.

ASD Atrial septal defect; INR International normalised ratio; LV Left ventricle; PFO patent foramen ovale; VSD Ventricular septal defect

MISCELLANEOUS

■ Allergy to a constituent of the tablets.

■ Haemolytic uraemic syndrome/thrombotic thrombocytopenic purpura. A past history of either of these poorly understood, related thrombotic syndromes is WHO 4, generally, especially if pill-related at outset. An isolated past history of an attack preceded by diarrhoea – as occurs with *E. coli* 0157 infection – would allow cautious use of COC (WHO 3).

■ Past benign intracranial hypertension (BICH) (*see Q 6.27*).

■ Amaurosis fugax: this transient complete loss of vision usually signifies transient retinal ischaemia, so obviously contraindicates the COC (WHO 4).

WOMAN'S OWN CONTINUING ANXIETY *RE* COC SAFETY, UNRELIEVED AFTER COUNSELLING

Note that several of the above (e.g. existing or possible pregnancy, undiagnosed genital tract bleeding, oestrogen-dependent neoplasms) are not necessarily permanent contraindications.

5.135 Relative contraindications – how are they assessed and how applied?

Here we have the impact not just of my judgement as compiler, but yours as prescriber! The art of medicine is nowhere better shown than in assessing how strong each of the contraindications at *Q 5.136* is (and that differs within the list – hence my use of the new WHO scheme of *Q 5.119* – as well as in different individuals), and then:

■ balancing the risk of each against the benefits to each pill taker

■ allowing for synergism between risk factors and the general teaching that two or more relative contraindications equal one absolute contraindication (see also *Box 5.1* (*Q 5.119*), note 2(b))

■ all in the light of everything relevant, like her probable fertility and her other contraceptive choices

■ and all, most emphatically, being discussed openly with the woman, so that she makes the final decision.

5.136 What are the relative contraindications to the COC?

■ See *Tables 5.10* and *5.11* (pp. 188 and 190). Risk factors for circulatory disease are all relative contraindications, mostly WHO 3: provided normally that only one is present, and not to so marked a degree that it alone would absolutely contraindicate this method. This category includes essential hypertension provided it is well controlled by treatment; also past toxaemia of pregnancy (pregnancy-related hypertension), which increases the risk of AMI in smokers (RCGP and

MICA studies) (*see Q 5.138* re HELLP syndrome). Warfarin treatment is usually WHO 3 (*Q 5.139*), and *see also Q 5.140 re* high altitude.

- Long-term partial immobilization (e.g. in a wheelchair). This is WHO 3 (*Table 5.10*). Complete flaccid paralysis of the lower limbs is viewed by some as WHO 4, especially if the BMI is > 30.

- Sex-steroid-dependent cancers in remission. Seek the specialist's advice: most will (appropriately in my view) permit COC use for melanoma in remission after treatment (whether or not diagnosed during pill taking). But the history of breast cancer is almost invariably considered an absolute contraindication (WHO 4) to the COC (*see Q 5.134*). Other options can usually be found.

- Oligo- and/or amenorrhoea should be investigated but the pill might subsequently be prescribed – WHO 2 – or even positively indicated (WHO 1; *see Qs 5.61–5.66*).

- Gallstones causing symptoms or being treated medically are WHO 3, but WHO 2 if asymptomatic or have been treated by cholecystectomy.

- Hyperprolactinaemia: this is now considered only a relative contraindication for patients under specialist supervision (WHO 3), as long as the woman is on dopamine agonist therapy (*see Q 5.65*).

- Very severe depression, if likely to be exacerbated by COCs (WHO 3). But unwanted pregnancies can be very depressing!

- Chronic systemic diseases. These are discussed further below (*see Qs 5.137–5.146*). In general they are weak relative contraindications, category WHO 2, mainly signifying extra counselling and above average monitoring. Examples in the stronger WHO 3 category are: porphyria cutanea tarda (*see Q 6.43*), Crohn's disease with major small bowel involvement (*see Q 5.145*), diabetes (*see Q 5.147*), chronic renal disease; and mild (not steroid-treated, in remission) SLE, although the presence of antiphospholipid antibody absolutely contraindicates the COC (*see Qs 5.135 and 5.146*). In these the common reason for special caution is that the condition might lead in various ways to an increased risk of circulatory disease. If that risk became established, as in a diabetic with evidence of arteriopathy, it would be an absolute contraindication WHO 4 (*see Q 5.136*). In the case of SLE and Crohn's there is also the risk of sex hormones causing deterioration of the condition. Splenectomy, for whatever reason performed (e.g. in the treatment of sickle-cell disease), is only a relative contraindication (WHO 2). However, the platelets should be monitored, initially at least annually, and a count rising to above 500 ± 109 per litre would absolutely contraindicate the oestrogen of the COC (WHO 4).

- Diseases requiring long-term treatment with enzyme-inducing drugs, which might reduce the efficacy of the pill (*see Qs 5.34 and 5.36*): provided the recommended regimen is followed, this is WHO 3.

■ Other relative contraindications now include:
   (a) if a young (< 40 years) first-degree relative has had breast cancer
        (WHO 2)
   (b) the presence of BBD (WHO 2) but WHO 3 if atypia (*see* Q 5.92)
   (c) during the monitoring of abnormal cervical smears (WHO 2)
   (d) during and after definitive treatment for CIN (WHO 2).

Women in groups (a) and (b) need recounselling after about 4–5 years' use.

CIN follow-up (i.e. groups (c) plus (d)) amounts to only a very weak relative contraindication, due to the data suggesting the COC is a cofactor for CIN, so it would be standard practice to continue the COC, with monitoring as advised by the laboratory.

5.137 On what criteria can one decide whether the COC can be used for patients with intercurrent disease?

First, there are some conditions that are positively benefited (*see* Qs 5.56 *and* 5.133) or at least not affected. There are persistent medical myths (*see* Q 6.77), and it is unfortunate that women continue to be unnecessarily deprived of the COC for the wrong reasons, like thrush, uncomplicated varicose veins, past amenorrhoea, current hypoestrogenic amenorrhoea (e.g. weight-related) or fibroids.

It is impossible to list every known disease or state that might have a bearing on pill-prescribing, but here are some useful criteria:

In general, discover first what the disease does in relation to known risks or effects of the COC. Does it cause changes that summate with adverse effects of the COC? Does it:

1 Increase the risk of arterial or venous thrombosis, anywhere? This includes consideration of restricted mobility.
2 Predispose to arterial wall disease or severe hypertension?
3 Adversely affect liver function?
4 Show a tendency to an important degree of sex hormone dependency, either by medical reputation (usually then a relative contraindication), or in that individual (absolute contraindication). If there was deterioration with previous administration of steroid hormones or during pregnancy, it means enough to be an absolute contraindication if the condition is serious.
5 Require treatment with an enzyme-inducing drug?

If (5) is true the pill can still be an option, but special conditions apply (*see* Q 5.36). If (1) to (4) apply there is the real problem of deciding whether the COC should be absolutely or (as at Q 5.136) relatively contraindicated (meaning not WHO 4 but WHO 3). Obviously the category will be WHO 4 if she has an added risk factor from *Table 5.10* or *5.11* such as smoking or obesity.

Note that the added risk obtaining in pregnancy can fully justify some increased risk due to the COC, at least in young and hence more fertile women, primarily because it is so effective. Its other benefits might also be highly relevant in some conditions. This is not so, however, for the list at *Q 5.134* (WHO 4, absolute contraindications). For them, remember injectables and IUDs/IUSs!

If none of the above criteria apply, then the condition could normally be added to the following list in *Q 5.138*.

5.138 Can you list those medical conditions in which the COC is broadly usable since there is no convincing evidence that deterioration might be caused or of any summation with effects of the pill?

According to current information, the following diseases all come into this 'Broadly usable' category (WHO 2):

Aids/HIV (*see Q 6.70*, although the category would change to WHO 3 if an enzyme-inducing antiretroviral drug were to be prescribed; and there are usually better contraceptive choices for these women; along with condoms); asthma; Gilbert's disease; treated Hodgkin's disease (if fertility preserved); hereditary lymphoedema; past HELLP syndrome once the pregnancy-related changes (hypertension, elevated liver enzymes, low platelets) have returned to normal; multiple sclerosis; myasthenia gravis; Raynaud's disease (unless the phenomenon proves to be symptomatic of a contraindicating condition); renal dialysis; retinitis pigmentosa; rheumatoid arthritis; sarcoidosis; spherocytosis; thalassaemia major; thyrotoxicosis and Wolff–Parkinson–White syndrome. Also most cancers under treatment, if hormone dependency or an increase in the risk of thrombosis are not suspected.

Despite the condition featuring above, in individual cases the prescriber should first review the checklist in *Q 5.137* and might need to consult with the hospital specialist(s) supervising treatment for the main disorder: to obtain their support to use the COC and also to guard against unforeseen drug interactions, etc. Such women need extra supervision within primary care as well (shared care). Note that reliable protection from pregnancy is often particularly important when chronic diseases are present.

There are of course many other illnesses in the textbooks, too numerous to mention here: the solution to prescribing queries is to evaluate each condition as described in *Q 5.137* above.

5.139 Can the COC be taken by some women with structural heart disease?

Yes, indeed. It is a myth that all such should be in category WHO 4. Every year a number of women – particularly after successful surgery, so-called 'grown-up congenital heart' or GUCH cases – conceive unwanted pregnancies using less effective methods because the COC was unnecessarily denied to them (see Leonard et al. 1966 *Heart* 76:60–62). Yet those with more severe disease may be at high risk in pregnancy. For example, maternal mortality is > 50% for women with pulmonary vascular disease. These women should never use the COC, but a woman with hypertrophic obstructive cardiomyopathy (HOCM), for example, will require intensive obstetric care, and yet would have no particular added risk through using a COC.

The criteria of Q 5.137 (chiefly whether there would be any added risk of arterial or venous thromboembolism) were discussed for a range of cardiac conditions by an *ad hoc* committee (of which I was a member), based at the Hammersmith Hospital in London during 2002–3. *Table 5.14* lists these, categorized as WHO 4, 3 or 2, as the committee classified them. Note the disclaimer (and other footnotes).

Note also that the committee decided that certain cardiac patients – even those who have had an arterial or venous thrombotic event – who are taking warfarin might be allowed the COC on a WHO 3 basis. This, as usual, means that another method such as Cerazette™, Implanon™ or an intrauterine method would actually be preferable. But if these are unacceptable, the COC is usable with careful supervision of the blood INR, the risk of thrombosis should be minimal though warfarin dose adjustments may need to be made to allow for any effect of the COC hormones to increase the INR, by impeding the metabolism of the warfarin (*see Q 5.45*). Whenever anticoagulation ceases, of course, WHO 4 applies. Much more useful information may be found in Table 5.14.

5.140 Is the combined pill best avoided at high altitude?

Sometimes, yes. This is certainly something to discuss with the woman concerned. The issue is not whether the COC causes altitude illness – not suggested by the evidence – but if it might increase associated risks. Acute mountain sickness can kill, through hypoxia leading to acute pulmonary oedema and cerebral oedema, and blood clots in the small arteries are a feature post-mortem. In milder attacks well short of that, which can occur if unacclimatized people ascend rapidly to above about 2500 m (> 8000 feet), there is an increasing risk of venous or arterial thromboembolism, including strokes. Although fibrinolysis is increased at altitude and during exercise, other circumstances in climbing are thrombogenic: dehydration through fluid loss or inadequate intake, trauma, immobility in tents when the weather closes in. Risk factors for developing altitude illness of all degrees of severity include the rate of ascent, the altitude at which the traveller will sleep and individual susceptibility (Barry and Pollard 2003 *BMJ* 326:915–19.)

Acetazolamide (Diamox™), which has been shown to improve climbing performance and prevent acute mountain sickness, acts as a mild diuretic and as a consequence of mild dehydration might exacerbate the thrombotic risk. Moreover, in high altitude pulmonary oedema (were it to occur) there is patchy pulmonary hypertension.

In summary, considering the principle of summation discussed at *Q 5.137*, going to altitudes above 2500 m has to be seen as in the category WHO 3 – in my view. If there were added risk factors from Tables 5.10 or 5.11, (pp. 188–191), WHO 4 would apply – after all, with more than one such risk factor the woman should not use the EE-containing pill even at sea level!

But for healthy trekkers following the guidelines in the above BMJ article – summarised as 'climb high and sleep low' – the COC would be WHO 2. Yet all should be informed of the possible minimal increase in risk of venous/arterial thrombosis.

From the practical point of view at high altitude, the COC is very useful to control menstrual bleeding, especially if tricycled. Yet BTB is a common problem for some women at altitude.

Autonomy is an important principle here: rock-climbing is orders of magnitude more dangerous than any risks modifiable by choice of contraceptive! The woman must have freedom to take an added risk but prescribers have autonomy too if they think the risk of COC unacceptable (i.e. WHO 4, rather than 3, for that individual after consideration of *all* the relevant risk factors.)

The Newsletter of the International Society for Mountain Medicine discussed this issue in April 1998.

5.141 Is there a continuing problem for those who live long term at high altitude?

In residents, after acclimatization there is a physiological polycythaemia that normally increases blood viscosity; but this alone would be only a weak relative contraindication (WHO 2) to EE in the combined pill.

5.142 What about long-haul aeroplane flights and thrombosis risk?

As the sole risk factor this is WHO 2 – the COC is broadly usable and need not, indeed should not, be stopped (the risks of pregnancy would be far greater!). However, although all commercial flights are pressurized to the equivalent of about 2000 m, there are now numerous case reports of pulmonary embolism and some deaths (with or without the pill). As at high altitude, some extracellular to interstitial fluid shift is common; mild ankle oedema results but more important is the likelihood of intravascular volume depletion and haemoconcentration. Other important factors are the maintained sedentary position – which is equally a risk of course during long car or coach journeys – coupled with a diuresis due to alcohol and caffeine, all perhaps superimposed on dehydration due to prolonged sunbathing on a Far Eastern beach just before boarding!

Evaluation of risk factors, especially for VTE (see *Table 5.10*, p. 188) is again essential. If the woman has a high BMI she should forget glamour and wear support hose. She also might consider stopping HRT just to cover the intercontinental flight. But normally as far as the pill itself is concerned, to quote my book *The Pill*:

There is no necessity to come off the pill – many flight attendants use it all the time. But follow their example and take some exercise during the flight: such as a brief walk around the plane every hour or so.

See also *Q 6.91*, concerning how to maintain COC efficacy when travelling west through numerous time zones.

5.143 Can the combined pill be prescribed to patients with sickle-cell disorders?

Yes is the answer for those with sickle-cell trait; the situation with regard to homozygous sickle-cell disease (SS and SC genes) is more uncertain. There is an increased risk of thromboembolic disease, especially strokes, in such women and pregnancy can precipitate a crisis. The COC imitates pregnancy and the oestrogen of the pill might in theory lead to superimposed thrombosis during the arterial stasis of a crisis. Therefore, until recently most manufacturers and many authorities have included the frank sickling diseases among absolute contraindications to the COC. However, studies in the West Indies and West Africa have shown that the COC ought now to be considered only a relative contraindication (WHO 2, especially when balanced against the great risks of pregnancy in sicklers). Injectables, especially DMPA, are usually an even better choice (*see Q 8.15*).

5.144 Can a woman who has made a complete recovery from a subarachnoid haemorrhage, and had her intracranial lesion treated, use the combined pill?

The COC is relatively contraindicated (WHO 3) assuming a close subsequent watch for hypertension, but the POP or an injectable would be preferable. This is because almost all women on the combined pill have a detectable slight increase in systolic and diastolic blood pressure, and one can never be certain that such a woman would not have some other weakness of a cerebral artery or angiomatous malformation.

5.145 Why are the inflammatory bowel diseases (Crohn's or ulcerative colitis (UC)) relative contraindications?

1   Both occur more commonly in COC takers in some studies. Crohn's (but not UC) is also strongly linked with smoking. However 300 pill takers with stable disease had no more flare-ups over time than non-takers (Cosnes et al. 1999 *Gut* 45:218–222). Hence the COC may be used (WHO 2, except as below).

2   In exacerbations of either illness there is a high risk of thrombosis, especially VTE. Therefore, the COC should be used only in cases not prone to severe hospitalized exacerbations, and if such occur the pill should be stopped at once and would be absolutely contraindicated so long as the disease remained severe (WHO 4).

3   Malabsorption: as contraceptive steroids are so well absorbed, mainly in the jejunum (which is unaffected), malabsorption of the COC is usually not a problem. However if there is major small bowel involvement by Crohn's, absorption could be affected and a nonoral method would be preferable (WHO 3) (*see also* Q 6.40).

5.146 Can the COC be used by women with systemic lupus erythematosus (SLE)?

Increasingly, this is being seen as an absolute contraindication (WHO 4) except in the mildest very stable fully investigated cases not on steroids, with close supervision (WHO 3 – but a progestogen-only method would be preferable). This is because:

1   There are now numerous case reports and some comparative studies describing the onset or flaring up of symptomatic SLE when oestrogen was given, either in the COC or even, interestingly, as hormone replacement therapy postmenopausally. SLE can deteriorate seriously with renal involvement for the first time during use of COCs, but not with progestogen-only therapy.

2   There is a recurring theme of recovery or improvement once the artificial oestrogen was discontinued.

3   Cases can develop the lupus anticoagulant/antiphospholipid antibody and once detected the COC is definitely contraindicated for fear of thrombosis.

Obviously each patient has to be taken on her own merits. But as progestogen-only pills and injections have been tried in SLE women with no significant increase in episodes of active disease, these are usually preferred to the COC.

5.147 Can the combined pill be used by patients with established diabetes mellitus (DM)?

Arterial disease is a major hazard for diabetics; hence ideally they should avoid oestrogen with its prothrombotic risks. A barrier method, or the POP (*see Q 7.44*), or Implanon™ or an IUD/IUS are all to be preferred.

In practice, however, some young diabetics are permitted use of an ultra-low-oestrogen combined pill (WHO 3) using a 'lipid-friendly' progestogen. Mercilon™ or Femodette™ with only 20 μg oestrogen would be good choices. Necessary criteria are:

1 Young, ideally under age 25, and preferably having had DM for a short time.
2 Free of any signs of complications of the disease, affecting arteries, nerves, kidneys or retina.
3 Free of the other conditions in *Table 5.11* (p. 190). It is vital that such a patient is not also a smoker, hypertensive or with a BMI above 30.
4 Perceived to need maximum protection against pregnancy and there is no satisfactory alternative. In short: WHO 3 at best, otherwise WHO 4.

Diabetics occasionally then need an increased dose of insulin, which is not in itself a problem. They should be on the COC for the shortest possible time, encouraged to have their family as young as their circumstances allow, and then be transferred to another long-term method – ideally IUD/IUS or possibly sterilization.

5.148 Can potential or latent diabetics take the COC?

Yes. Caution used to be advised because the early pills did impair glucose tolerance and create hyperinsulinism. However, the RCGP study and others have shown absolutely no increase in the incidence of late-onset-type DM among current or ex-pill-users. Moreover, the more recent lowest-dose COCs do not even raise plasma insulins significantly. None of the following need therefore be considered as contraindications: a strong family history of DM (maturity onset); gestational diabetes; birth of a baby weighing more than 4.5 kg (10 lb).

Such women are just supervised a little more closely than usual and need particular advice to avoid obesity.

5.149 If a young woman suffers a thrombosis in an arm vein after an intravenous injection, does this mean a predisposition to thrombosis? Should she avoid the COC (WHO 4), in future?

The answer is no. The episode would be due to a chemical thrombophlebitis. This is not associated with any tendency to venous thrombosis elsewhere in the body.

5.150 In what way does the possession of blood group O influence prescribing policy?

Women with blood group O have been shown to have a lower risk of thrombosis than those with other blood groups. The protective effect probably applies to arterial as well as venous disease. Knowledge of her blood group might therefore be helpful in a positive way, when prescribing to a woman who is otherwise not an ideal pill user. For example, one might be happier to prescribe the COC to a 34-year-old smoker if she were known to be blood group O rather than A.

MIGRAINE HEADACHES, WITH AND WITHOUT AURA

5.151 What is a working definition of migraine and why is it so important in pill prescribing?

Whole chapters have been written just on this definition; please read the article by Anne MacGregor and myself (1998 *British Journal of Family Planning* 24:53–60). Migraines are here simply defined as unpleasant headaches that 'stop the person doing things', usually one-sided, accompanied by nausea and/or photophobia/phonophobia.

 Studies have shown an increased risk of ischaemic stroke in COC users. There is evidence that this risk is further increased in migraine sufferers, especially with other arterial risk factors like smoking. Less well evidence based but probably important (so prescribers need to be cautious, pending further data) are certain features of the women or of the headaches that might help to focus the risk of this rare catastrophe in a pill taker. While trying to 'catch' such women, the recommendations below have been devised (and should be interpreted) in such a way as not to exclude unnecessarily too many women from a useful contraceptive, thereby adding in the risks of pregnancy.

5.152 What are the clinically significant symptoms of migraine with aura (formerly classical or focal migraine)?

The timing is crucial: they should begin before the headache itself, evolving over several minutes and typically lasting around 20–30 min. There might be a gap of up to 1 h from resolution of aura before the headache begins or headache might start as aura resolves. Visual symptoms occur in 99% of true auras:

■ A bright rather than dark loss of part or whole of the field of vision, on one side in both eyes (homonymous hemianopia). Note that the complete loss of vision (amaurosis) in one eye is very different from aura. It would require (even more) urgent action, as it might be due to retinal artery or vein thrombosis: stopping the COC forthwith plus urgent referral to an ophthalmologist.

■ Teichopsia/fortification spectra are often described, typically a bright scintillating zig-zag line gradually enlarging from a bright centre on one side, to form a convex C-shape surrounding the area of lost vision (bright scotoma).

The above are the main symptoms, visual in nature. The other sensory symptoms occur in about one-third of auras, are confirmatory and rarely occur without visual aura:

■ Unilateral sensory disturbance, typically in the form of pins and needles (paraesthesia) spreading up one arm or affecting one side of the face or the tongue; the leg is rarely affected.
■ Disturbance of speech (usually nominal dysphasia).
■ Motor disturbance (e.g. loss of motor function of a limb) is very unusual and more likely to indicate an organic lesion (*see* Q 5.154), not migraine with aura.

Note the absence in the above list of photophobia or symmetrical blurring or 'flashing lights' or any other symptoms that occur during headache itself. Relevant symptoms are generally asymmetrical, meaning that they are 'focal' or interpretable as due to (transient) cerebral ischaemia.

Furthermore, aura symptoms must not be confused with *premonitory symptoms* which occur in some women 1–2 days before migraine, with or without aura: sensitivity to light or sound, food cravings, fatigue, poor concentration, yawning and pallor.

5.153 How should one take the history of migraine with aura?

By asking the woman to describe a typical attack from the very beginning, including before there was any headache. Listen to what she says and match it with Q 5.152, but *at the same time watch her carefully*. A most useful sign that it is likely to be true aura is, if, when asked to describe what they see, the patient draws a zig-zag line in the air with a finger to one or other side of her own head.

Note that aura can sometimes occur without any headache following. If the aura description is clear and unequivocal, it has the same significance as it would have if a headache followed (*see* Q 5.154).

5.154 What important symptoms or features are not typical of migraine with aura, and how should they be managed?

These are:

■ *sudden onset* or much longer duration, for some hours, of the same symptoms as in Q 4.148

■ a *black scotoma*, or amaurosis fugax (loss of vision in one eye)
■ *motor loss*, or sensory loss affecting the whole of one side of the body or the lower limb only.

These suggest possible cerebral thromboembolism or a transient ischaemic attack (TIA) and still mean the COC should immediately be stopped. But as with loss of consciousness or epilepsy they (unlike a straightforward history of migraine with focal aura) also signify urgent referral to a neurologist.

It is reported also that it is possible in scuba divers to confuse with migraine the symptoms of compression sickness (which of course requires urgent transfer to a decompression chamber).

5.155 So what are the absolute contraindications? (to commencing or continuing the COC, i.e. WHO category 4)

1 Migraine with aura during which there are the neurological symptoms of Q 5.152 preceding the headache itself. Should they occur, the artificial oestrogen of the COC should normally be stopped and thereafter avoided to minimize the risk of thrombosis causing permanent ischaemia, i.e. a thrombotic stroke.

2 All other migraines – even without aura – that are unusually frequent/severe. 'Status migrainosus' describes attacks lasting more than 72 h, which contraindicate the COC absolutely unless they resolve completely after treatment for medication misuse (see below).

3 All migraines treated with ergot derivatives, due to their vasoconstrictor actions.

4 Migraines without aura occurring regularly during pill-taking *plus* additional arterial risk factors or relevant interacting diseases (e.g. connective tissue diseases linked with stroke risk).

Figure 5.13 comes from the article Anne MacGregor and I wrote in 1998 and which was published in the *British Journal of Family Planning* (24:53–60). The additional risk factors in the figure are WHO 2 ones from *Table 5.11* (p. 190), including age over 35. They usually need to be more than one in number for migraines without aura to enter the category WHO 4. However, one added risk factor could suffice if it was very 'strong' (WHO 3), e.g. essential hypertension requiring treatment (*see* Q 6.9).

5.156 What action should be taken apart from stopping the COC?

Above all, organize with the woman an acceptable effective alternative contraceptive method! It is not a 'pill or nothing situation'.

In all the above circumstances any of the progestogen-only, oestrogen-free hormonal methods can be offered – immediately: similar headaches might continue but now without the potential added risk from prothrombotic effects of the ethinylestradiol. Particularly useful choices are

DMPA, Cerazette™, Implanon™ and the LNG-IUS (*see Q 9.145*) or a modern copper IUD.

5.157 So when is migraine a 'strong' relative contraindication to the combined pill (WHO category 3)?

1 See *Fig. 5.13*. This means primarily migraine without aura where one WHO 2 (not 'severe') risk factor for ischaemic stroke is present. A good example of this is age over 35, even as the only risk factor. The reason for caution comes from considering how the attributable risk rises with age. According to Lidegaard's Danish data (in which women with aura were not excluded but most subjects had migraine without aura, occurring at least once per month):

The background annual risk of thrombotic stroke for women at age 20 is 2 in 100 000. Even with migraine > once per month, plus taking COC, this rises to 10 in 100 000. But at age 40, background risk is 20 in 100 000, rising to 56 in migraineurs (same attack frequency) and, with the same risk ratio (1.8) as for younger women, adding the COC makes 100 in 100 000 total incidence. And that is without being able to quantify the extra risk of focal aura.

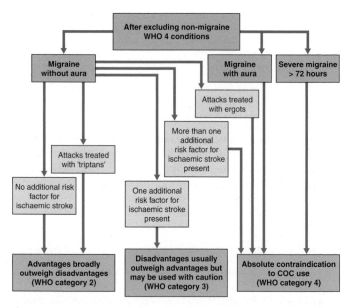

Fig. 5.13 Flow diagram for COC use and migraine. Q 5.155.

Another WHO 3 example would be a 20-plus cigarette smoker in her 20s with frequent/severe migraines without aura occurring during days of pill-taking – because the (low) background incidence at 20 would have to be multiplied by a relative risk of 5 or 6 through having migraine and also taking the COC.

2   Past brief history of typical migraine with aura, more than 5 years earlier before the COC or only during pregnancy. This is WHO3: the COC may be given a trial with regular supervision. Such women should be fully aware of the focal neurological symptoms listed in Q 5.152 and be given a specific warning that if they were to recur they should stop the pill at once.

WHO category 3 always means caution/counselling. Along with general advice about controlling/watching for new risk factors, and the specific advice below about important possible future changes in her headache symptoms (*see* Q 5.152), the opportunity should be taken to discuss alternatives to the COC: particularly new options like modern IUDs and IUSs.

5.158 When would migraine be only a WHO 2 risk, and how would you counsel such women?

In my opinion, the COC is 'broadly usable' in all the following cases:

1   Migraine without aura, and also without any arterial risk factor from *Table 5.11* and still under age 35. It is in fact disputed whether migraine without any aura is truly a risk factor at all for thrombotic stroke. If these or other 'ordinary' headaches occur particularly in the PFI, tricycling the COC might help (*see* Q 5.31).

2   Use of a triptan (e.g. sumatriptan) in the absence of any other contraindicating factors.

3   The occurrence of a woman's first-ever attack of migraine without aura while on the COC. It should be stopped if she is seen during the attack, but provided there were none of the features listed at Q 4.149, the COC can be later restarted with the usual counselling/caveats below.

> The counselling of all such women (WHO category 3 and 2) must include specific instruction to the woman regarding those changes in the character or severity of her headache symptoms which means she should stop the method and take urgent medical advice. These symptoms are listed in Q 5.152, and in more lay terms also appear – for all pill takers to read and keep for reference in the FPA's current combined pill leaflet.

5.159 Which COC brands or regimens are best for headaches and migraines without aura ('common' migraines)?

There are insufficient data regarding which brands, or even about 'second' versus 'third' generation pills, but monophasic pills are generally preferred to triphasic pills (fully described in *Qs 5.179–5.184*). The latter are not good for women with a tendency to any variety of headaches because the extra fluctuations of the hormone levels might act as a trigger. In addition, in any woman whose headaches tend to happen in the PFI, it can be enormously helpful to prescribe the tricycle regimen, but again with a monophasic pill (*see Q 5.31*).

INDIVIDUAL VARIATION IN BLOOD LEVELS OF SEX STEROIDS: THE IMPLICATIONS FOR TREATMENT OF THE SYMPTOM OF BREAKTHROUGH BLEEDING (BTB)

5.160 As women vary, if the first pill brand does not suit what guidelines are there to help to individualize the second or subsequent pill prescription?

Some women do react unpredictably and several brands might have to be tried before a suitable one is found. Some are never suited. This is hardly surprising. Individual variation in motivation and tolerance of minor side-effects is well recognized, and the management is fully discussed later. But as we shall see there is also marked individual variation in blood levels of the exogenous hormones and in responses at the end-organs, especially the endometrium.

To give a brief summary of what follows, prescribers should try to identify early in the use of the COC method, if necessary over a series of visits, the lowest dose for each woman that does not cause the annoying symptom of BTB. This should minimize adverse side-effects (both serious and minor) and also reduce the measurable metabolic changes. This approach does not impair effectiveness.

5.161 What are the implications of individual variation in absorption and metabolism for the blood levels of the exogenous steroids in the average pill user?

1   Blood levels, whether of EE or of all the progestogens that have been studied, vary at least 10-fold between women who are apparently similar, taking the same formulations and sampled exactly 12 h after their last tablet was swallowed (*Fig. 5.14*). The pharmacokinetic AUC varies less, but still about three-fold. This is due to individual variation in:
    (a)   absorption
    (b)   metabolism, in the gut wall and in the liver (*see Qs 5.33 and 5.34*)

Titration of COC dose

Zone of high blood levels
(↑metabolic impact?)

'Ideal' zone

Bleeding threshold

Zone of BTB

Fig. 5.14 Schematic representation of the approximately 10-fold variability in peak blood levels of both contraceptive steroids, and the rationale of suggested titration against the bleeding threshold. Q 5.161.

(c) degree of binding to transport proteins especially SHBG in the blood plasma, which themselves are variably altered by different pills

(d) the efficiency with which normal EE is reformed and reabsorbed by the activity of the large bowel flora (*see* Q 5.34).

2 In addition to variable blood levels between women, there is a superimposed variation in target organ sensitivity. This is very difficult to assess and complicates matters further (*see* Q 5.175).

3 Then there is a further five- to ten-fold fluctuation in any woman between the peaks after absorption and the troughs when the next daily tablet is taken. This saw-tooth pattern is shown in *Figs 5.2* and *8.1* (*see* Q 8.5). *Figure 7.3* also conveys one of the presumed advantages of slow-release systems of administration: relatively constant daily blood levels.

5.162 What is the relevance to pill-prescribing of this great variation in blood levels and AUC between different women taking the same formulation, as in *Fig. 5.14*?

First, as already discussed fully above (*see Q 5.38*), there is pretty good evidence from research on enzyme inducers that women whose blood levels are low tend to suffer problems with endometrial stability (chiefly BTB). They might even conceive (especially if they ever lengthen the PFI).

5.163 What about those women with relatively high circulating blood levels of artificial steroids? What evidence is there that side-effects can be correlated?

It is a very tenable hypothesis that metabolic changes and both major and minor side-effects of the COC are more common and more marked in those women whose blood levels are exceptionally high. In support, pill takers in a US study who developed clinical hypertension were statistically more likely to have high blood levels of EE than control takers of similar pills without any rise in blood pressure.

5.164 Is it feasible to measure the levels of either the oestrogen or progestogen in body fluids?

This is not yet practical as a clinic procedure, although a simple testing kit for levels in the saliva or urine would be useful.

5.165 Without blood level measurements, how might one attempt to 'tailor' the pill to the individual woman?

I believe that one can, to a degree, but not by the approach that used to be recommended, namely attempting to base the choice on assessed features of that woman's normal menstrual cycle. This was, in my view, always illogical when one recalls that all COCs remove the normal cycle and replace it with an artificial one. That being so, it is surely preferable to make the replacement cycle as good as it can be for all. The aim is that it should, after adjustments during follow-up (*see Qs 6.21 and 6.22*, and *Tables 6.1* and *6.2*), eventually be 'better' than each woman's normal cycle, rather than a slavish imitation of it.

I therefore promote the 'tailoring' approach that follows, designed to discover with the woman's cooperation the 'smallest' pill that gives her adequate control of her cycle.

5.166 In *Fig. 5.14*, what does absence of BTB mean?

On the hypothesis of *Q 5.163*, it could mean two very different things. Absence of BTB means either that the woman has ideal blood levels of the artificial hormones or that they are higher than necessary for the desired effect of contraception – with plausibly a greater risk than necessary of causing unwanted effects.

5.167 How then might we avoid giving the women who tend to the higher blood levels (or larger AUC) a stronger pill than they really need?

By attempting during follow-up to give each woman the 'smallest' (lowest dose) pill her uterus will allow, without bleeding. This can mean titrating downwards, trying a pill lower in the same ladder – if not already tried and found to cause BTB.

5.168 What if BTB does occur? Does she need a higher dose or different formulation?

Maybe! A higher dose pill (or a phasic or gestodene variety, *see Qs 5.178 and 5.179*) might be appropriate. But, first and foremost, important alternative causes of the bleeding must first be excluded (Table 5.15). I am aware of a young woman who was seen by a number of different doctors and nurses during 1991, complaining of BTB. They kept trying different brands without success until someone passed a speculum and, tragically, found an inoperable (adeno) carcinoma of the cervix. She had had a reportedly negative cervical smear 1 year previously but this was no excuse for the failure to examine.

Moreover, 'missed pills' should not be one's first thought when COC users present with spotting or BTB: among women positive for *Chlamydia* about 13% in a 1993 US study by Krettek had spotting as a symptom, compared with only 5% of uninfected pill takers.

Note carefully all the other possibilities in *Table 5.15*; also *Q 5.31 re* BTB in later packets during tricycling.

5.169 What other 'Ds' can be added to those in *Table 5.15*?

Since the last edition, during my lectures around the world a number of others have been suggested with varying degrees of seriousness, from the floor. More causes of BTB:

- ■ D for doctor-caused (poor instruction/advice).
- ■ D for dud pills: iatrogenic causes (which have really happened) include wrong prescriptions for POPs and HRT products instead of the COC. Overdue date (time-expired product) or other cause of damaged product is another possibility!
- ■ D for diathesis/dyscrasia: a coincidental bleeding disease could first manifest itself this way.
- ■ D for drink: alcohol and other non-therapeutic substances, i.e. drugs, chiefly because their abuse is a likely cause of default (liver enzyme induction by alcohol is not thought to be important).

TABLE 5.15 Checklist in cases of possible 'breakthrough bleeding' (BTB) in pill-takers

A *note of caution*: first eliminate other possible causes!

The following checklist is modified from the book by Sapire (see Further Reading):

Disease – EXAMINE the cervix. It is not unknown for bleeding from an invasive cancer to be wrongly attributed to BTB. *Chlamydia* often causes a blood-stained discharge due to endometritis

Disorder of pregnancy causing bleeding (e.g. because of recent abortion, trophoblastic tumour)

Default – missed pill(s). Remember that the BTB may start 2 or 3 days later and be very persistent thereafter

Drugs – especially enzyme inducers, see Qs 5.34 and Q 5.38 – cigarettes are also relevant (see Q 5.169)

Diarrhoea with VOMITING – diarrhoea alone has to be very severe to impair absorption significantly, see Q 5.25

Disturbance of absorption – likewise has to be very marked to be relevant, e.g. after massive gut resection.

Diet – gut flora involved in recycling EE can be reduced in vegetarians. Could theoretically be a factor but no obvious increase in BTB risk in vegetarians has been noted clinically

Duration too short – minimal BTB that is tolerable might resolve after 2–3 months, see Q 5.172. See also Q 5.32 re BTB during tricyling (possible need to 'bicycle' instead)

Finally, after the above have been excluded:

Dose – if she is taking a monophasic, try a phasic pill (Qs 5.172, 5.179–5.182)
    – increase the progestogen or oestrogen component (Qs 5.172 and 5.173)
    – try a different progestogen

Cigarettes are also now clearly linked (Oxford/FPA and Rosenberg studies, *American Journal of Obstetrics and Gynecology* 1996 174:628–632) to BTB, both in the pill cycle and in the normal cycle. This is thought to be the effect of increased catabolism of oestrogen through constituents of tobacco smoke.

INITIAL CHOICE OF PREPARATION, AND EARLY FOLLOW-UP

We are now in a position to consider how best to put the above facts and principles into practice. The objective is that each woman receives the least long-term metabolic impact that her uterus will allow, i.e. the lowest dose of contraceptive steroids that is just above her own bleeding threshold.

5.170 What is the normal choice for the first pill prescription?

As previously stated there is no proven 'best buy'. In general one does not choose the more complicated triphasics (*see Qs 5.179–5.184*) or 20-µg pills when future compliance is suspect. Pills known to have a relatively high rate of BTB are also best kept for trial later, when a new user is better able to cope (but all users must be advised about BTB in case it should occur, because forewarned is forearmed; *see Q 6.96*).

Microgynon 30™ in its ED ('Every Day') version is my own first choice for a healthy first timer for the reasons fully described in *Q 5.12 and Q 5.6ff.*

5.171 Which women might need consideration of a stronger formulation (50–60 μg) from the outset?

Those women who are known to have reduced bioavailability of the COC:

1 Women on long-term enzyme-inducing drugs (*see Qs 5.34–5.36 and 6.27*).
2 Rarely, women with established malabsorption problems (e.g. massive small bowel resection).

In addition:

3 Some women who have had a previous contraceptive failure with the COC, yet claiming perfect compliance or having missed no more than one tablet. But unlike (1) and (2), most of these should be given a standard formulation or the same (monophasic) as they previously had, only now tricycling the packets plus a shortened PFI after every third pack (*see Q 5.27*).

5.172 What pill should follow if BTB is unacceptable after 2–3 months' trial and there is no other explanation?

Provided that the other causes in the list in *Table 5.15* have been carefully excluded, if BTB occurs and is unacceptable early on, or persists beyond about three cycles, the next strongest brand up the 'ladder' in *Fig. 5.12* can be tried. In general, gestodene-containing COCs have a good reputation for cycle control. Phasic pills might come into their own here, especially if the cycle control problem includes absent WTB.

If after trying lower-dose options BTB can only be prevented by a 50-μg oestrogen pill or pill combination (*Q 5.173*), for that particular woman the latter need not be considered a 'strong' brand. I explain this to women as in *Q 5.39*.

The answer to Q 4.167 is different for BTB late in a sequence of tricycling: if this applies, *see Q 5.32*.

5.173 If cycle control is a big problem, can one prescribe two pills, for example one Marvelon™ plus one Mercilon-20™ daily, to construct a 50-μg desogestrel product?

Yes, I would support this, but in selected cases with due caution as for other situations outside the strict terms of the summary of product characteristics

(SPC). Whenever more than one tablet is swallowed per day, this is an unlicensed use of a licensed product and the 'named patient' criteria must be fulfilled (see Appendix A, p. 535).

Although evidence based, this could be a little more difficult to justify than with long-term users of enzyme-inducer drugs, who have been proved regularly to have lower bioavailability of the COC. If, remotely, in these circumstances a thrombotic or other serious CVS event occurred it might be more difficult to establish that there had not been another cause for the bleeding problem – perhaps at the end-organ (*see Q 5.175*) – and hence that 'too much' oestrogen was not being given by the two pills a day regimen.

5.174 Later on, if there is good cycle control in an established asymptomatic COC user, should one try moving down the ladder?

At the time of repeat prescription, the possibility of trying a lower-dose brand (if available) should always be considered. Otherwise one will never know whether they might not be equally suited to a lower and probably safer dose. If no lower dose exists, both prescriber and taker of the pill can have the satisfaction of knowing that metabolic risks and hence probable risk of side-effects have been minimized within the context of marketed products.

5.175 Low blood levels of the artificial hormones usually cause BTB – but is all BTB caused by low blood levels?

No. It is true that BTB is not a totally accurate marker of blood levels, and indeed variability in BTB or WTB with the same blood level could be caused by variation at the end-organ (the endometrium). This is indubitably true, and probably explains much of the light BTB common in the first one or two cycles and the late tricycle bleeding discussed in *Q 4.32*.

But women find BTB annoying in any event. Why give more drug than the minimum to prevent the annoying symptom? The dose administered should be only just above (and not enormously above) the bleeding threshold: whether mediated by low blood level or an unusually susceptible end organ. Hence titration downwards in those without BTB is still logical. But caution is essential in the reverse situation, as stressed already at *Q 5.168* and *Table 5.15* – remember particularly to check for *Chlamydia*!

5.176 Should women with BTB be advised to take additional precautions? Can they rely on their COC?

It has been suggested that attempting to find the best choice of pill by titrating downwards at follow-up, in the way described above, will lead to breakthrough conceptions. Yet pill takers who conceive rarely report having had BTB beforehand. That conceptions rarely occur unless pills are (also) missed is, I believe, for the following reasons:

1 It is a tribute to the fact that even the current low-dose pills are amazingly effective, with back-up contraceptive mechanisms (notably the progestogen 'block' to cervical mucus penetration by sperm) operating even if breakthrough ovulation should occur.
2 It seems that (fortunately) BTB is an early warning – usually occurring when there is more circulating artificial steroid than the minimum to permit conception – in compliant women. (It might well be true, though, that BTB implies a reduced margin for error, so these women ought to be more careful than usual about not lengthening the PFI, *see Qs 5.15–5.18*).
3 It is likely that the bleeding from the uterus itself temporarily enhances the anti-implantation contraceptive mechanism.
4 While present, BTB probably reduces coital frequency!

5.177 How would you summarize this policy?

All we want to do is give the lowest metabolic impact to the woman that her endometrium will allow. I would stress, however, that this prescribing system is based on the hypothesis of *Fig. 5.14*, which has not yet been rigorously tested. I would ask the reader to judge its plausibility and my view that it should be followed, pending the discovery of any better scheme.

5.178 What should be the second choice of pill if there are non-bleeding side-effects?

See *Qs 6.21 and 6.22* and *Tables 6.1* and *6.2*.

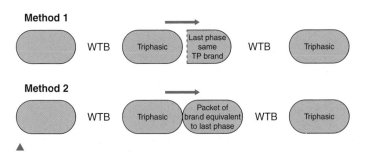

Fig. 5.15 How to postpone periods with triphasic pills. Q 5.177. *Note*: for Synphase™ just run the packets on. Use this figure in conjunction with Table 5.16. Q 5.184.

THE PROS AND CONS OF PHASIC PILLS

5.179 What are phasic pills and what are their advantages?

Their main claimed advantage is that they tend to give a better bleeding pattern for a given (low) dose of hormones, using the given progestogen. For example, Logynon™/Trinordiol™ gives an average daily dose of 92 µg of LNG (combined with 32.4 µg of EE). If this low dose of progestogen were used in a daily fixed-dose regimen, the incidence of BTB would probably be unacceptable.

Unexpectedly, the same has not been demonstrated for the gestodene-containing triphasics (see *Table 5.13*), when compared with their actually slightly lower-dose monophasic equivalents! However, all the gestodene combined pills are reported to give better cycle control than the levonorgestrel- or norethisterone-containing triphasics, particularly in the early months of use.

All except one triphasic (Synphase™) imitate the normal menstrual cycle to some extent, in particular by there being a higher proportion of the progestogen to the oestrogen in the second half of the pill-taking cycle. Histologically, this leads to the production of an endometrium that appears more like the normal secretory phase, with more gland formation and the presence of spiral arterioles. This improved histology probably lies behind the good WTB that occurs (some patients complain it is too good!).

5.180 What about the other postulated advantage, that the approximation to the normal cycle will itself lead to a reduction in long-term side-effects?

That is unlikely I think, although not impossible. On the contrary, some of the beneficial effects – which seem to relate to the very fact that the pill cycle produces more stable hormone levels and is not the same as the normal cycle (*see Q 5.58*) – might also be reduced. As yet, we just do not know.

5.181 What are the disadvantages of phasic OCs?

These can be listed as follows:

1   An increase in the time required to explain the pill packet to the user.
2   An increase in the risk of pill-taking errors, maybe particularly by teenagers – although some companies have made the newer packaging much more 'user-friendly'.
3   A reduction in the margin for such errors, particularly in view of the low dose being taken in the very first phase right after the 'contraceptively dangerous' pill-free time (*see Qs 5.15 and 5.24*).

4 Some women complain of symptoms that imitate the premenstrual syndrome, such as breast tenderness, in the last phase of pill taking before the withdrawal bleed.

5 They are obviously not a good choice for women with (aura-free) migraines or anyone prone to headaches or mood changes or any symptom that tends to be precipitated by hormone fluctuations.

6 In the UK they are extra expensive to the NHS because the pharmacist or dispensing doctor is paid a separate dispensing fee for each of the three phases – and even for the placebo phase of Logynon ED™!

7 A small problem with postponing withdrawal bleeds (*see* Q 5.184), and for the same reason they are not suitable for tricycling (*see* Q 5.31).

8 Studies in Holland, Australia and New Zealand have all found that triphasics are definitely over-represented, among the COCs reportedly in use, by pill takers presenting with unwanted 'breakthrough' conceptions. The reasons might include compliance problems due to complexity of the packaging and also relatively lower innate efficacy – see answer (3) above.

5.182 So for whom might phasic OCs be chosen?

1 The main indication is for cycle control with low dose, especially to get a good withdrawal bleed. (Note, however, that in both the norethisterone and gestodene pill ladders the phasics are not actually quite the lowest dose products.)

2 Upon request, if the woman likes the idea of 'imitating the menstrual cycle'; they usefully increase choice if side-effects occur with monophasic products.

5.183 What are your views specifically about BiNovum™ and Synphase™?

1 BiNovum™ in my view is a brand that has almost no place now that TriNovum™ is available. TriNovum™ gives a lower mean daily progestogen dose (750 µg instead of 833 µg), gives at least as good cycle control and has much better packaging.

2 Synphase™ might be useful for women experiencing BTB in the middle of the packet of a fixed-dose brand, especially Ovysmen™/Brevinor™. It is the only triphasic pill that has the highest progestogen to oestrogen ratio in the middle phase. However, in comparison with Trinovum™ there is a negligible reduction in mean daily progestogen (714 µg rather than 750 µg).

5.184 How can a woman postpone the withdrawal bleed on a phasic pill?

There is no problem with Synphase™. As with fixed-dose pills (*see Q 6.84*), two packets can simply be taken in a row without the usual 7-day break. But if this is tried with one of the other phasic brands, BTB is likely (although not certain) to occur early in the new packet because of the abrupt drop in progestogen from the higher level in the last phase of the previous packet.

There are two possible solutions (see *Fig. 5.15*). Contraceptive efficacy will be maintained throughout either scheme:

1 Tablets from the last phase of a 'spare' packet can be taken, thereby giving 7, 10 or 14 days' postponement according to the phasic brand in question.
2 Alternatively, the woman can follow immediately with a packet of the 'nearest' fixed dose brand up the same ladder in *Fig. 5.12* and *Table 5.13* (i.e. the nearest equivalent to the final phase of her phasic pill). To be specific, this means using one of the brands listed in *Table 5.16*.

To avoid any possible confusion, this procedure of *Fig. 5.15* is not in the least necessary if the women has missed pills late in her packet. In that case the advice in *Q 5.19* is all that is required to maintain efficacy. If she has a bleed early in the new pack she was expecting that anyway.

TABLE 5.16 Postponing 'periods' with phasics	
Name of phasic*	**Brand to follow* to delay WTB using method 2 of Figure 5.15**
Logynon™	Microgynon™
Tri-Minulet™	Minulet†™
TriNovum™	Norimin™
Binovum™	Norimin™
Synphase™	Synphase™

*Or the identical equivalent by another manufacturer from Table 5.13 – the alternatives are Trinordiol™, Ovranette™, Triadene™ and Femodene™
†There would be a small risk of a BTB episode here since Minulet™ has 25 µg less gestodene than phase 3 of Tri-Minulet™

The combined oral contraceptive – follow-up arrangements and new routes of administration

6

DEALING WITH OTHER SIDE-EFFECTS AND EVENTS DURING PILL USE

CENTRAL NERVOUS SYSTEM

GASTROINTESTINAL SYSTEM

6.1 What are the main aspects of pill monitoring, once (so far as is possible) the 'safest' pill brand has been identified for the individual?

After careful selection and counselling, the list of what can (and should) be done during long-term monitoring is short – but important. In summary:

1 Start by warmly greeting the pill taker and asking her how she is. Give her space to mention her own concerns. If she has any type of bleeding side-effects *see Qs 5.160–5.184*. Non-bleeding side-effects are discussed below (*see Qs 6.19 and 6.20* and following).

2 Ask at each visit about headaches and particularly about any change in associated symptoms (*see Q 5.152*). Advise in advance about all the warning symptoms in *Q 6.13*, including those relevant to migraine.

3 Look for the onset of any new cardiovascular risk factors – or intercurrent disease with the same implications (*see Q 5.137*) – especially if one is already present (e.g. arrival of age 35 in all smokers).

4 Look for the warning signs (*see Q 6.13*), primarily:
   (a) a rise in blood pressure (*see Q 6.7 and Table 5.11*)
   (b) the onset of or change in character or worsening of migraines (*see Qs 5.151–5.159*) – the migraine sufferer needs to be prospectively advised (i.e. more specifically than just the list at *Q 6.13*)
   (c) sharp pleuritic pain in the chest, current or recent, is unlikely to be pleurisy – consider the rare possibility, especially in a new pill taker, of the early symptoms of pulmonary embolism.

4 Arrange routine (preferably 3-yearly) cervical cytology, with a bimanual examination only when clinically indicated (*see Q 6.3*).

5 Advise on breast awareness (without it becoming a nerve-racking ritual) along with a good leaflet. The pill taker should know that you will be prepared to examine her on clinical grounds, i.e. if she ever notices some change in her breasts, but routine professional breast examination has no evidence-base and no linkage whatever with any hormone methods.

6 Advise about special situations, notably immobilization, long-haul air flights, high-altitude holidays, major surgery and the treatment for varicose veins (*see Qs 6.14 and 6.15*).

7 Weight is *not* routinely measured, only if relevant to BMI assessment (*Q 5.120*).

6.2 Which pill takers can be seen at reduced frequency, and by whom?

In my opinion, everything depends on whether the pill taker is one of the 'safer' women or not (*see Qs 5.136 and 5.137*). The prescriber should mentally classify the pill taker into one of the two groups – a form of triage really – on which follow-up arrangements depend.

'AMBER LIGHT' GROUP

Women with any of the recognized relative contraindications (primarily those in WHO 3) or with any important chronic illness should normally be seen by the doctor: with a low threshold for more frequent visits, perhaps 1–3 months after the first prescription; and it would be unlikely that the gap between checks would increase to more than 6-monthly thereafter. The reason is simple, they are the ones in whom the cardiovascular risks are focused: the heavy smokers have an inbuilt times ten or more greater risk of having a heart attack than any risk-factor-free woman (*see Q 5.101* and *Table 5.8, p. 169*).

Even so, the COC is such a safe product that it could be entirely appropriate for a family planning trained nurse to care for many women in this category, i.e. as described immediately below, just more frequently, following an agreed protocol.

'GREEN LIGHT' GROUP

These ordinary 'safer' women are still seen 3 months after the first pill prescription, or any change of brand, for blood pressure (BP) check and symptom assessment, as well as to answer any queries. Subsequent visits have traditionally been 6-monthly but the frequency in this low-risk group can be further reduced: I now advise that if the BP is stable in a healthy migraine-free woman after 12 months, annual checks are sufficient. WHO even suggests this annual check policy with the prescription of 13 cycles of treatment starts from the outset. But this risks missing an early adverse effect such as hypertension, migraine with aura or, more remotely, VTE with premonitory symptoms in the leg or chest.

It is good practice and an appropriate use of scarce resources for the follow-up checks to be delegated to the practice nurse, so long as she is fully and appropriately trained in reproductive health. There must be an agreed protocol specifying when (e.g. at what BP level) she should call in the doctor.

Both nurses and doctors should recognize that pill takers in this 'green light' group are very different from the first group, and are very unlikely to suffer a serious adverse effect after the first year (when the majority of the rare idiopathic VTEs tend to occur).

6.3 Ideally, shouldn't all pill takers have a full pelvic examination at least annually?

No, this is part of medical mythology. Bimanual examinations (BMEs) can identify two main things, tenderness and enlargements. Although most of the disorders listed in *Q 5.69* might in theory be picked up by a careful BME, everything mentioned is actually *less* likely to happen in pill takers anyway, compared with, for example, the partners of intermittent condom-users! Those are the ones at the greater risk of ovarian cysts (benign or malignant), fibroids, endometriosis, ectopics, even pelvic infection. Arguably, it would be more logical to persuade them to come in, and be examined this way, if you can, rather than the pill takers!

Obviously, BMEs should be done in each woman as indicated on clinical grounds for that individual, and the cervix screened according to guidelines.

6.4 How often should the breasts be examined?

This examination also, whether at the first or a follow-up visit, should be done solely on robust clinical grounds, including any request from the woman herself for a check, usually of some change she has noted on either side. Otherwise it is irrelevant that the woman is a pill taker and clinicians must be prepared to defend themselves against an allegation of a 'TUBE' (totally unnecessary breast examination)!

6.5 How frequently should BP be measured, and why is it so important?

BP should be measured before treatment and thereafter at 3 months, then 6-monthly and then, after at least 12 months; and if it is essentially unchanged from the pretreatment visit, it can be checked annually thereafter in women free of all relevant risk factors or diseases (*see Q 6.1*). Studies have shown that (with one possible exception requiring further study as discussed in *Qs 6.7 and 5.100*) the COC generally causes a measurable increase in both systolic and diastolic BP. A tiny (few millimetres) increase occurs in most women and a large increase in a few (estimated at up to 1% with modern pills):

1 Moderate hypertension: defined internationally as BP equal to or above 160/100 mmHg. This is WHO 4 because it increases the risks of most varieties of arterial disease and can even become irreversible. (Malignant hypertension has, rarely, been attributed to the COC.) If truly pill-induced the hypertension is fully reversible if the pill is discontinued.

2 Mild hypertension: BP 140–159/90–99 mmHg – even this should be taken seriously (WHO 3), especially if there are other circulatory risk factors (*see Qs 5.120, 6.7*).

3 Although not technically hypertension at all, I would classify as WHO 2 the situation in which the BP has gone up from the baseline normal for that woman before she started the COC, to anything higher (up to the 139/89 mm Hg cut-off level for WHO 3).

As generally taught, the classification as above, and any decisions arising from it, should not be based on isolated readings. Repeating the measurement after a period of rest for the woman and a second observer are ideal.

6.6 At what levels of BP should the pill be stopped?

It used to be agreed in the UK that repeated readings above 160/95 mmHg would always be too high, both for starting and continuing with the COC. However, WHO is slightly more permissive, stating that a raised level that, when repeated does not exceed 159 systolic or 99 diastolic, is WHO 3 for the COC, but that 160/100 or above is WHO 4. Therefore, pending further guidance, I now use these internationally agreed levels.

6.7 When should a rather small rise in BP, perhaps not out of the normotensive range, nevertheless lead to a consideration of change of method?

Behind this question are the studies that show that hypertension acts as a marker for an increased risk of arterial disease. Studies of large populations (by life insurance companies) have shown that raised BP is associated with a small but measurable reduction in life expectancy, even in women. While it is not certain that pill-induced mild hypertension has the same significance as the idiopathic variety, it would be prudent to assume that it does. Faced, therefore, with a 33-year-old, heavy-smoking woman with a BP repeatedly hovering just below 140/90 mmHg and knowing that before pill-taking it was, say, 110/70 mmHg, one would prefer she switched to another method of birth control right away rather than continuing to the upper limit of 35 years.

BP levels that are above the WHO 3 lower limit of 140/90 mmHg often indicate changing to a POP (see *Chapter 7*) but a new possibility in the younger age group would be to try the new drospirenone-containing product (Yasmin™, *see Qs 5.100, 6.63*).

6.8 So can the BP be used as an ongoing test of liability to arterial disease?

This is what I am suggesting. In other words, for years pill-prescribers have longed for a simple clinical test, for example, a reagent that could be added to a woman's urine in the clinic and would turn it green if she could safely continue with the COC and red if she should discontinue. It is my view that we have that test already – not perfect, but usable in the same kind of way. A rise in BP is like a red or at least pink test, implying that the woman (especially if she already has a risk factor) has now entered a category at increased risk of arterial disease.

6.9 Can patients actually on hypotensive treatment be legitimately given the COC?

This is WHO 3 in my view, and POP or an injectable would be better choices among hormonal methods. But the COC (e.g. Yasmin™ for the reasons above) might be acceptable with good BP control and careful monitoring in a young, non-smoking woman who accepts the extra risk, will use no other method of birth control, and after full consultation with the physician supervising control of her hypertension.

> This presupposes that the woman's hypertension is not pill related (which would be WHO 4). It would not be acceptable for a woman whose hypertension was induced by the COC (and readily reversible by simply stopping it in favour, say, of the POP), then to be given antihypertensive drugs to enable her to stay on it. There can be few occasions when treating the side-effects of one drug by other powerful drugs can be anything but bad medicine.

6.10 What types of migraine indicate that the combined pill should be stopped?

See Qs 5.151–5.158. To recap, these are:

■ any change in the character of migraine to include the focal neurological symptoms of aura (*see* Q 5.152), symptoms that are usually explicable in terms of (although not necessarily actually caused by) transient cerebral ischaemia
■ migraines that are exceptionally severe during days of pill-taking and last more than 72 h
■ migraine without aura plus more than one additional risk factor for stroke
■ concurrent treatment with an ergot alkaloid.

In these categories the oestrogen of the combined pill should be stopped forthwith, and usually for ever. This is for fear that the additional thrombotic risk might result in a thrombotic stroke. But all other contraceptives are options: the POP and injectables can be started right away.

6.11 What if a woman's first ever migraine without aura attack occurs while taking the COC? Should she stop the method?

The manufacturer's SPCs say yes to this. If there is any concern that the symptoms might be thromboembolic, in my view COCs should be stopped pending a clear diagnosis. If this rare possibility is carefully excluded, COCs may be continued or recommenced; however on a WHO 2 basis (*see Q 4.158*) she must as usual be warned in simple terms about the important symptoms to watch out for in future (*see Q 5.152*).

6.12 What about 'ordinary' headaches that occur on the COC?

These are not a contraindication, more in the nature of a common, more or less tolerable, side-effect and one for which the woman might or might not ask help. If so, it is well worth ascertaining whether the headaches tend to occur in the pill-free week. If they do, the tricycle regimen, using the lowest acceptable fixed-dose formulation, leads – at worst – to the woman experiencing only four or five headaches a year instead of 13! (*see Q 5.31*).

As the trigger for such headaches seems often to be oestrogen-withdrawal, another option worth consideration is the use of 100-μg patches of estradiol daily, through the pill-free interval.

6.13 What symptoms should lead pill users to take urgent medical advice (potential major problems)?

Pill users should be told to:

1 transfer at once to another effective method of birth control, *and*
2 come under medical care without delay, pending diagnosis and treatment, if any of the following should occur (this list is a form of revision of the pill story so far!):

 (a) severe pain in the calf of one leg – possible deep venous thrombosis (DVT)
 (b) severe central pain in the chest or sharp pains on either side of the chest aggravated by breathing – could be MI or pulmonary embolism
 (c) unexplained breathlessness with or without the coughing up of blood-stained sputum – could be pulmonary embolism
 (d) severe pain in the abdomen (*see Q 6.41*)
 (e) any unusually severe, prolonged headache, especially if it is the first ever attack or gets progressively worse, or is associated with the symptoms at (f) to (i) below (*see Qs 5.151–5.158*)
 (f) a bad fainting attack or collapse, with or without focal epilepsy
 (g) weakness or paraesthesia suddenly or gradually affecting one side or one part of the body
 (h) marked asymmetrical disturbance of vision, especially a bright scotoma in a visual field, without as well as with a migraine headache following
 (i) disturbance of the ability to speak normally (nominal aphasia)
 (j) a severe and generalized skin rash – could be erythema multiforme.

Potentially, most of the above are thrombotic or embolic catastrophes in the making; but very often there will prove to be a much less serious explanation or one that is not pill related.

Clinical signs that might not be complaints but still demand urgent action (including stopping the COC) are:

(k) the onset of jaundice (*see Qs 6.34 and 6.35*)

(l) high blood pressure (i.e. above 160/100 mmHg, *see Qs 6.5 and 6.6*).

The pill should also normally be discontinued forthwith if immobilization is necessary after an accident, or emergency major or leg surgery is required (*see Qs 6.14–6.18*).

IMPLICATIONS OF SURGERY

6.14 Should a combined pill user discontinue treatment before elective major surgery?

This is WHO 3–4; it all depends on the nature of the surgery. My opinion on this is a little more cautious than some pronouncements (e.g. the THRIFT Consensus Group 1992 *British Medical Journal* 305:567–574). If it is major surgery, lasting more than 30 min and involving immobilization thereafter, i.e. mainly in bed for at least 48 h, or less major but associated with hypotension or prolonged immobilization thereafter, or any surgery involving the legs, the COC should:

1 be discontinued at least 2 (preferably 4) weeks before the operation (many coagulation factors are back to normal by 2 weeks but there is insufficient evidence to state that 2 weeks' discontinuation would always suffice)

2 not be recommended until at least 2 weeks after full mobilization. This restart can be a 'quick start' (*see Q 6.17*): there is no need to wait for any menstrual bleeding.

The reason for this advice is the well-established increased risk of DVT postoperatively, and the potential for this to be increased by the prothrombotic changes caused by oestrogens (Vessey et al 1986 *British Medical Journal* 292:526–528) estimated the risk of clinical VTE postoperatively as 0.96% on low-dose pills and 0.5% for non-takers. Given these figures, a policy of stopping the COC has the potential to prevent about 500 VTEs and up to 10 deaths in every 100 000 major operations.

For the reason that they are oestrogen free, the above rule does not apply to the POP, nor to progestogen-only injectables/implants, which can be continued without a break during major surgery. Indeed, they can be an appropriate choice to cover the time on a waiting-list (*see Q 6.17*).

6.15 Should the COC be stopped for a minor operation such as laparoscopic sterilization?

This is definitely unnecessary (WHO 2) because the risk of postoperative DVT is vanishingly small after such minor surgery. The same applies to dental extraction. 'Iatrogenic' pregnancies seem frequently to be caused this way.

However, as thromboembolism occurred after 3 of 438 laparoscopic cholecystectomies in a 1993 report from Sydney (one was fatal), it would be best to avoid COC use prior to complex laparoscopies.

6.16 What about minor leg surgery, such as operative arthroscopy, or ligation of varicose veins? Or injection treatment for leg veins?

These are quite another matter. Oestrogen-containing therapy should be discontinued at least 2 weeks before either such surgery or sclerotherapy, and avoided for the duration of leg bandaging thereafter.

6.17 What contraception is suitable before and after relevant surgery? And how should the switches from and back to the COC be managed?

Progestogen-only methods are all appropriate. A good choice might be Cerazette™ (*see Q 7.11ff*) – or injectable DMPA (*see Q 6.14*). The first *injection* can be given at any time in the woman's pill-taking cycle, after which she just finishes the current packet. A new packet of her usual pill can be started as early as 2 weeks after full mobilization, without waiting for the expiry of the 12-week duration of the injection, whether she has amenorrhoea or if irregular bleeding is a problem. After all, DMPA and the COC are quite often given together to control irregular bleeding (*see Q 8.48*).

This restart of the COC can be a 'quick start': there is no need to wait for menstrual bleeding. If the method used to 'cover' the surgery has been abstinence and there is any expectation of imminent ovulation, it might be wise not to rely solely on the COC for the first 7 days. (But this would be unnecessary if her surgery and convalescence were fully covered by an anovulatory contraceptive such as Cerazette™ or an injectable).

6.18 What should be done if a patient who is a pill taker is admitted as an emergency for major surgery or orthopaedic (fracture) treatment with immobilization?

In these circumstances the risk of DVT is high, especially if she is overweight. The COC should be discontinued at once and careful consideration given to the use of subcutaneous heparin prophylaxis. This would be particularly important for urgent major gynaecological, orthopaedic and cancer surgery.

Do not forget to ask the young girl on traction, after falling from her boyfriend's motorbike, to stop taking her (combined) pills. Indeed, the immobilization involved in treating a leg fracture after a skiing accident, even as an outpatient, can be sufficient for many continental orthopaedic surgeons to recommend heparin prophylaxis. This might be overcautious in an outpatient but such a leg-immobilizing fracture is at least a WHO 3 situation: so stopping the COC and perhaps switching short-term to a progestogen-only contraceptive is preferable while the leg is in plaster.

DEALING WITH OTHER SIDE-EFFECTS AND EVENTS DURING PILL USE

6.19 What general points can be made about the so-called 'minor' side-effects?

1 First and foremost, avoid any hint of being dismissive or patronizing: such symptoms frequently do not seem minor to the woman affected!

2 Many of them are common in the general population, hence it is difficult to be sure that the COC is to blame in an individual case.

3 The frequency of complaint depends on many factors, including anxiety about possible harm due to the therapy.

4 Many side-effects can be classified under two main headings:
   (a) Those related to cycle control. The common problem of BTB and spotting should first be evaluated as described in *Qs 5.168 and 5.169*, then managed as in *Qs 5.170–5.177*. Pill-related BTB can benefit from use of a higher dose product, a different progestogen, or possibly a phasic pill.
   (b) Those that are also common in pregnancy.

6.20 Which are the common, often pregnancy-mimicking minor (unwanted) side-effects often attributed to the COC?

Not all these are also more common in pregnancy. In some cases the link with the COC might not be causal. Beneficial minor side-effects are included within the list in *Q 5.56*. The order below is alphabetical:

Common:

1 acne (usually benefited, but can worsen with levonorgestrel pills)

2 breast enlargement and bloatedness with fluid retention

3 cramps and pains in the legs

4 cystitis and other urinary infections

5 depression and loss of libido

6 gingivitis

7 hair loss (or gain, *see Q 6.66*)

8 headaches

9 nausea
10 vaginal discharge (non-specific) and cervical 'erosion'/ectopy
11 weight gain.

Less common:

1 breast pain (*see Qs 6.54 and 6.22*)
2 chloasma (*see Q 6.66*)
3 photosensitivity
4 galactorrhoea (*see Q 6.54*)
5 superficial thrombophlebitis.

Some more serious conditions reported in pill takers are similarly more common in pregnancy. For example, some immune disorders (*see Q 6.22*); chorea, cardiomyopathy, pemphigoid gestationis, haemolytic uraemic syndrome and cholestatic jaundice; not to mention hypertension and venous and arterial thrombosis.

Subsequent questions (*see Q 6.23–Q 6.71*) consider side-effects by body system (**excluding the circulation because thromboembolism, hypertension and arterial disease already been dealt with in Chapter 5**). Thereafter, if the woman wishes to continue with the pill method, Tables 6.1 and 6.2 along with *Qs 6.21 and 6.22*), suggest possible changes of formulation, which can then be tried to control her symptom(s).

6.21 Which next pill? Are there any guidelines if a patient complains of any minor side-effect and wishes to continue the method?

Beware! Before rushing to change formulations, never forget that there might be another, non-pill-related, explanation for any side-effect, and that a side-effect might be caused or highlighted because of anxiety or a psychosexual problem (see the Preface). This applies particularly to this and the next question, and the linked Tables 6.1 and 6.2. With modern COCs, an emotional or psychosexual explanation becomes more probable (although not invariable) if a woman keeps returning with a wide assortment of side-effects after only taking a few tablets, and nothing ever seems to suit.

On first principles, first take a history and, as appropriate, examine. If the side-effect involves abnormal bleeding, see *Table 5.15* and *Qs 5.168 and 5.169*. Thereafter, for both BTB and absent WTB, she might benefit from a phasic pill or being moved 'higher up the ladder' (*see Q 5.172*).

Phasic pills might be worth changing from, however, if the symptoms are showing cyclical variation, for example breast tenderness, PMS-like

---

TABLE 6.1   Which second choice of pill? a: relative oestrogen excess

Symptoms	Conditions
Nausea	Benign breast disease
Dizziness	Fibroids
Cyclical weight gain (fluid)	Endometriosis
'Bloating'	
Vaginal discharge (no infection)	
Some cases of breast fullness/pain	
Some cases of lost libido with no depression – especially if taking an anti-androgenic oestrogen-dominant product such as Yasmin™/Dianette™ (Q. 6.25)	

- ◼ *Treat with progestogen-dominant COC such as Loestrin-30™, Microgynon-30™, Eugynon-30™ (but with caution regarding lipids)*
- ◼ BUT *remember*, symptoms might not have a pill-related cause.

TABLE 6.2   Which second choice of pill? b: relative progestogen excess

Symptoms	Conditions
Dryness of vagina	Acne/seborrhoea
Some cases of:	Hirsutism
Sustained weight gain	
Depression	
Loss of libido if associated with depressed mood (Q 6.24)	
Lassitude	
Breast tenderness	

- ◼ *Treat with oestrogen-dominant COC, such as Ovysmen™/Brevinor™, Marvelon™ or Yasmin™, or Dianette™ (an acne treatment that is also contraceptive, containing 35 mg of EE combined with 2 mg cyproterone acetate). Caution is necessary, in that oestrogen-dominance might link with a slightly higher risk of VTE, see Q. 5.110.*
- ◼ Remember as in Table 6.1, the above symptoms might have a non-pill-related cause.

symptoms (cyclical irritability, etc.). Monophasic pills, perhaps sustained for more than one packet consecutively (tricycling), can be of real benefit here.

For all other minor side-effects there are two empirical rules and two more specific ones. The empirical rules are:

1 Reduce the dose where possible (first of the oestrogen, if possible, then of the progestogen).
2 Alternatively, switch to another progestogen ladder (see *Fig. 5.12*). For the more specific rules, *see Q 6.22*.

6.22 What are the more specific rules?

1 For side-effects or conditions that have become associated (through clinical experience and sometimes by formal research) with a relative excess of the oestrogen, prescribe a more progestogen-dominant COC.
2 Conversely, for symptoms that have become associated with the progestogen, prescribe an oestrogen-dominant COC. This policy is summarized in *Tables 6.1 and 6.2*. But be aware that these tables have a rather weak evidence base: if we are honest we have to admit that most changes of pill to improve symptoms are ultimately on a trial-and-error basis!

CENTRAL NERVOUS SYSTEM

6.23 Is depression more common among pill takers than controls, and how can it be managed?

In the RCGP study it was shown that for every 130 depressed pill users there were 100 who were non-OC-using controls. This implies that only 30 of the 130 could really blame the COC, even in the much higher doses then given. But there are some who are free from depression when off treatment, with recurrence when rechallenged. In a proportion, altered tryptophan metabolism leads to lowered pyridoxine levels. In these it was suggested in the 1970s that pyridoxine might be beneficial (use less than 100 μg daily to avoid reversible peripheral neuropathy): in a study from Wynn's unit, 50 μg daily was given, taking up to 2 months to be effective. This work needs repeating with more modern pills. It is more common practice to try a change of progestogen or change of method, with or without antidepressant therapy.

Depression could also be secondary to other pill side-effects (e.g. headaches). But the Oxford/FPA Study (1985) ruled out any link between the COC and 'serious' psychiatric illness, which includes severe depression needing hospital referral.

6.24 How does the COC affect libido?

Loss of libido is reported particularly among those who are also depressed. Many extrinsic factors might explain this, including self-fulfilling prophecy due to what has been alleged about the COC or frustrated desire for a child. However, there are certainly some cases where there is a real physiological effect of the hormones and complete recovery when another method is used.

Contrariwise, in some women libido is actually increased on the COC because the method is so reliable, non-intercourse-related, and often reduces premenstrual tension. This might explain why female-initiated sexual activity late in the pill cycle was found to be more common than late in the normal cycle.

6.25 How should one manage the complaint of loss of libido?

1   First, the pill might be irrelevant to the problem. Discuss fully psychosexual aspects of the relationship, and the marital and family circumstances, and offer referral for counselling as appropriate.
2   Second, check whether part of the problem is soreness or dryness – which could be caused locally by thrush, or a vulval skin eruption, or suturing following delivery.
3   Use of a water-soluble lubricant may help.
4   Finally, changing to a different pill might help: in my experience, if depression is the main problem, and seems clearly temporally related to the pill, it is helpful to move to a lower progestogen dose/more oestrogen-dominant formulation. However, loss of libido, usually without depression, in users of pills using cyproterone acetate (Dianette™) or drospirenone (Yasmin™) might relate to their being anti-androgenic progestogens, and improves on switching to a (less oestrogen-dominant) levonorgestrel or norethisterone product.

6.26 How does the COC affect epilepsy?

The condition is not initiated by the COC. The attack rate is often reduced, although rarely it might be increased. Hormone fluctuations are unhelpful, so avoid triphasic COCs (*see* Q 5.181). Liver enzyme-inducer antiepileptic therapy is one of the few indications for at least a 50-μg dose of ethinylestradiol along with tricycling (*see* Qs 5.36–5.39). Moreover, regardless of therapy, if fits are commonly initiated around the pill-free time, tricycling a monophasic might reduce their frequency.

6.27 If epileptics and others on chronic enzyme-inducing treatments are on the pill, how should they be managed?

First, please read *Qs 5.15–5.40* before this answer.

As this situation is WHO 3, first offer another contraceptive altogether. Injectables are a good option (*see* Q 8.11), as is the intrauterine route, especially the LNG-IUS (*see* Q 9.151).

If the pill is strongly preferred, I used to advise shortening the PFIs as well as the increased dose mentioned above. But it simplifies compliance to eliminate most of the PFIs using the tricycle regimen (*see* Q 5.31). This also appears to improve epilepsy control, although no comparative trial has been published. After three or even (if BTB is not a problem) four consecutive packets, the woman should still shorten the PFI: arbitrarily to just 4 days. Diary cards might be helpful.

If the woman subsequently complains of BTB, exclude another cause (*see Q 5.168*) and consider taking the break earlier, either when triggered by the bleed or by bicycling (*see Q 5.32*).

If all else fails and another contraceptive is not acceptable, the next step can be – cautiously – to try an even higher dose, for example two tablets of 30- or 35-µg fixed-dose pills. If necessary, the combined oestrogen content of the two pills per day can be increased to 90 µg (maximum), titrated against the BTB. In this way the usual policy of giving the minimum dose of both hormones to be just above the threshold for bleeding (*see Qs 5.168 and 5.170*) can be followed. The epileptic can be reassured that she is 'climbing a down escalator' (*see Q 5.39*).

Caution is necessary when enzyme inducers are withdrawn because it takes some weeks for the liver's level of excretory function to revert to normal (*see Q 5.40*).

6.28 What about headaches and migraines?

These very important CNS-related subjects have already been covered under 'risk factors' (*see Qs 5.151–5.159*) and 'monitoring' (*see Qs 6.10–6.12*).

6.29 How can the pill affect the eyes?

If any acute visual disturbance occurs, the woman should be told to stop the pill at once, pending further investigation:

1 At worst, acute loss of vision in one eye (black scotoma) could be caused by retinal artery or vein thrombosis or haemorrhage. Amaurosis fugax is the term given to a transient blackout of the vision of one eye, usually due to transient often thromboembolic retinal ischaemia. The COC should be stopped and avoided thereafter (WHO 4) along with urgent hospital referral.

2 Loss of a field of vision (bright scotoma). This must be taken seriously, even though not caused by an eye problem, because it may relate to migraine with aura or rarely a TIA.

3 'Benign' intracranial hypertension (BICH). This is a rare condition of unknown aetiology, causing raised intracranial pressure and papilloedema with headache and impairment of visual acuity – usually in young women, 90% of whom have a significantly raised BMI. Urgent hospital admission is essential for imaging to exclude a tumour and for medical treatment (initially with acetazolamide) and consideration of cerebrospinal fluid (CSF) shunting to reduce intracranial pressure or

eye-saving optic nerve sheath fenestration. The weak association with the COC and with other contraceptive hormones (e.g. Norplant™) is probably coincidental. However, as the condition is certainly not 'benign' with regard to the eyesight – there is a risk of permanent visual-field loss if it is treated late or recurrent – it is generally considered an absolute contraindication (WHO 4) to starting or continuing the COC. This would also apply if the eventual diagnosis was cerebral vein thrombosis, as applies in some cases. Exceptionally, the COC could be used (WHO 3) if the condition was established to be (tetracycline) drug-induced and there was no obesity.

4 Blurring of vision with photophobia can be a normal manifestation during migraine without aura.

6.30 What about the pill and contact lenses?

An increased likelihood of discomfort or rarely corneal damage among contact lens users taking the COC was reported with the old hard lenses (and stronger pills). It is believed to be caused by a slight degree of corneal oedema. With modern soft lenses and low-dose pills this problem is now uncommon. If it occurs, the woman should see her optician and a brand containing the lowest possible dose of both steroids should be tried. Rarely, women have to make a straight choice between their contact lenses and this contraceptive method.

6.31 Does the pill cause or aggravate glaucoma?

There is no evidence of any effect, even among those with a family history: although of course intraocular pressure rarely rises significantly during the peak childbearing years.

GASTROINTESTINAL SYSTEM

6.32 Does the COC cause nausea or vomiting?

Nausea can occur, particularly in the first cycle. Pill takers can usually be reassured that, although it might recur after the PFI with the first pills of the next packet, nausea usually affects fewer or none of the first pills in each subsequent pack. Vomiting is most unusual, but if within 2 h it could interfere with absorption of a tablet and hence affect cycle control and efficacy (*see* Q 5.25).

Both symptoms are oestrogen-related and are thus not so frequent with modern pills. They are more common in very underweight women, and in them may be intolerable, starting with the very first tablet and with every COC tried. More usually perseverance is rewarded. Use tablets with 20 μg of oestrogen – or oestrogen-free (i.e. the POP). Nausea can also be helped by taking the pill at night rather than in the morning.

Vomiting starting for the first time after several months of trouble-free pill-taking should not be attributed to the pill. Consider pregnancy for one thing.

6.33 How often is weight gain on the COC truly due to it, and how can it be minimized?

The fear of this is one of the things that most puts young women off the pill. Yet clearly not all weight gain is caused by the pill, particularly in its modern ultra-low dose versions; it is often blamed unfairly, as confirmed in a recent systematic review (Gallo et al. 2003, Cochrane Library). It might help to quote Endrikat et al. 1995 (*Contraception* 52:229–235). Among 228 users of a 20-μg gestodene-containing product (Femodette™), after 12 cycles from baseline as many had actually lost as had gained weight:

- weight gain of more than 2 kg in 12.7%
- unchanged or within ± 2 kg, 73.7%
- loss of more than 2 kg in 13.6%.

The first group ($N = 29$) would be bound to blame the pill for their weight gain, yet it is unlikely to be truly pill-attributable, as there were actually more ($N = 31$) contented (and so very likely less vocal) weight-losers!

Also very relevant to allegations about the pill and weight is that many women start the pill while still in their teens. A steady increase in weight during adolescence is the norm, regardless of pills.

There is also a kind of cyclical weight gain that is oestrogen linked (*see* Q 6.22) and due to fluid retention. This is more noticeable in some than others, tending to be shed with a diuresis in the pill-free week. Yasmin™ containing the weakly diuretic drospirenone is likely only to help those with this fluid-related type of weight gain.

Moreover, mean weights among adult women (and men) tend to increase year-on-year, as has been shown in several different Northern European studies of the 1990s.

Apart from appropriate advice about diet and (often most relevantly in an increasingly sedentary society) exercise, a lower-dose brand or different progestogen can be tried before necessarily trying a different method.

6.34 How should jaundice in a COC-user be managed?

First, the pill should be stopped immediately because it has additive effects on liver metabolism. If some form of infectious hepatitis is diagnosed, the COC is temporarily WHO 4 and normally not restarted until at least 3 months after the liver function tests have returned to normal.

Abnormal liver function tests caused by any other mechanism (e.g. cirrhosis) contraindicate the method (WHO 3–4 according to severity), although the POP is usable (*see Q 7.52*).

6.35 How often is jaundice caused by the pill?

Rarely. Cholestatic jaundice is more common among COC-users and also in pregnancy. A COC-related past history is WHO 4, reducing to WHO 3 if there is only a pregnancy history (with appropriate forewarning and rapid stopping of the hormones upon any recurrence). Gilbert's disease is incidental and benign with no impairment of liver function (WHO 2).

6.36 Does the COC cause gallstones?

The increased risk of this condition among COC users is significant only during the early years of pill-taking. This suggests that the risk applies primarily to predisposed women. Studies of bile biochemistry have shown that contraceptive steroids can accelerate cholelithiasis.

6.37 If a woman has had definitive treatment for gallstones can she use the COC?

If the treatment was medical the COC would be best avoided (WHO 3) because of the risk of recurrence. If the woman has had definitive surgical treatment by cholecystectomy, the COC is permitted (WHO 2).

6.38 Is acute pancreatitis linked with the COC?

Yes, in part perhaps through the link with gall-bladder disease. Most of the sporadic cases had cofactors like obesity, alcohol abuse, hypertriglyceridaemia or lipid problems, and there have been very few reports associated with modern low-dose pills.

If a woman suffers an attack of this condition on the COC artificial oestrogen is contraindicated (WHO 4) if the triglyceride levels are high or perhaps WHO 3 if they are not. Helpfully, her triglycerides will probably fall if she transfers to any progestogen-only method.

6.39 What are the presentation and management of COC-related benign liver tumours (see Q 5.96)?

They present with abdominal pain and an upper abdominal mass, and sometimes with a life-threatening haemoperitoneum. The treatment is surgical removal. Subsequently both the COC and progestogen-only methods should be avoided (*see Qs 5.96, 5.134, 7.51*).

6.40 Is the COC, like cigarettes, linked with Crohn's disease?

This example of inflammatory bowel disease is discussed in *Q 5.145* and also in a 2003 guidance paper from the Faculty FF PRHC (Journal of Family Planning and Reproductive Health Care 29: 127–135). They conclude that 'a pathogenic role for the COC is unsubstantiated'.

In the UK, pre-existing Crohn's is seen as WHO 2 or 3 for the COC depending on severity (*Q 5.145*). During severe exacerbations of any inflammatory bowel disease the risk of thromboembolism puts the COC into WHO category 4.

6.41 What is the differential diagnosis of abdominal pain that could be related to COC use?

1 Thrombosis of major intra-abdominal vessels such as the hepatic veins or a mesenteric artery or vein.
2 Gallstones (*see Q 6.36*).
3 Pancreatitis (*see Q 6.38*).
4 Liver adenoma (*see Q 6.39*).
5 Acute porphyria *see Q 6.42*).

Much more commonly, the pain will have an unrelated aetiology!

INBORN ERRORS OF METABOLISM

6.42 Why is the COC contraindicated in the acute porphyrias, and what advice should be given to those with latent porphyria (in their genome) but who have not suffered an attack?

Both combined pills *and* progestogens alone can provoke attacks of acute porphyria. All who have had an acute attack – especially if that was itself triggered by either of these hormones – are therefore in category WHO 4 for both hormones.

Those who are asymptomatic but have the inherited enzyme defect and excrete excess porphobilinogen in their urine are also in WHO 4 for the COC. But the progestogen-only method of emergency contraception (*see Q 10.28*) can be used – cautiously – provided the risks are fully explained and accepted (WHO 3): special caution is necessary if the woman is in her teens or early 20s because these are the ages at which first attacks of acute porphyria are most common.

The POP can also be tried with considerable caution in latent cases if no other contraceptive is acceptable (WHO 3). Anecdotally, I have treated a latent acute porphyria case successfully with the POP after she had twice had no symptoms with the levonorgestrel-only emergency method. But injections (and arguably implants) should never be used because, unlike tablets, they cannot be stopped rapidly if a first attack actually is provoked.

6.43 Should the COC be avoided by women with non-acute porphyrias?

This is a complex subject and further advice for individual cases can be obtained from the Porphyria Service of the Department of Medical Biochemistry at the University Hospital of Wales in Cardiff, which stresses that the acute hepatic porphyrias are the main problem, and that the other porphyrias are not in WHO category 4 for synthetic oestrogens and progestogens: generally, they would be in WHO 2. However, oestrogens have been blamed for the pathogenesis of porphyria cutanea tarda, and patients who have been treated should be warned that they might relapse and need further treatment if the COC were used (i.e. it is in category WHO 3).

RESPIRATORY SYSTEM

Beware of the label 'pleurisy', which Vessey showed was twice as likely to be given to a COC-taker as to a non-user. If unexplained pleuritic chest pain or dyspnoea occurs (especially in a COC taker recently returned from holiday after a long-haul flight) this is pulmonary embolism until proved otherwise (*see Qs 6.1 and 6.13*).

6.44 Does the COC promote allergic rhinitis or asthma?

There is some tenuous evidence of a causal association between COC use and these conditions, particularly the former (*see Q 6.69*). But many with both complaints continue to use modern COCs with apparent impunity.

Professor Farmer, in his 1999 GP database study, showed – unexpectedly – a doubled risk of VTE in patients with asthma. This is most likely explained by diagnostic bias (asthma being a condition involving so much contact with physicians) but needs further study.

URINARY SYSTEM

6.45 What is the link between COC use and urinary tract infections?

Several studies have shown that such infections are more common in COC-users than in controls. Women on the pill might have more frequent intercourse, thus increasing their risk of so-called 'honeymoon cystitis'. But some studies have also shown an increased incidence of symptomless bacteriuria in COC-users, resolving when the pill is stopped. This suggests a causal link, so in recurrent cystitis it might sometimes be worth transferring to another method (but normally avoiding the diaphragm among female barriers, *see Q 4.51*).

REPRODUCTIVE SYSTEM – OBSTETRICS

6.46 What are the risks to the fetus if the woman continues to take the COC during early pregnancy?

In animal research, sex steroids can certainly be teratogens. Diethylstilbestrol is a non-steroidal oestrogen that can harm the human fetus, often with very delayed manifestations; and the complex literature about deliberate hormone use (e.g. the former hormone pregnancy tests) in early pregnancy includes some studies that suggest an increased incidence of rare congenital abnormalities.

The copious literature is largely reassuring about the COC. The rate of birth defects in the Oxford/FPA and RCGP studies following COC exposure in pregnancy was no higher than expected in any group of women having a planned baby. In a major study of 1370 abnormal babies in Connecticut there was no increase in COC use during the pregnancies compared with the mothers of normal infants. Studies of national birth defect registers in Hungary and Finland also strongly suggest that pill use in pregnancy has no effect on visible malformations, although multiple births are more common.

The rule that a pregnant woman should avoid all drugs, especially in the first trimester, remains the ideal. But the situation envisaged by the question is not uncommon – can the woman be given any kind of risk estimate? She can certainly not be promised a normal baby. Quite apart from the uncertainty about rare anomalies, at least 2% of all babies show an important abnormality. Bracken (1990) found a relative risk from COC use of 0.99 (i.e. no detectable change) for all important malformations, in a meta-analysis of 12 prospective studies. This agrees with the large population-based case–control studies.

Note that there should be no added risk at all after failed postcoital hormone treatment, which is given before implantation (*see Q 10.19*).

6.47 Is there any residual fetal risk for ex-pill-users?

Here the balance of the published work is heavily tilted towards absence of risk. In 1981 an expert scientific group of the WHO declared categorically that there was no evidence of any adverse effects on the fetus of pill use prior to conception. The only residual anxiety relates to the fact that alterations in mineral and vitamin levels have been observed in OC-users (*see Q 5.98* and *Table 5.7*). These can take a few weeks to revert to normal and supplementation with vitamins (most importantly folic acid) at and after conception has been shown to reduce the risk of neural tube defects in women with a previously affected baby.

6.48 Should women stop the COC well ahead of conception?

Some authorities advise that they should discontinue the pill and use a mechanical method of contraception for two to three cycles. This has not been proved to help, although it should certainly do no harm. Ultrasound scanning has lessened the importance of this for dating of the pregnancy. Although most authorities do not consider them important, some couples do find it reassuring that there are no detectable changes from normal in vitamin and mineral metabolism by about 2 months post pill. The FPA pill leaflet no longer recommends waiting for one or more natural periods before trying to become pregnant.

A woman who conceives sooner than any arbitrary time should, in the light of *Q 6.47*, be very strongly reassured. Avoiding drugs and cigarettes is far more important! Along with an adequate, balanced diet, the Chief Medical Officer recommends a daily dose of 0.4 mg folic acid as routine prophylaxis against neural tube defects, starting before conception.

Specialist advice should be obtained before conception, if a woman on antiepileptic therapy plans a baby.

For trophoblastic disease, *see Q 5.77*.

REPRODUCTIVE SYSTEM – GYNAECOLOGY

6.49 How does the COC affect the symptoms associated with the menstrual cycle?

Beneficially in most respects (see the summary list in *Q 5.56*). Regular bleeding patterns are the norm but if there is irregular bleeding it is important to remember all the non-pill causes of BTB (*see Qs 5.168 and 5.169, Table 5.15*)!

Premenstrual syndrome was less common overall in the RCGP study but any prescriber knows that some individual pill takers do complain of a similar symptom-complex towards the end of each packet, with fluid retention, breast tenderness and depression/irritability predominating. These symptoms seem to be more common on phasic pills, and less frequent in users of Yasmin™. However, overall they remain more frequent in (so-called) normal cycles than in monophasic pill-taking cycles, especially if two or more packets are taken in succession (*see Qs 5.31 and 5.133*).

Similarly, most women notice the menstrual flow to be both lighter and less painful, but a minority who normally have light menses actually report the reverse.

BTB, absent WTB on the COC and secondary amenorrhoea after COC use are cycle symptoms considered elsewhere (*see Qs 5.10, 5.61–5.67 and 5.160–5.177*).

6.50 What is the effect of COCs on pelvic infection, functional ovarian cysts and fibroids?

These effects appear to be beneficial, overall (*see Qs 5.59, 5.60, 5.96 and 5.133*).

6.51 What effect does the combined pill have on endometriosis?

This condition is sometimes treated but more often maintained in suppression after initial definitive surgical or medical treatment by a progestogen-dominant COC such as Eugynon-30™ or Microgynon-30™, on a continuous or tricycle basis (*see Q 5.31*).

There is also a definite clinical impression that it is less common among current users of combined OCs, and this has received some confirmation by the RCGP and Oxford/FPA but protection among ex-users is not clear and the reverse has even been shown in other studies. Perhaps a potential benefit is not aided by the regular PFIs and bleeds of normal pill-taking, unlike the continuous or almost continuous regimens used therapeutically (and increasingly as a woman's choice).

The most significant gynaecological effect of the COC of course is a benefit: protection against cancers of the ovary and endometrium (discussed in *Qs 5.57, 5.75, 5.76*).

6.52 Does the COC cause vaginal discharge?

Do not attribute this to the pill without first eliminating other causes:

1   Cervical erosion (now better known as ectopy). This was definitely more common in the prospective studies based on COCs containing 50 μg or more of oestrogen. It still occurs, although less frequently, on modern pills and requires treatment only if the woman complains.
2   On the other hand, some women (especially if taking very progestogen-dominant pills) complain of vaginal dryness.
3   It is still generally believed that thrush (candidiasis) is more frequent in COC users. Yet a paper with the title *The pill does not cause 'thrush'* was published in the *British Journal of Obstetrics and Gynaecology* in 1985. The journal would never have allowed such a title if this study of over 1300 women attending three departments of genitourinary medicine in England had been the slightest bit equivocal! Other recent studies are confirmatory. This is perhaps because current low-oestrogen pills have less pregnancy-mimicking effect on the glycogen content of vaginal cells. In practice, it should certainly not be assumed that modern pills are to blame in any case of recurrent thrush and the condition is therefore WHO 1 for the COC method.
4   *Trichomonas vaginalis*: COCs seem to provide some (as yet unexplained) protection against this, but none against the transmission of other STIs.

6.53 Does the COC affect other vaginal conditions?

There is a suggestion from research in the USA that the COC protects against the rare toxic shock syndrome. No effect of the pill either way has been reported on the incidence of bacterial vaginosis.

THE BREASTS

6.54 What effects does the COC have on the breasts?

For benign breast disease, see Q 5.96, and for breast cancer see Qs 5.81–5.93. Most women notice an increase in size of their breasts and some change in texture. These effects might be acceptable but breast tenderness is not. It can occur in susceptible women with any pill formulation but seems particularly associated with the last phase of phasic brands.

Galactorrhoea among pill takers is rare and needs investigation (plasma prolactin). A pituitary adenoma or microadenoma should be definitely excluded before labelling this as a minor side-effect (which it can sometimes be).

6.55 Should the combined pill be used during lactation?

In my view and that of the WHO, the answer is a definite 'no'. Breastfeeding is WHO 4 for the pill on several counts. First it is an 'overkill' because practically 100% contraception can be obtained by the combination of lactation with the POP (see Q 7.16). Second, the COC frequently reduces the volume and quality of milk, and third, a larger dose of hormone is being given to the breast-fed infant than would be the case with the POP.

MUSCULOSKELETAL SYSTEM

6.56 If given to young, postpubertal girls, will the COC cause stunting of growth? Indeed, are any other adverse effects more likely in very young teenagers than in the older young woman?

Given in high dose to young female animals, oestrogen alone can lead to premature closure of the epiphyses. However, there is no evidence that a daily dose of 30 μg or even 50 μg of EE, especially when taken with progestogen, has any effect on the potential height in postpubertal girls. Menstruation normally starts when adult weight and height have mostly been achieved. Pill taking should always be delayed until menstruation is established.

Young teenagers need good counselling, if the COC is to be prescribed at all. The risks they run are great, affecting so many aspects of emotional development, their future ability to have stable relationships, their total sexual and reproductive health (see Qs 11.3, 11.10, 11.11). But these are the risks of early sexual activity. No proven risks (or benefits) specific to the COC are known to be greater when it is started at 13 than at 23. So the strictly pharmacological considerations are not different from those for a woman in her early 20s. However, in amenorrhoeic teens, the oestrogen content of the COC might be therapeutic, in assisting the achievement of peak bone mass.

6.57 Is the COC associated with carpal tunnel syndrome, primary Raynaud's disease, chilblains, and cramps in the legs?

Associated, yes, these have been described: but causation is less certain. Raynaud's phenomenon might be a manifestation of a contraindicating condition (such as a connective tissue disorder, which might itself promote arterial disease), so the symptom must be investigated.

Otherwise, if these problems are troublesome it is worth a trial of discontinuation of the COC; but it can also be continued if the patient so desires.

6.58 How should one assess the complaint of leg pains and cramps?

Careful assessment and examination are important. If bilateral, the symptom is less likely to be significant but look for water retention, varicose veins, chilblains or associated Raynaud's phenomenon.

If unilateral, DVT must be excluded. If in doubt the pill should be stopped and the patient referred for further investigation. Her contraceptive future depends on an accurate diagnosis being made.

6.59 How does the COC affect arthritis and related disorders?

A reduction in rheumatoid arthritis risk has emerged in some studies but not others. The consistent finding is a protective effect against severe manifestations of the disease in current COC-users (Beerthuizen 2001 *Gynaecology Forum* 6:18–19). This makes it WHO 1, a good choice for most with this condition.

Tenosynovitis and a form of allergic polyarthritis can occur but causation has not been proved (*see Q 5.146* for SLE).

CUTANEOUS SYSTEM

6.60 Which skin conditions can be improved by COCs – and by which COCs?

Acne, seborrhoea and sometimes hirsutism can be benefited by any of the oestrogen-dominant COCs (whereas there is little or no benefit when there is progestogen dominance, *see Qs 6.21 and 6.22*). In the UK, only one pill brand (Dianette™) has a specific indication with respect to these conditions, see below.

6.61 What is different about drospirenone, the progestogen used in Yasmin™?

Yasmin™ is a new (2002) monophasic combined oral contraceptive marketed by Schering. Each tablet contains 3.0 mg drospirenone and 30 μg of EE. Drospirenone differs from other progestogens in COCs:

- It has diuretic properties due to antimineralocorticoid activity. This might help to oppose the salt and fluid-retaining effects of EE and so help symptoms like bloatedness (*see Q 6.63*).
- Yasmin™ has also been in a small trial, compared with Microgynon-30™, to induce a very small (statistically significant) lowering of mean BP.
- Drospirenone acts as an antiandrogen, so the combination is an alternative to Dianette™ for the treatment of moderately severe acne and PCOS.
- Drospirenone with EE is an oestrogen-dominant combination and so cannot be expected to have the lower risk of VTE associated with the functionally antioestrogenic levonorgestrel (*see Q 5.110*) of, for example Microgynon™. But the actual comparative VTE risk of Yasmin™ is so far unknown.

6.62 Compared with other modern pills, does Yasmin™ truly have an advantage with respect to weight gain?!

See Q 6.33 for the minimal effect on body mass of alternatives. A European multicentre, randomized trial does indeed show statistically lower body weight changes as compared with the desogestrel-containing Marvelon™. However, most authorities interpret this decrement in weight as due only to diuresis, so in long-term use there is a maintained slight (about 1%) reduction of total body water compared with controls. After allowing for this diuretic effect over the two years of the study, there was the same gradient of weight gain with both the products studied. This is most likely to be just the normal background increase (*Q 6.33*) and so not caused by either COC!

6.63 Given the above and considerations of cost, what criteria should normally be applied for using Yasmin™?

Yasmin™ is to be welcomed as a new choice for appropriate women, as an alternative to Dianette™ (unlike the latter, it is not marketed primarily for its acne/hirsutes benefits) and Marvelon™, which is clinically recognized as the best 'mainstream' pill for acne. It is relatively costly.

Interestingly, this product adds some new WHO 4 conditions for pills: it should not be used in patients at risk of high potassium levels (i.e. renal insufficiency, hepatic dysfunction and adrenal insufficiency). After assessing this and all the usual COC contraindications, in my view, Yasmin™ is a useful 'second line' COC as follows:

■ A clear indication for oestrogen/antiandrogen therapy (significant acne, PCOS).

■ During COC follow-up, as a useful oestrogen-dominant second choice for empirical control of minor side-effects, particularly those associated with fluid retention such as bloatedness and cyclical breast enlargement. Whether it is better than other COCs for PMS-type symptoms remains to be established (*see Q 5.133*).

■ Raised BP: the level being such as to make the clinician consider a change from the current formulation of combined pill – but COC still clinically usable, i.e. BP increased, but only to 140/90 which is the upper limit of WHO 2 for raised BP, or maybe a little above. Such a switch to another COC, rather than another method, would only be if the BP were well below the 160/100 level, which is seen as WHO 4 (*Q 5.119 and Table 5.11*). Cerazette would be a good alternative if the BP were not to respond adequately.

■ Last and definitely least, what about weight? If the BMI is already > 30 the BNF rightly recommends a less oestrogen-dominant formulation with levonorgestrel or norethisterone. Otherwise, anxiety about weight gain, if coupled with a history of acne or of probable fluid retention with earlier pills, might occasionally justify Yasmin™.

6.64 Where does Dianette™ feature now we have Yasmin™? Is it to be seen primarily as an effective treatment for acne and hirsutism?

Dianette™ is an antiandrogen/synthetic oestrogen combination (cyproterone acetate (CPA) 2 mg with EE 35 μg) for the oral treatment of moderately severe acne and moderate hirsutism in women, especially when due to PCOS (*see Q 5.65*).

These are its indications but it is also a reliable anovulant and often gives good cycle control as well. It has similar rules for missed tablets, interactions with drugs (including antibiotics), absolute and relative contraindications, and requirements for monitoring as COC. But it is **not** indicated for use solely as an oral contraceptive. It can be free of charge to the woman if the prescription is marked 'for contraception' or the symbol for 'female' (♀).

Dianette™ is definitely an oestrogen-dominant product, as shown by its desired effect in PCOS of permitting EE to raise SHBG. So it must be expected to allow the oestrogen similarly to have relatively greater effects in a prothrombotic direction than a levonorgestrel product would (see above); and indeed Vasilalus et al. 2001 (*Lancet* 358:1427–29) found a four-fold increase in VTE risk compared with levonorgestrel pills. So the CSM advice (BNF 2003) is that Dianette™ is contraindicated in women with a close FH of confirmed idiopathic VTE i.e. WHO 4 in all circumstances (cf *Table 5.11* for ordinary COC).

There has been no good head-to-head RCT of Yasmin™ versus Dianette™, but indirect evidence suggests Yasmin™ would have almost identical effectiveness for the conditions for which Dianette™ is indicated.

With either product caution is essential because so many prospective users with PCOS do have high BMIs (30–39, WHO 3). However, the added benefit due to being a therapy and not just a contraceptive might be held in many cases to justify some added risk (i.e. implying, despite the high BMI, a maintained benefit–risk difference).

6.65 What is the recommended maximum duration of treatment with Dianette™?

The SPC recommends 'withdraw when resolution [of the acne or hirsutism] is complete' but repeat courses can be given if the conditions recur.

There is a concern that prolonged high-dose treatment with CPA can cause benign and malignant liver tumours in rats, and hepatotoxicity has been described with the much higher 50-mg-plus doses used by dermatologists and for prostate cancer therapy. There is some reassuring evidence, however, from the MILTS study, that the 2 mg dose as in Dianette™ does not increase the risk of such tumours above that for all the other COCs (and which is very small, *see* Q 5.95).

Resolution of acne is usually within a year, yet in my experience patients develop a very strong 'brand loyalty' to their Dianette™. The quoted SPC statement implies that we should encourage them to switch when their condition is controlled to an oestrogen-dominant COC (commonly to Marvelon™, reassuring clients that this is usually sufficient as maintenance therapy). If they do not tolerate the alternative they might well accept Yasmin™, which indeed might nowadays be used instead of Dianette™ from the outset.

It is also acceptable ultimately to return to and continue with Dianette™ for much longer than 1 year, assuming the woman accepts the unlikely, but possible, hepatic and prothrombotic risks.

6.66 Which skin conditions are more common in COC users?

1   *Chloasma/melasma*: this 'pregnancy mask' can develop in women on the COC after exposure to sunlight, just as in pregnancy. The condition can be very slow to fade after the pill is stopped. Mild degrees can be masked by careful use of cosmetics and tolerated if exposure to sun can be

reduced. The condition can also occur/recur with the POP or other progestogen-only contraceptives, hence a non-hormonal method might have to be chosen.

2 *Photosensitivity*: in prospective studies this problem tends to be reported more often in COC takers than controls. Very rarely it might be the first manifestation of one of the porphyrias (usually non-acute type, *see Q 6.43*). Once acquired, like chloasma it tends to be permanent even if the pill is discontinued.

3 *Pemphigoid (herpes) gestationis*: if this serious skin condition occurs it absolutely contraindicates the COC (WHO 4).

4 *Hirsutism*: is unlikely to be truly caused by the COC, but may be helped by an oestrogen-dominant/antiandrogenic product, especially Yasmin™ or Dianette™.

5 *Loss of scalp hair*: there may be a true link but not a long-term, pill-related problem. Head hair density is always the resultant of the telogen (resting) and anagen (growth) phases. In pregnancy, and similarly in some women on the COC, a greater proportion than usual of the hair is synchronized into the growth phase. This is fine at the time but can lead to a noticeable synchronized loss some time later – as is often reported in the puerperium.

6 *Telangiectasia, rosacea, neurodermatitis, spider naevi, erythema multiforme, erythema nodosum, eczema, and possibly other skin disorders*: all these have been described but not established, as possibly causally associated or exacerbated by COCs, in a minority of women (*see Q 5.136* for a discussion of melanoma).

6.67 What action should be taken if such skin problems present in a COC taker?

First, consider discontinuing the COC. Severe conditions such as erythema multiforme or pemphigoid gestationis would normally mean future avoidance of this method. If the condition has an immune/allergic basis it is usually unclear whether the COC steroids are the actual allergens (*see Q 6.71*). According to the views of the woman herself, therefore, and any dermatologist involved, if the condition is relatively mild (e.g. erythema nodosum) she can be cautiously rechallenged with a low-dose COC, perhaps containing a different progestogen, or with the POP. Recurrence would suggest another method.

6.68 Does the COC cause gingivitis? Any other oral problems?

Hypertrophic gingivitis is a rare but well-recognized complication of COC use. Lesser degrees are more common, as in pregnancy. Symptoms are minimized by good oral hygiene. 'Dry socket', a painful state after tooth extraction, is also said to be more common in COC users.

ALLERGIES AND INFLAMMATIONS

6.69 What effect does the COC have on immune mechanisms?

Several studies on immunoglobulins have suggested that artificial sex steroids can modify immune mechanisms. The effects are of a similar nature to, but less marked than, those associated with pregnancy. A study from France, however, in which antibodies to EE were reported in patients suffering from venous thrombosis, has not been confirmed.

The RCGP study, in particular among the prospective studies, showed an increase in inflammations and some disorders that are believed to have an immune basis. However, as shown in *Fig. 6.1* these are partly balanced by a well-established protective effect against thyroid over- and underactivity, and probably rheumatoid arthritis (*see Q 6.59*). Once again, as with both malignant and benign tumours (see *Figs 5.8* and *5.9*), combination OCs seem to be capable of causing both beneficial and adverse effects within the same medical field. Causative associations are not all proven by any means and the magnitude of the effects described in *Fig. 6.1* is mostly small; but we badly need more information.

6.70 Does use of the COC promote transmission of HIV infection? Or make AIDS more likely after infection?

Studies among prostitutes in Nairobi were the first to suggest an increase in the likelihood of seroconversion to HIV positive if the COC were used, but a truly causative link has not been established. Effective contraception is obviously important for any woman known to be HIV positive, as well as

Some apparent associations of COC use with immune disorders/inflammations

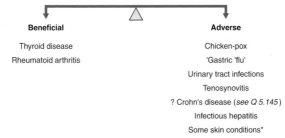

Beneficial	Adverse
Thyroid disease	Chicken-pox
Rheumatoid arthritis	'Gastric 'flu'
	Urinary tract infections
	Tenosynovitis
	? Crohn's disease (*see Q 5.145*)
	Infectious hepatitis
	Some skin conditions*

*See text, Q 6.66

Fig. 6.1 Immune disorders/inflammations and the pill. Q 6.69.

regular condom use. For compliance reasons the LNG-IUS or DMPA are usually better choices than the COC. They do not appear to worsen the prognosis.

6.71 Do women sometimes become allergic to the COC hormones, or in COC users is there an increased tendency to react to other allergens?

Anecdotal data exist to suggest that either can occur. For example, in vitro studies of blood lymphocytes suggested hypersensitivity to mestranol in two cases (one of erythema multiforme, one of erythema nodosum). However, I have had a case of erythema nodosum who was able to go back on the same brand of COC without suffering any recurrence.

SPECIAL CONSIDERATIONS: WHEN TO COME OFF THE PILL?

6.72 Are there benefits to be gained from taking breaks from COC use? Is duration of use of any relevance?

From the point of view of preservation of fertility, the answer is a categorical no on both counts (*see Qs 5.68 and 5.69*). In relation to all the examples of circulatory disease, duration of use has now been found to have no effect (*see Q 5.101*).

Even if, intuitively, it is still felt best to limit total duration of use, breaks will be of no value; unless they are so long as to have a real influence on total accumulated duration of use (*Fig. 6.2*).

▲

Fig. 6.2 Breaks and accumulated duration of use of the COC. Q 6.72. The blocks represent segments of pill-taking duration (in which the only breaks taken are the pill-free weeks). Note how a woman who takes 6-monthly breaks every 2 years still accumulates 10 years of total duration in 12 years.

It is worth reminding any woman with this concern that during 10 years she has in fact taken 130 breaks! Not that this is essential of course: appreciating that she would be taking more hormone dose per year, she might have chosen to tricycle (see *Table 5.2, Qs 5.30 and 5.31*).

Metabolic risk markers show no apparent progression beyond 2 years' continuous use. It could even be argued that repeated restarting of the COC might be more harmful than the relatively steady-state situation that is maintained during sustained use.

The main problem with breaks of several months at a time was well shown in a study in which, during a planned break of just 6 months, 25% of young women had unwanted pregnancies.

6.73 What if she is hard to convince that a break will not benefit her?

Of course we should never force anyone to continue: if a woman wants to make a break then what matters most is to arrange an effective and satisfactory alternative. But so often the notion is not hers at all, but comes from a friend or a magazine and, if so, *Q 6.72* might help to reassure her about continuing.

6.74 What about duration of use and cancer risk? (*see Qs 5.71–5.95*)

Some studies show beneficial effects on cancer of the ovary and endometrium and others show possible harmful effects on cancer of the liver, cervix and breast. In each of these opposite categories both the beneficial and the adverse effects described are usually found to be greater with increasing duration of use! (The exception is breast cancer, where age and recency of use are the important factors, *see Q 5.85*). So the advantages of increased duration of use would help to balance the disadvantages. Short breaks are again unlikely to be relevant, see *Fig. 6.2*.

It is currently impossible to state with certainty whether the good effects of pill use outweigh the adverse effects on cancer overall (*see Q 5.73*) – although they might do so – and it is equally impossible to assess accurately the changes on both sides of the equation caused by increased duration of use (*see Q 6.75 and Table 6.3*): the pros and cons seem roughly in balance.

6.75 How much should age per se influence prescribing, with regard to both cardiovascular system risk and cancer?

CVS RISKS AND AGE

Here opinions have changed since the first edition of this book, triggered by the landmark decision of the FDA's Fertility and Maternal Health Drugs Advisory Committee in October 1989. Their recommendation, subsequently endorsed by the FDA itself, was for:

TABLE 6.3 Management by age, smoking and duration of COC use

A: Age and COC use

	Age (years)				
	30	**35**	**40**	**45**	**50–51**
Smoker	Review	Change method	(COC contraindicated for contraception in UK practice) (POPs and HRT usable)		
Non-smoker	–	Review	Review	Review	Change method, or no method now if post menopause

B: Accumulated duration of use

	Duration (years)				
	5	**10**	**15**	**20**	**25⁺**
Smoker	Review	Second review	?Change method	Change method	–
Non-smoker	–	Review	Review	Review	Review

Note:
Regardless of smoking, all with a relevant family history (or other risk factor) for breast cancer should review use regularly as years go by, in the light of best available data (see Q 5.91 and 5.92) and in the context of new contraceptive choices now available.

The removal of all age limits on the use of (combined) oral contraceptives by healthy non-smoking women – i.e. free of all risk factors.

Was this a cavalier decision, flying in the face of previously agreed practice? I think not, because:

1 non-smoking pill takers are actually much 'safer' than we used to think
2 modern prescribing and monitoring are more structured and careful
3 the pills themselves are believed to be safer
4 above all, we now have a much better appreciation of the benefits of the COC to gynaecological and some aspects of general health for women, most particularly older women (*see Qs 11.38 and 11.39*).

In short, even though the cardiovascular risks (and breast cancer risks, see below) do increase with age, the benefits increase at least as much and the risk–benefit ratio until the average age of the menopause is therefore probably unchanged. But only at their own request for healthy and ideally migraine-free non-smokers!

After age 51 (mean age of menopause) fertility is so low that I recommend using a less strong contraceptive than the COC anyway (*see Q 11.53*).

> The important issue of how to diagnose the menopause when it is masked by the COC or other hormones is discussed in *Qs 7.62–7.64, 8.47, 11.43–11.47.*

CANCER RISKS WITH AGE

These show a general increase with age; and the 1996 CGHFBC 'model' for breast cancer risk shows that the pill-attributable 24% increment applied to an increasing background risk suggests proportionally more cases as the pill is used by older women (*see Q 5.91*). (The reassuring 2002 study from CDC (*see Q 5.86*) gives insufficient information on pill users who continue through to the menopause.)

But the COC protects against cancer of the ovary and endometrium and probably the large bowel, the incidence of which rises particularly over age 40. The extent of this balancing of the risk is difficult to quantify.

Fortunately, there are several equally effective new options for older pill users (banded copper IUDs, IUSs, implants).

6.76 If a smoker really does give up cigarettes at age 35, can she continue to take the COC? And if so, until what age?

There are no good data about this important question, for both practical and ethical reasons. Ex-smokers are a rare breed and their cardiovascular morbidity would need examining prospectively with and without continuing to take the pill. We can extrapolate to some extent from the British Regional Heart Study of 7735 men, which reported that in ex-smokers of up to 20 cigarettes a day no excess risk of ischaemic heart disease (IHD) was observed in those who had quit 6–10 years prior to the screening, compared with never-smokers. However, heavy ex-smokers (> 20 per day) still had a significantly higher risk after 11–20 years.

Other studies show a marked early decline in risk of IHD, due to loss of the acute metabolic effects of smoking, but they suggest in men that it takes 10 years to return to the levels seen in never-smokers. If this delay is due to early coronary atheroma generated by years of smoking, one must be concerned about the prothrombotic effects of EE in any COC (*see Q 11.41*).

According to a 1990 report from the US, in women ex-smokers '…the increase in risk of a first myocardial infarction dissipated after 2–3 years'.

This is more rapid than among the British men, but it does not establish safety if COCs had been taken and continued to be taken. The ex-heavy-smoker cannot be reassured like the risk-factor free woman about continuing with the pill until her menopause (*see Q 6.75*); and in my view as also shown in *Table 5.11* (p. 190 and *see Q 5.123ff*) for such ex-smokers continuing pill use above age 40 does become WHO 3 rather than WHO 2.

SOME REVISION QUESTIONS

6.77 What are the medical myths about prescribing the pill?

The list in *Table 6.4* is not exhaustive but includes some important examples currently believed by some healthcare professionals.

TABLE 6.4 Pill myths	
Myth – Do not prescribe the COC in the following circumstances:	**Actuality – The COC is: (WHO 1) unless otherwise stated)**
Wish to optimize fertility	Beneficial (Q 5.69)
Fibroids	Beneficial (Q 5.96)
Current amenorrhoea, after investigation	Usually beneficial (Q 5.65)
Past amenorrhoea, resolved	Neutral (Q 5.67)
Recent menarche (menstrual cycles established)	Neutral (Q 6.56)
History of gestational diabetes (watch weight)	Neutral (Q 5.148)
Thrush	Neutral (Q 6.52)
Recent trophoblastic disease (hCG now normal)	Neutral (Q 5.77)
Sickle-cell trait	Neutral (Q 5.143)
Thalassaemia	Neutral (Q 5.138)
Epilepsy (allowing for drug interactions)	Neutral (sometimes beneficial) (Q 6.26)
Mitral valve prolapse	WHO 2 (Table 5.14)
Sickle-cell anaemia	WHO 2 (Q 5.143)
Any migraine (non-focal, tolerable, no change)	WHO 2 (Q 5.159)
Cervical neoplasia (preinvasive)	WHO 2 (Q 5.80)
Wish to minimize *overall* cancer risk	Not certain, but avoiding COC probably increases this risk (Q 5.75)

6.78 What are the pill myths relating to continuing use of the method?

TABLE 6.5 Pill myths	
Myth	**Actuality**
1 There should be a break from pill use every few years	False (Q 6.72)
2 Duration of pill use should never be more than 5 (or 10) years at a time	False (Qs 6.72–6.74)
3 The pill should be stopped in all women reaching 35 years	Smokers (or if risk factors) (Q 6.75)
4 The COC should be stopped before all surgery	Only for major or leg surgery (Q 6.14)
5 Stop COC if there is prolonged absence of withdrawal bleeds (to preserve fertility)	Irrelevant (Q 5.10)

There are also myths which many doctors share with pill-takers about 'missed pills' (see Qs 5.18, 6.88 and 10.23)

6.79 In what important situations do doctors commonly forget to enquire whether the patient is on an oestrogen-containing pill?

1 Emergencies: involving surgery, immobilization of a leg for fracture or confinement to bed.
2 When elective arrangements are made for a major operation or for surgery or sclerotherapy for varicose veins.
3 When any potentially interacting drugs are prescribed, particularly when neurologists change antiepileptic drug regimens.
4 When arranging any laboratory test, especially of the blood. The results of many tests can be modified by the COC (see *Table 5.7*, p. 164).

NEW DEVELOPMENTS: NEW ROUTES OF ADMINISTRATION OF COMBINED HORMONES WITH OESTROGEN

There are no less than three new routes for these hormones currently appearing or shortly anticipated:

6.80 What is EVRA™?

EVRA™ is a transdermal patch delivering ethinylestradiol (EE) with norelgestromin, the active metabolite of norgestimate. The daily skin dose of 150 µg norelgestromin and 20 µg EE produces blood levels in the range of those after a tablet of Cilest™ but without either the diurnal fluctuations or the oral peak dose given to the liver. Pending more specific research information, all the absolute and relative contraindications and indeed most of the above practical management advice in Chapters 5 and 6 about the COC apply, with obvious minor adjustments, to this new product. It appears to be relatively oestrogen-dominant, with a bleeding and non-bleeding side-effect profile very like Cilest™ itself – plus about 2 percent of women in the trials had local skin reactions which led to discontinuation.

The patch has excellent adhesion even in hot climates and when bathing or showering; the incidence of detachment of patches was 1.8 % (complete) and 2.9 % (partial). In the pooled analysis of 3 pivotal studies (Zieman M et al 2002 *Fertility and Sterility* 77 (2) Suppl 2: S13–18) the Pearl index for consistent users of EVRA™ was similar to the oral pills – and less than 1 per 100 woman-years. Interestingly, in the clinical trials one-third of the few failures occurred in the 3% weighing above 90 kg. Whether this was because of greater dilution of the dose given in more total body water, or somehow related to their extra subcutaneous adipose tissue, is unknown. But in my view this apparently reduced effectiveness contraindicates EVRA™ for such women (who are at least WHO 3 for VTE risk at that level of likely BMI anyway…).

Maintenance of EVRA™ efficacy

■ Avoid use at all if body weight > 90 kg
■ Each patch is worn for 7 days, for 3 consecutive weeks followed by a 'patch free week' and in one of the RCTs this regimen was shown to aid compliance. There is 2 days 'margin for error' for late patch changes. One would therefore expect better user-efficacy for those who are forgetful, but:
■ As with the COC it will still be essential never to lengthen the contraception-free (patch-free) interval. If this interval *exceeds* 8 days for any reason (either through late application or the first new patch detaching and this being identified late), I advise extra precautions for the duration of the first freshly applied patch (i.e. for 7 days). This should be after immediate emergency contraception if there has been sexual exposure, during the preceding patch-free time.
■ There would of course be the possibility of offering it in a 'tricycle' way, as with the COC – meaning the consecutive use of say nine or twelve patches before the break. By analogy with the COC this would be more effective for forgetful users and give fewer bleeds, but with more hormone intake per month and at added cost. And since the labelling in the SPC specifies menstrual postponement for just one cycle, this is use of a licensed product in an unlicensed way: so it should be on a 'named patient' basis (see Appendix A).

■ Absorption problems through vomiting/diarrhoea, and tetracycline by mouth, have no effect on this method's efficacy, but:

■ During any short term enzyme inducer therapy, and for 28 days after this ends, additional contraception is still advised as for COCs – plus elimination of any patch-free intervals during all this time.

6.81 What news is there about systemic contraception by the vaginal route?

Workers in Brazil and Israel in the early 1980s showed that a standard pill (LNG 250 μg plus EE 50 μg), as formulated for oral use, was effective when taken vaginally. Symptoms such as nausea were less frequent, although it is possible that this was partly due to achieving lower blood levels of oestrogen.

Except in South America, where the above version has been marketed since 1999 as Lovelle™, vaginal pills have not become popular, partly because daily compliance remains necessary as for oral pills.

6.82 So when can we expect NuvaRing™ in the UK?

Probably in 2004 or 2005, but this is always difficult to predict because of local commercial factors. Already available in some European countries and the US, this is a combined vaginal ring that releases etonogestrel (3-keto-desogestrel) 120 μg and EE 15 μg per day. It has proved very popular in studies, with excellent cycle control and very few contraceptive failures.

As described in *Q 8.69ff*, vaginal erythematous patches of uncertain origin were discovered during a study of a levonorgestrel-releasing ring at the Margaret Pyke Centre during 1991–92. Fortunately these have not been shown any more frequently in users of NuvaRing™ than in controls. Expulsions were a problem recognized by some women, however, usually during defecation.

NuvaRing™ is normally retained (although there is an option of removing it for the duration of sexual activity) for 3 weeks and then taken out for a withdrawal bleed during the fourth. In many ways it therefore equates to 'Mercilon™ via the vagina' and has the same contraindications and a similar side-effect profile. Alternatively, like EVRA™, it could be used continuously (three or four rings in a row, analogous to tricycling, *see Qs 5.28–5.31, 6.80*).

6.83 When will we see the monthly combined injectable contraceptive (CIC) Lunelle™ in the UK?

This again is difficult to predict: it appears likely to be delayed until a planned self-injector system is perfected, possibly by 2005 or 2006.

Lunelle™, otherwise known as Cyclofem™ (25 mg DMPA with 5 mg estradiol cypionate in 0.5 ml aqueous volume) is injected intramuscularly into deltoid, thigh or buttock. Subsequent doses ought to follow every

28–30 days but must be no sooner than 23 days and no later than 33 days. Regular monthly bleeding lasting about 5 days is expected about 2 weeks after each dose as the oestrogen dose falls.

It has proved effective, fully reversible and popular in the Americas, especially among 'Latino' populations. Cycle control is usually good.

The contraindications, and most side-effects in comparative studies, are as expected for COCs, aside from a trend for more weight gain to be reported.

Watch this space!

 PATIENT QUESTIONS

SOME QUESTIONS ASKED BY USERS ABOUT THE COC

6.84 I am told thrombosis has to do with clots – I have clots with my periods so does this mean that I can't use the pill?

Far from it! Clots with the periods just means that they are heavy, and could well improve dramatically if you went on the pill – the COC would usually do this more reliably than any POP.

6.85 Can I postpone having a pill-period?

Certainly. The bleeding you get between packets of pills is actually entirely caused by you when you take a 7-day break between packets. It is really a 'withdrawal bleed' rather than a proper period and there is no reason why from time to time you should not run two packets on to each other so there is no break and therefore no bleeding. The rules are a little different, however, for so-called phasic pills (*see* Q 5.184).

It is of course an option to have very infrequent pill-periods as in the so-called tricycle regimen (*see* Q 5.31 and *Fig.* 5.4 (p. 120)) – provided you accept the fact that this means taking more of the hormones per year.

6.86 Do I always have to see periods at weekends?

Certainly not. If it happens to have worked out that your periods are tending to come at weekends on any type of COC, all you need to do is to start your next packet about 3 days early one month (meaning you only have a 4-day break), to move your withdrawal bleeding to midweek (*see* Q 5.51).

6.87 My 'period' is much lighter than normal, almost absent in fact and a different colour – does this matter?

No, anything from quite average sort of bleeding through to nothing at all can be normal for the response of an individual woman's womb to the stopping of the pill's hormones. Should you have no periods at all 2 months in a row you should take prompt advice to eliminate the possibility of pregnancy and also to discuss whether you should start the next packet. This action should be taken even if you have only missed one withdrawal bleed after a month during which you missed pills, had vomiting, severe diarrhoea or treatment with an interacting drug.

(Many other questions are asked about issues related to bleeding on the COC, whether normal, abnormal, or absent. These can be answered by reference to *Qs 5.10, 5.32, 5.38, 5.51, 5.62–5.67, 5.170–5.184, 11.17(18–26)*.

6.88   Is it safe to make love in the 7 days between pill packets?

Yes: but only if no pills have been missed (by forgetting, stomach upset or drug interaction) towards the end of the previous packet, and also only if you do in fact start another packet after the pill-free week (*see Qs 5.15–5.24 and 11.17(16)*). Beware, particularly when you come off the pill for any reason. You *never* have seven contraceptively safe days following any last packet of a course of the pill. This might be especially important to remember if you are stopping the pill because of sterilization (of you or your partner).

6.89   Which are the most 'dangerous' pills to be missed – presumably in the middle of the month?

Not so, the middle of the month is the least bad time to miss pills, although you should not make a habit of missing any. The worst pills to be missed are any that result in lengthening of the pill-free time (*see Qs 5.15, 5.18, 5.24*). Never be late starting your next packet! This is something lots of people don't even consider as missing a pill.

6.90   I want to switch from taking the pill every evening to morning pill-taking. How should I do this?

Ideally this should be done by taking two tablets 12 h apart on one day, *not* leaving a 36-h gap. If you want to make the change with the start of a new pack it would be important to take the first new pill early, after 6.5 days, rather than leaving 7.5 days between the last pill of the old and the first of the new packets (see *Fig. 5.1* and *Q 5.15* for the reason why!)

6.91   Are there any problems in pill taking for flight crews or long-haul air travellers?

It is easy to become confused about regular pill taking because of passing through different time zones. The effectiveness problem is when flying due west because the new bedtime pill might be late – hours more than the official 24 h after the preceding one. One solution is a watch that gives the time in the departure city as well as local time, and to continue to base pill taking on the time where the journey began.

On arrival at a new destination pill users should always err on the side of taking a pill too early rather than late.

Suppose you fly to London from Auckland and normally take your pill at bedtime, if you then switch to taking it at the London bedtime you could have a 36-h interval between tablets. This increases the risk of pill-failure (although not much for the COC it would be completely unacceptable for ordinary POPs, *see Qs 7.12–7.21*). With both types of pill it increases the risk of irregular or breakthrough bleeding (BTB). So what should you do?

■ To recap, while on the flight or during any stopover you should continue taking your tablets at the correct hour based on your departure time zone. Nothing else needs to be done.

■ Upon arrival, as the journey was westbound, after your regular COC (or POP) has been taken at 24 h on the departure time basis, take an extra tablet (use the last one in that pack) at the next London bedtime. This will be after 12 more h in the Auckland to London situation, but only 8 h later if the trip was London to Los Angeles, for example. Not a problem.

■ And if the journey was eastbound, taking that day's pill at the correct local time will shorten the actual pill-taking interval and this is always contraceptively safe.

■ If this is done no extra precautions are needed and, with both types of pill, the risk of either BTB or breakthrough conception should be negligible.

6.92 My skin has got worse on the pill, yet I was told it should get better – why is this?

It all depends on the severity of your acne and which pill you have been given. The recommended ones are at *Q 6.22* (see *Table 6.2*, p. 245).

6.93 Does using either the COC or the POP delay the menopause?

No. This occurs as a result of an inexorable process of egg loss, which seems to be unaffected by anything, including never having babies and pill-taking. It even occurs at the same time as it otherwise would in women who as a result of surgery have been left with only one ovary. But it can be brought on earlier by a hysterectomy.

6.94 Can I take antihistamines for hayfever and the pill?

The ones given by your GP, or that you can buy in the chemist, seem to cause no important change in the effectiveness of your pill. Other medicines might do, however (*see Qs 5.33 and 5.34*, *Table 5.3*, p. 126), and the warning sign of an interaction can be bleeding during tablet taking. Always tell any doctor, dentist or hospital that you take the pill.

6.95 Is it true that you are more likely to get drunk if you are on the pill?

Some research published in 1984 suggested this because it showed that alcohol leaves the body more slowly in pill users than in non-pill-users. Subsequently, other researchers in Australia found the opposite – that pill takers recovered from the effect of alcohol more quickly than non-takers!

But the take-home message about which there is no argument is that all women should be extra careful about alcohol. This is because their smaller livers make it have a bigger effect than in men, both short-term and long-term (meaning that the risk of liver damage is greater in women).

6.96 What are the take-home messages for any new pill taker?

1 Your FPA leaflet: this is not to be read and thrown away, it is something to keep safely in a drawer somewhere for ongoing reference along with the PIL in your pill pack.

2 The pill only works if you take it correctly: if you do, each new pack will always start on the same day of the week.

3 Even if bleeding like a 'period' occurs (breakthrough bleeding), carry on pill-taking. Ring for advice if necessary. Nausea is another common early symptom. But both usually settle as your body gets used to the pill.

4 Lovemaking during the 7 days after any packet is only safe if you do go on to the next one: otherwise (if you are stopping the pill for any reason) start using condoms after the last pill in the pack.

5 Even if your 'period' (withdrawal bleed) has not stopped yet, never start your next packet late. This is because the pill-free time is obviously a time when your ovaries are not getting the contraceptive, so might anyway be beginning to escape from its actions.

6 For what to do if any pill(s) are more than 24 h (one day) late, see Q 5.17.

7 Other things that can stop the pill from working include vomiting and some drugs (see Qs 5.25, 5.33–5.42).

8 See a doctor at once if the things listed in Q 6.13 occur. And feel free to come back for any reasons of your own as well, including any symptoms you would like dealt with.

9 As a one-off manoeuvre you can shorten one pill-free gap to make sure all your future withdrawal bleeds avoid weekends.

10 And you can avoid bleeding on holidays, etc. by running packs together. (Discuss this with whoever provides your pills if you want to continue missing out 'periods' long term, see Q 5.31).

11 Good though it is as a contraceptive, the pill does not give adequate protection against STIs. Whenever in doubt, especially with a new partner, use a condom as well.

12 Always feel free to telephone or come back (maybe to the practice nurse) for advice or help at any time.

The progestogen-only pill

7

BACKGROUND AND MECHANISMS

EFFECTIVENESS

BACKGROUND AND MECHANISMS

7.1 What are progestogen-only pills (POPs)?

In the UK these pills contain a microdose of one of four progestogens (*Table 7.1*). They are taken on a continuous daily basis, 365 days a year.

7.2 Which POPs are in current use?

See *Table 7.1*. POPs have accounted for no more than 10% of the UK oral contraceptive market, although this is set to change with the arrival of Cerazette™ (*see Q 7.10*). They have much to commend them, especially in the older age group.

7.3 How much is known about the POP method?

The short answer is: still remarkably little. No large cohort studies are in progress and case–control studies have not been attempted because of the low prevalence of use. Hence we are largely forced to draw on the few metabolic and clinical studies available; and otherwise to extrapolate from available data on the combined pill (adjusting in an admittedly arbitrary way for absence of artificial oestrogen and presence of a particularly small dose of the progestogen).

7.4 What is the mode of action of POPs?

This is summarized in *Table 7.2*. The main action has previously been thought to be the alteration in the cervical mucus. But there is also a considerable effect on ovulation in most women and in most cycles – at least 50–60% of the time – and more in older women. Ovulation might be abolished completely, resulting in amenorrhoea, but even without this there are varying degrees of interference with the ovulatory process, as described in *Q 7.5*.

TABLE 7.1 Progestogen-only pills in the UK			
Name	No. of tablets per packet	Progestogen	Dose (μg)
Norgeston™	35	Levonorgestrel	30
Neogest™	35	Levonorgestrel	37.5*
Micronor™/Noriday™	28	Norethisterone	350
Femulen™	28	Ethynodiol diacetate	500
Cerazette™	28	Desogestrel	75

*Plus 37.5 μg of inactive isomer.

TABLE 7.2 Various progestogen delivery systems

	COC	EVRA™	POP (old type)	NET-EN	DMPA	Cerazette™	Implanon™
Administration	Oral	Transdermal	Oral	i.m.	i.m.	Oral	Subdermal
Frequency	Daily	7-day patches	Daily	2-monthly	3-monthly	Daily	3-yearly
Oestrogen dose	Low	Low	Nil	Nil	Nil	Nil	Nil
Progestogen dose	Low	Low	Ultra-low	High	High	Low	Ultra-low
Blood levels	Daily peaks & troughs	Steady	Daily peaks & troughs	Initial peak then decline	Initial peak then decline	Daily peaks & troughs	Steady
First pass through liver	Yes	No	Yes	No	No	Yes	No
Major mechanisms							
Ovary: ↓ Ovulation*	+++	+++	+	++	+++	+++	++
Cervical mucus: ↓ sperm penetrability	Yes	Yes	Yes	Yes	Yes	Yes	Yes
Endometrium: ↓ receptivity to blastocyst (a weak effect)	Yes	Yes	Yes	Yes	Yes	Yes	Yes
Consistent use failures/100 WY	0.2–3	0.6–0.9	0.3–4	<2	0–1	0.2–0.9	0–0.07
Menstrual pattern	Regular	Regular	Often irregular	Irregular	Very irregular	Often irregular	Often irregular
Amenorrhoea during use	Rare	Rare	Occasional	Common	Very common	Common	Common
Reversibility							
Immediate termination possible?	Yes	Yes	Yes	No	No	Yes	Yes
By woman herself at anytime?	Yes	Yes	Yes	No	No	Yes	No
Median time to conception from first omitted dose/ removal	c.3 months	c. 3 months	c. 2 months	c. 3 months	c. 6 months	c. 3 months	c. 2 months

*By two mechanisms – no pre-ovulatory follicles formed, plus no LH surges occur.

i.m, intramuscular; 100 WY, 100 Woman-years.

Note: Cerazette™ contains same active agent as Implanon™ (desogestrel being a pro-drug for etonogestrel) and shows other similarities.

It must therefore be understood at the outset that the hormonal environment of a previously cycling woman on the POP is the result of the direct effect of the exogenous progestogen and an amount of ovarian activity, which varies – both between women and between cycles. This explains the very varied menstrual pattern that is observed and is also relevant to other side-effects.

7.5 What effects can the POP have on ovarian function?

In individual women, or in the same woman in different menstrual cycles, the effects vary. Although the patterns have been described in four groups, this is for convenience. The situation is better described as a spectrum running from no interference with the ovarian cycle through to complete quiescence of the ovaries and no follicular or luteal activity.

In a short-term study (1980) of a POP with just 300 g of norethisterone (the UK's Micronor™/Noriday™ contains 17% more NET), Swedish workers have described four main groups in this continuum (percentage of cycles in parentheses):

1 Cycles showing almost no change from normal, with apparently normal ovulation, minimal shortening of the luteal phase and progesterone levels within normal limits (40%).
2 Normal follicular phase but marked shortening of the luteal phase, with lower progesterone levels for a shorter time (21%).
3 Follicular activity with higher peak oestrogen levels than usual but no ovulation and no progesterone production. Ultrasound scans of the ovaries in POP-users, most probably coming mainly from this group as described by the Swedes, show the formation of abnormal follicles or functional cysts, which might be single or multiple (23%).
4 Diminished follicular activity, low oestrogen levels, no ovulation, no corpus luteum formation and no endogenous progesterone production. Ultrasound scanning confirms quiescent ovaries (16%).

> The POP is often given during lactation (see Q 7.54). The endocrine findings are then as in group 4, signifying the same efficacy as the COC but (except uniquely in the case of Cerazette™) often shift at the time of weaning variably towards those of group 1, as expected, with an increasing risk of ovulation.

7.6 How do the changes described in the last questions show themselves in the menstrual pattern and affect the risk of contraceptive failure?

1 A majority of the women experiencing cycles of the type in group 1 above will have regular periods. They are not immune to breakthrough

bleeding (BTB), however, probably because of direct effects of the artificial progestogen on the endometrium. Here ovulation is the norm, the pharmacological effects on the pituitary/ovarian axis are minimal; but this means that they are also the group with the highest risk of breakthrough pregnancy. They are relying chiefly on the mucus and perhaps sometimes the endometrial effects for contraception (*Fig. 7.1*).

2 Groups 2 and 3, which show varying degrees of cycle disturbance, short of complete abolition, merge with each other and are therefore together in the middle column of *Fig. 7.1*. It is from among these women that extrafrequent or erratic, irregular bleeds will be reported: the endometrium no longer receives adequate endogenous progesterone and many of those in group 3 also have increased oestrogen stimulation from the increased follicular activity. The bleeding pattern is a result of this abnormal ovarian activity and the (rather rapid) fluctuations each 24 h in the level of exogenous progestogen. It would appear that it is in cycles showing the patterns of groups 2 and 3 that symptomatic or asymptomatic functional ovarian cysts can be formed. The risk of breakthrough pregnancy is considerably less than in group 1, probably almost nil because such a cycle is anovular (although the woman could always have a group-1-type cycle in another month).

3 In group 4, at the extreme of the continuum, there is either complete amenorrhoea or intermittent, very light bleeding. The latter is caused by irregular shedding of the endometrium, receiving less oestrogen than usual and just the daily exogenous progestogen administration (in a saw-tooth pattern, like all oral medications, *see Q 8.5*). The risk of contraceptive failure here, with or without erratic bleeds, is nil. It is of course also the norm for POP-taking during lactation, and is common during any use of the anovulant Cerazette™ (*see Q 7.11*).

7.7 What, then, does amenorrhoea on the POP mean?

First, it can certainly be caused by pregnancy and this must be excluded in the usual way. Once that explanation is ruled out, paradoxically the women experiencing prolonged episodes of amenorrhoea are the ones not ovulating and so actually at least risk of conception. It is from among the group 1 POP-using women, who are experiencing regular periods and being regularly reassured thereby, that the majority of unplanned conceptions occur. *See also Q 7.66* for a discussion of the possible risks of sustained amenorrhoea.

7.8 Are any particular POPs more likely to cause erratic periods or amenorrhoea?

As has to be said about so many aspects of POP use, the possibility of differences between the POPs has been inadequately studied. The Swedish studies quoted in *Q 5.5* were not able to demonstrate any correlation

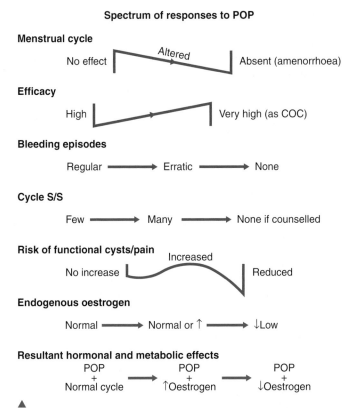

Fig. 7.1 Spectrum of responses to the progestogen-only pill. Q 7.6. *Note:* the metabolic effects are minimal anyway in *all* the groups, across the spectrum. See also Qs 7.5, 7.35, 7.39.

between doses given or measured blood levels of the artificial progestogen and the types of ovarian reaction or the bleeding profile – even though the blood levels also showed wide patient-to-patient variation (*see* Q 7.9). So it appears that the main factor is the degree to which the end-organs, especially the ovary and the uterus, are susceptible to the effects of the POP in the blood.

7.9 In POP-takers, is there the same variability in blood levels of the steroids as described for the COC (*see Q 5.162*)?

Yes. There is the same enormous variation between women who are apparently similar taking the same POP and having their blood levels estimated at the same time after their last tablet was ingested. But variation in target-organ sensitivity appears more important (*see Q 7.8*) in causing bleeding side-effects.

There is also (as for COC-users) the fact of variation, again about ten-fold, between the peak and trough blood levels each day within the same woman. This aspect is discussed in *Qs 5.15 and 8.1* (*Figs 5.2 and 8.1*).

7.10 How does the enterohepatic cycle operate for the POP?

As in *Fig. 5.5* (*see Q 5.14*), after the artificial progestogen is absorbed, liver metabolism creates metabolites that re-enter the lumen of the bowel via the bile. But the action of the bowel flora does not result in reformation of active progestogen. Hence the achieved circulating levels of the POP are normally not dependent on hydrolysis by the intestinal flora and subsequent reabsorption of the progestogen; so antibiotics can have no effect on POP blood levels. However, enzyme-inducing drugs can reduce the blood levels and affect efficacy, just as they do with the COC (*see Q 7.28*).

7.11 What is Cerazette™, the desogestrel POP?

This useful new product containing 75 µg desogestrel 'rewrites the textbooks' about POPs, mainly because it regularly blocks ovulation (group 4 in *Q 7.5*). This makes it somewhat like 'Implanon™ by mouth' and indeed it is useful as a way of advance testing the acceptability of Implanon™. (This gives somewhat of a 'handle' only on the non-bleeding hormonal-type side effects however.)

Despite good evidence of anovulation in 97% of cycles, the CSM did not approve the proposed 12-h advice for defining a missed Cerazette™ POP – it judged that insufficient data were presented to establish this difference from other POPs (*see Q 7.21*). An international study is now planned, recruiting women who are instructed to miss pills by 12, 24, 36 h, etc. during very careful monitoring of cycles of Cerazette™ and POP use, measuring ultrasound and blood markers of ovulation.

As with all progestogen-only methods, irregular bleeding remains a very real problem, indeed that is one area showing no great advantage in a comparative study with LNG 30 µg users (Collaborative Group on Desogestrel POP 1998 *European Journal of Contraceptive and Reproductive Healthcare* 3:168–178). The drop-out rate for changes in bleeding pattern showed no difference but there was a useful trend for the more annoying frequent and prolonged bleeding experiences to lessen with continued use and at one year around 50% had either amenorrhoea or only 1–2 bleeds per 90 days. Despite this higher incidence of (more acceptable) amenorrhoea than with existing POPs, Cerazette™, like Implanon™ still appears to provide adequate, follicular phase levels of estradiol.

In summary, it might well become a first line hormonal contraceptive for many women, given that:

1 It must be free of all the risks attributable to EE, plus no effects on BP were reported in the above study. Hence it can be used in many cases where the COC is WHO 4 or 3 but a pill method with comparable efficacy is desired.

2 It also ablates the menstrual cycle like the COC but again without using EE. So, in those who do not get unacceptably frequent or prolonged uterine bleeds, it has potentially beneficial effects on menstrual disorders, especially dysmenorrhoea, menorrhagia and PMS.

3 It could also be a good alternative anovulant method when there is a past history of ectopic pregnancy.

In the rest of this chapter and elsewhere in the book, the abbreviation POP, if used unqualified, refers to all POP products other than Cerazette™.

EFFECTIVENESS

7.12 What is the overall effectiveness of the POP?

As usual, reliability depends greatly on the motivation of the woman. An overall rate of 0.3–4/100 woman-years can be quoted for standard POPs, the higher rate occurring when patient compliance is poor, and particularly at very young ages, as discussed in Q 7.16. The lower rate applies particularly during lactation (see Q 7.54). Cerazette™ had a consistent-user Pearl failure rate of just 0.17 per 100 woman-years (CI 0.0–0.9) in the premarketing study (in non-breastfeeders). This is a rate normally obtainable only in studies of *combined* pills.

7.13 What is the influence on the effectiveness of age?

In the Oxford/Family Planning Association (FPA) study there was a marked influence of age on standard POPs (*Table 7.3*) – Cerazette™ was not available for testing. The failure rate falls from 3.1/100 woman-years for the age group 25–29 to 0.3 above the age of 40. Possible explanations are:

1 The usual influence of declining fertility with age, shown for example also for the IUD (see Q 9.11).

2 Related to (1), it is well known that the prevalence of abnormal menstrual cycles increases with increasing age, and this is likely to predispose to abnormal ovulation (and the woman's POP cycles therefore being in groups 2–4, as discussed in Q 7.5). Although not reported, it would be expected that the older women in the Oxford/FPA study had a greater incidence of irregular bleeding and amenorrhoea; whereas the younger women would tend to have ovarian cycles that were more 'resistant' to the effect of the exogenous progestogen, and hence

more would be ovulating and at greater risk of conception. They would necessarily be relying solely on the other two main effects of the method (on the mucus and endometrium).

3   Older women tend to have less frequent intercourse but this is less true now as many 40 year olds have embarked on new relationships.

4   The younger women were possibly less consistent in their pill taking.

7.14 Do other factors affect the effectiveness of POPs? What about body weight?

The Oxford/FPA study was unable to show any statistically significant difference between the failure rate according to which particular POP brand was used, although appreciable variation was noted. Cigarette smoking also did not appear to be of importance.

BODY WEIGHT

The Oxford/FPA study did show a trend to higher pregnancy rates with increasing weight. Although not statistically significant, this has to be taken seriously because it is not implausible biologically (see below). Moreover, there was significance in similar analyses of data for other progestogen-only methods that rely on achieving very similar blood levels.

With both the levonorgestrel-releasing vaginal ring (*see Q 8.69*) and Norplant™ (*see Qs 8.59–8.68*), specifically in trials of the higher-silica polymer 373 (an older subcutaneous implant that had a higher failure rate overall), the pregnancy rate was positively correlated to increasing weight. The ring in particular is such a similar method that I feel that the weight effect has to be considered real for the POP also, until a larger POP study or meta-analysis settles the issue. See also the Kovacs data in *Q 7.17*.

The bottom line for me is that there is as yet no proof that body mass is not important in the effectiveness of the POP. However, its influence is likely to be much less important in users of the anovulant Cerazette™, as with the COC (see the next question).

TABLE 7.3 Progestogen-only pill – user-failure rates/100 woman-years Oxford/FPA Study (1985 report) – all women married and aged above 25, any duration of use

	Ages (years)			
All ages	**25–29**	**30–34**	**35–39**	**40+**
0.9	3.1	2.0	1.0	0.3

NB: These figures are different from those given in Table 1.2, because they are based on nearly twice as many woman-years of observation.

7.15 Why does the body mass effect on efficacy show up with some low-dose progestogen methods and not with the combined pill and injectables?

In reality the interesting observation is the absence of a weight effect with the latter two products, though similar data are now emerging about other combined methods (*Q 6.80*). Note the emphasis here on mass or weight, not BMI. Dilution of the administered drug in the greater amount of 'water of distribution' (apparent distribution volume) existing in a bigger person – whether they are tall or short – is expected for any drug. It is the basis, after all, for usually reducing adult doses when giving drugs to children.

My explanation for the absence of an observable effect so far with the COC and injectables is that they have too high a safety margin as effective anovulants (coupled with their adjunctive contraceptive effects), in users of whatever weight, for this trend to be detectable in studies of a realistic size. The doses given by the progestogen-only methods of *Q 7.14* (the ring and polymer 373 implant), however, are nearer the minimum for efficacy so something like weight can exert a detectable influence on the failure rate, and the same probably applies to standard POPs. But it is *not* expected to apply to Cerazette™ because it is an anovulant and hence ought to behave like the COC with regard to body mass, even if it is high.

7.16 What are the implications of the above findings with regard to efficacy?

1   In lactation: the combination of full breastfeeding and the POP equates to almost 100% contraception (*see Qs 7.23, 7.54*). Cerazette's™ extra effectiveness is unnecessary and comes at added cost. Even the young woman who is overweight would be most unlikely to conceive – until weaning begins anyway.

2   For older women: the main implication of these findings is the remarkable efficacy of the method. As these are precisely the women who might need to transfer from the COC (see *Table 5.10*), it is useful to be able to tell a woman over 40, quite truthfully, that her chances of conceiving if she is regular taker of the old-type POP are the same as for a 25-year-old taking a modern combined pill. (The Oxford/FPA study gives method-plus-user failure rates of around 0.3 in both instances.)

3   For the young: unfortunately, the Oxford/FPA study did not include women under the age of 25. However, extrapolating from *Table 7.3*, the expected failure rate in teenagers is likely to be quite high, say 4/100 woman-years, especially as compliance tends to be less good in the young. Some studies that included women in their twenties have shown acceptable failure rates of 1–2/100 woman-years. So with careful selection and education of users the POP is certainly on the list of options for the

young. But Cerazette™ would be my preferred choice now for all teenagers who desired a POP.

4   For the overweight (*see Qs 7.14 and 7.15*): pending more data, I personally feel we should warn women weighing above 70 kg (11 stone) of the possibility of a higher failure rate than those quoted in *Q 7.12*. If nothing else is suitable and the woman is not breastfeeding, the use of two POPs per day could be considered, but not in the over 45s. They are after all compounds with a very safe therapeutic margin. But this is unlicensed prescribing (see Appendix A). Hence my own preference now is to consider high body mass as a positive indication for using a single daily Cerazette™.

7.17 For those users who are still ovulating, how long does the contraceptive effect on the cervical mucus last, following each dose?

As illustrated in *Fig. 7.2*, following one tablet the effect appears maximal about 4 h later, but in this one study there was some return of sperm penetrability around 24 h. Regular POP taking seems to abolish this, so one can assume that the cervicouterine fluid is difficult for sperm to traverse throughout the 24 h.

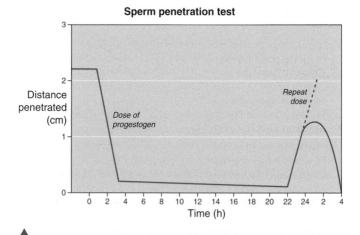

Fig. 7.2 Sperm penetration of cervical mucus after progestogen. Q 7.17. *Note*: minimum reduction in sperm penetration occurs between 4 h and 22 h after a single dose of megestrol acetate (0.5 mg). Unlike the rest of the figure, the effect of a repeat dose is presumed, not experimental (redrawn from Cox 1968 The precoital user of minidosage progestogens. *Journal of Reproduction and Fertility Supplement* 5:167–172, Figure 1).

Figure 7.2 actually derives from some work in the late 1960s using the POP megestrol acetate (0.5 mg). Similar data are available for levonorgestrel but these studies badly need repeating with more modern investigative techniques, and for Cerazette™ (which is still thought to use the mucus effect as back-up to its mainly anovulant action).

In a study of the POP by Kovacs in 2000 (Br J of Family Planning 26:165–6), the expected effect of a LNG-containing POP in reducing sperm penetrability of the cervical mucus was undetectable in only three women: they were all very obese with body masses greater than 75 kg, confirming the greater water of dilution concept discussed in *Q 7.15*.

Scanning electron microscope (SEM) studies have shown a characteristic tight mesh of microfibrils in mucus obtained from women using various microdose progestogens – when the progestogenic effect is maximal. However, in cycling women (group 1 in *Q 7.5*), if the mucus is sampled at midcycle as little as 36 h after the last tablet was taken the SEM appearances are already nearly back to the normal open mesh of oestrogenic mucus that sperm can readily penetrate. The contraceptive effect of the POP on mucus can thus certainly be assumed to disappear by 12 h if a woman is late taking a tablet.

7.18 What endometrial effects have been described in POP users?

As with other tissues, observations differ according to the variable amount of endogenous ovarian activity superimposed on the direct effect of the progestogen (*see Q 7.5* and *Fig. 7.1*).

That said, blockade of progesterone receptors occurs and characteristic changes have been described in the histology of the endometrium on both light and electron microscopy. Uterine glands diminish both in number and in diameter. These and associated biochemical effects are believed to reduce the likelihood of successful implantation.

7.19 How important is the endometrial effect, how long does it take to develop and how readily is it lost?

The answers to all these questions are largely unknown. The mucus effect has been more fully studied and the endometrial effect is generally considered much less important as a back-up contraceptive mechanism.

7.20 For maximum efficacy of the POP, how and when should it be taken?

As implied by *Fig. 7.2*, and the answer to *Q 7.17*, the answer to 'how?' is 'extremely regularly'. Indeed, I always tell prospective POP users that the POP is 'a package deal'. In other words, 'here is your packet of pills, now set a dedicated alarm on your mobile!' Women who are not breastfeeding are encouraged to take their tablets at precisely the same time each day. There is very much more leeway during full lactation (*see Qs 7.6, 7.23, 7.54*) because ovulation is then inhibited and the situation is not unlike taking the COC. This must also be the case with Cerazette™, although not so stated in its SPC.

7.21 What rule do you recommend for missed POPs?

It has proved difficult to reach international agreement on the matter of 'missed POP rules'. This is not too surprising in view of:

- the spectrum of effects of this method on different women and in different cycles (*see Q 7.5*)
- the lack of data about the relative importance of the end-organ contraceptive effects in *Table 7.2*
- the different situation applying during breastfeeding (unless otherwise stated the discussion below applies outside of 100% lactation).

There is good agreement among the authorities on one point: as the mucus effect is so quickly lost, extra precautions should begin if a woman is more than 3 h late in taking her old-type POP (27 h since the last tablet).

The difficult part of the advice is: for how long should loss of contraception be assumed? From 1985 to 1992 in the UK the FPA recommended in its instruction leaflets that an additional contraceptive method should be used just for the next 48 h. From 1993 to 2003 the FPA leaflets have specified 7 days (see below). From 2004 onwards the leaflets, following the advice of WHO in its important document *Selected practice recommendations* (downloadable from *www.who.int/reproductive-health*) have returned to the earlier wording for the management of a late or missed tablet, namely:

- take one pill as soon as possible
- return to regular daily pill-taking
- abstain from sex or use additional contraception for the next 2 days.

7.22 When should emergency postcoital contraception be considered in addition, if POP tablets are missed?

For old-type POPs this decision should be based on the mucus effect, i.e. emergency pills should be offered for any unprotected intercourse that occurred after the 3 h delay and which might lead to loss of the mucus effect, but before two pills had been taken to restore it (*see Q 10.23(6)*). The usual careful quizzing about the *earliest* exposure would apply, and a minimum 2 days of extra precautions should then follow, as in the new WHO advice.

7.23 How should the advice differ if ordinary progestogen-only pills are missed during lactation – or if Cerazette™ is the pill?

During lactation, ovulation in POP users is inhibited while there is sustained amenorrhoea; particularly during the first 6 months postpartum when (if the lactational amenorrhoea criteria are observed) lactation even without the POP is 98% effective (see *Fig. 2.4*). Missing a POP is then equivalent to missing a COC in midpacket (*see Q 7.21*). Cerazette™ almost certainly has at least 12 h leeway for pill-taking on its own, even without the added contraceptive effect of breastfeeding, despite the fact that for the time being we are advised by the SPC to suggest that extra precautions start after 3 h delay.

Until the Cerazette™ advice changes, and because breastfeeding (along with the POP) varies in its intensity, it can do no harm to recommend as normal practice in both cases that: extra contraception is initiated (now at least only for 2 days!) after 3 h delay. In my view (but this is not in the current SPC so Appendix A must apply) some individuals, after discussion, might be told they can operate on the basis of up to 12 h. It would be exceptional ever to find it necessary to offer emergency contraception to fully breastfeeding POP-users with amenorrhoea whose offspring is not yet 6 months old, or to Cerazette™ users if they have missed a couple of tablets.

7.24 How long does it take to establish efficacy when starting the POP?

The contraceptive effect on the mucus develops very rapidly (see *Fig. 7.2*). We do not know the minimum time needed to establish the antiovulation or anti-implantation effects. However, with a first-day start and hence taking at least seven pills before the earliest likely fertile ovulation, any POP-induced interference with it ought theoretically to be as great as it will be in later cycles. So no extra precautions are now advised with a first-day start of any POP and this seems adequate.

7.25 What, therefore, are the recommended starting routines?

See *Table 7.4* and its important footnotes.

7.26 What advice should be given to a woman who vomits a tablet and fails to replace it successfully within 2 h?

She should take extra precautions as well as taking her tablets for the duration of the vomiting and for 2 days thereafter. If intercourse took place when the mucus effect was likely to have been reduced through vomited pills, emergency contraception should be considered, as for missed POPs (*see Q. 7.22*). But that would nearly always be unnecessary during full lactation, or if the pill concerned was Cerazette™.

7.27 Should any action be taken if a POP-user requires antibiotic treatment?

Yes if the antibiotic is an enzyme inducer! This means only rifamicins (e.g. rifampicin) and griseofulvin. Otherwise no action is required because, as

TABLE 7.4 Starting routines with the POP or Cerazette™

	Start when?	Extra precautions?
Menstruating	1st or 2nd day of period	No
	Any time in cycle ('Quick start')	Yes[†]
Postpartum		
(a) No lactation*	Day 21 (see text and Q 11.22)[‡]	No
(b) Lactation*	Day 21, or later (see Q 7.56)	No
Induced abortion/ miscarriage	Same day or next day	No
Post COC	Instant switch	No
Post DMPA	Instant switch before or at 12 weeks since last injection	No

*Bleeding irregularities minimized by starting at or after the 4th week.
[†]Provided there is reasonable certainty that there is no chance of an early pregnancy (in amenorrhoea see Q 11.22) can start POP any time plus 2 days' extra precautions. WHO advises the latter only for starts that are later than day 5.
[‡]See Q 11.22 re starting artificial hormones later on, during postpartum amenorrhoea.

explained in *Q 7.10*, ordinary broad-spectrum antibiotics can have no effect on the blood level of the active exogenous progestogen.

7.28 Should the POP be avoided by women using enzyme-inducing drugs?

Enzyme inducers do lower progestogen as well as oestrogen blood levels and the failure rate of any POP (including Cerazette™) would therefore be expected to increase. Extra precautions should be advised during and for at least 7 days after any short-term treatment – and much longer after rifampicin (*see Q 5.37*). (The drugs concerned here are in *Table 5.3*, *Q 5.34*, to which should be added bosentan – another enzyme inducer, but only used for treating pulmonary hypotension, so would be WHO 4 for the COC.)

Long term, a better hormonal option might be an injectable. If the POP is preferred on a WHO 3 basis, my advice is that the dose be increased, normally to two POP (or Cerazette™) tablets per day. Even then the woman should be warned that the efficacy of such a regimen is not well established. And, as usual, because this is not supported by the SPCs, the 'named patient' criteria should be observed (see p. 000).

As in COC users, St John's wort is contraindicated (see *Table 5.3*, p. 126).

7.29 Can the small dose of progestogen influence other drugs?

Because the effect of the COC on other drugs is usually negligible (*see Q 5.45*), the lower dose in the POP can certainly be disregarded.

ADVANTAGES AND BENEFICIAL SIDE-EFFECTS

7.30 What are the advantages of the POP?

1 Acceptable efficacy, in the range of 0.3–4/100 woman-years. Higher efficacy applies to Cerazette™ and with all POPs in older women for whom COCs might be contraindicated.

2 No epidemiological proof, so far, of increased risk of either circulatory or malignant disease but *see Q 7.36*. Again this is not certain because of inadequate study; plus any (good or bad) effects may very well vary between women because of the variable impact of the POP on the hypothalamo–pituitary–ovarian axis.

3 Avoidance of all side-effects in which artificial oestrogens are implicated.

4 Minimization of any side-effects in which progestogens are implicated.

5 Minimal alteration in all metabolic variables that have been measured (*see Qs 7.39–7.46*).

6 Good general tolerance: especially suitable for women who complain of side-effects with other hormonal methods, or in whom the latter are contraindicated.

7 Most minor symptoms of the COC (such as weight gain, nausea, headaches and loss of libido) are not a problem.

8 Return of women's fertility on discontinuation more rapid than after the COC.

9 The tiny dose means minimal effect on lactation, and levels of the artificial steroids within breast milk seem to be negligible.

10 No harmful effect from overdose, even when taken by a child.

7.31 Do the beneficial effects listed in *Q 7.39* also apply to the POP?

1 Some do – most of the contraceptive benefits, for example.

2 Some women report improvement in symptoms of the menstrual cycle, notably premenstrual symptoms and dysmenorrhoea. Others report the reverse (*see Qs 7.32 and 7.69*). Cerazette™ (*see Q 7.11*) is more likely than other POPs to improve such gynaecological symptoms, and indeed might substitute usefully for the COC in treating all the conditions 1 to 6 listed in *Q 4.129*.

3 Protection against pelvic infection is extremely probable through the mucus 'barrier' effect, though not yet proven for the POP (*see Qs 5.59 and 8.13*).

4 For the remaining items, including the cancers, listed in *Q 5.56* there is so far no evidence to suggest that the beneficial effect applies to old-type POPs. And functional ovarian cysts are more, not less, frequent (see below).

MAIN PROBLEMS AND DISADVANTAGES

7.32 What are the main problems of the POP?

1   The need for obsessional regularity in pill taking (*see Q 7.20*). This is believed to be less critical on Cerazette™ and during full lactation.

2   Alteration of the menstrual pattern is the main problem, except in breastfeeders. The reasons are explained in *Q 7.5*. According to that Swedish study, one can predict to some extent the type of change that the POP will produce. Women whose own normal cycles had long follicular/short luteal phases were more likely to be in group 4 on the POP (tending to have episodes of amenorrhoea). Those with regular or short cycles – who had relatively short follicular but normal length luteal phases – were more likely to enter group 1 and have the more regular bleeding.

In general, the duration and volume of flow might change and there could be intermenstrual episodes. Alternatively, the woman might develop amenorrhoea.

All in all, cycle irregularity (especially frequent/prolonged bleeding) is the most common reason for abandoning the method – with Cerazette™ also. Yet a woman can be told that irregularity or oligo- or amenorrhoea mean the method is probably more effective in her particular case (*see Q 7.6*). Another disadvantage therefore is that:

3   Precisely in those women with the most acceptable, regular cycles, the risk of pregnancy is greatest.

4   Acne is a not uncommon complaint with the old-style POPs.

5   A small number of women develop symptomatic functional ovarian cysts (*see Q 7.34*), causing pain that can sometimes be severe enough to imitate an ectopic pregnancy.

6   Pregnancies in POP users are more likely to be ectopic than pregnancies occurring in the general population. As for the IUD (*see Qs 9.29 and 9.31*), it is not thought that the POP actually increases the risk of ectopics in a population of POP users; indeed the reverse is true.

7.33 What is the risk of ectopic pregnancy? Why do ectopics occur in POP users?

When compared with sexually active non-pregnant controls, studies have shown a reduced risk of ectopic pregnancy in POP users. This is to be expected because the method often interferes with ovulation, and with fertilization. Ectopics can only happen if normal ovulation occurs, followed by fertilization, i.e. the risk relates only to a subgroup of group 1 in *Q 7.5*. Moreover, the effect of the POP on cervical mucus should reduce the risk of tubal damage from pelvic infection.

However, the likelihood of any breakthrough pregnancy that (rarely) actually happens being ectopic is increased. Possible explanations include the following:

1   A selection effect, exactly as described for the IUD (*see Q 9.30*), if there is pre-existing tubal damage and fertilization occurs. The numerator of ectopics is reduced, but if the denominator of POP 'breakthrough' pregnancies is reduced even more, the relative frequency of ectopics among the conceptions will increase.
2   Progestogens can modify tubal function. Overall, contractility and the rate of ovum transport are decreased, the latter probably from a reduction in the number of ciliated cells, but the significance to ectopic risk is not established.

Of the two, the first explanation is thought by far the more important (*see Qs 9.30–9.31*). Like the COC, Cerazette™ ought to reduce the risk of ectopics to vanishingly low levels. For a past history of ectopic, *see Q 7.52*.

7.34 How frequent are functional ovarian cysts among POP users?

In a study by the Margaret Pyke Centre, functional ovarian cysts (FOCs) as diagnosed by ultrasound occurred in as many as half the POP users (12/21), compared with four out of the 21 controls. Most of these were asymptomatic but seven women – all of them POP users – complained of some pain; one required admission for rest and analgesia.

It is also clinical experience that some POP users are diagnosed as cases of ectopic pregnancy (menstrual irregularity plus one-sided pain and a tender mass) but laparoscopy shows only a functional cyst, or evidence that one has recently ruptured.

7.35 What is the cause of FOCs?

The precise causation of FOCs remains undefined. They are clearly due to an abnormality of ovulation (sometimes luteinization of an unruptured follicle), which is succeeded by accumulation of fluid. On the basis of the groups defined in *Q 7.5*, one would expect the frequency to be no different from a control population in group 1, and actually reduced in the group with quiescent ovaries: group 4. Yet they still occur in Cerazette™ users: four symptomatic cysts were reported out of 979 women in the study quoted in *Q 7.11*.

7.36 Does the POP affect neoplasia risk?

Little is known, for the reasons discussed in *Qs 5.72 and 7.3*. The UK National Case Control Study (1989) found a possible protective association with breast cancer, whereas the CGHFBC suggested an increased risk similar to that which they described for the COC (*see Q 5.84*). So the jury is still out: if there is any real influence of the POP on carcinogenesis (in the breast or elsewhere) it will be subject to two important considerations:

1   Any effects will be (slightly) beneficial on some cancers, adverse on others (as for the COC, *see Q 5.73*), and usually related in each case to duration of use.
2   Intuitively, the effects are likely to depend in part on the amount of interaction with the woman's menstrual cycle, i.e. her 'group' in Q 7.5.

For the present, one can truthfully tell any woman that no POP study to date has shown a statistically significant increase in the risk of cancer. Even less is known about Cerazette™ in this respect.

7.37   What effect does the POP have on trophoblastic disease?

See Q 5.77 for a discussion of the reasons why, in the UK, it is advised that the COC (and also for the time being all POPs and any other contraceptive hormones) should normally not be used until hCG levels are undetectable.

7.38   What is the influence of the POP on benign tumours, such as benign breast disease and fibroids?

There is no evidence that any of the tumours mentioned in Q 5.96 are affected by use of any POP – but no conclusive evidence of no effect, either.

7.39   What are the effects of the POP on metabolism?

Although this has been slightly better studied than the epidemiology, there are few good studies of modern POPs. Moreover, the studies can be faulted on at least one of the following counts:

1   Inadequate attention to confounding: meaning that the changes seen might be due to characteristics of the woman for whom a POP was chosen, rather than the POP itself.
2   Lack of attention to the different metabolic responses to be expected, according to whether the users respond to the POP as in the groups 1, 2, 3 or 4 in Q 7.5. *Figure 7.1* shows that the resultant metabolic effects might well vary from (in group 1) those of the normal menstrual cycle with normal ovarian oestrogen plus a small effect from the POP, to the situation (group 4) where the progestogen is opposed by relatively little endogenous oestrogen production.

Despite these limitations, the overall findings of the metabolic studies are very reassuring, as discussed in the next questions.

7.40 What are the effects of the POP on coagulation and fibrinolysis?

1   Studies have shown that the POP, unlike COCs, has no important measurable adverse effect on blood clotting, platelet aggregation or fibrinolytic activity.

2   One interesting study looked at prostacyclin and thromboxane levels. Among COC users, prostacyclin levels were decreased (favouring platelet aggregation). There was no change in the POP group, however, and in the latter, particularly among women using levonorgestrel alone, the thromboxane concentrations were depressed. As thromboxane enhances platelet aggregation, this could even indicate a decreased risk of thrombosis in POP users.

7.41 Presumably, the POP can therefore be used by women with a definite past history of thromboembolism, even if COC related?

Yes, definitely (*see Q 7.49*). But most SPCs for POPs still do not say this!

The norethisterone products are particularly interesting. Past thrombosis is stated to be a 'contraindication' to the POP Noriday™ (which contains 350 µg of this progestogen) and the data sheet recommends it is discontinued at least 4 weeks before elective operations. However, if you turn over just a few pages in the ABPI SPC *Data Sheet Compendium* (1999) you discover that Utovlan™ contains norethisterone 5 mg, which is regularly used for gynaecological indications such as menorrhagia, in doses up to 15 mg daily. Yet past thromboembolism is (rightly, in fact) not included as a contraindication and there is no mention at all about stopping the drug before major surgery! How come, when the same manufacturer's norethisterone is being given in 45 times the dose in Utovlan™ as in the Noriday™ POP, about which the SPC creates anxiety about a past thrombosis history?! I rest my case.

7.42 What are the effects on blood lipids, especially high-density lipoprotein-cholesterol (HDL-C)?

The POPs currently available seem to have little effect on all the main aspects of lipid metabolism; but in one or two studies the important subfraction HDL_2-C was slightly depressed with POPs containing either levonorgestrel or norethisterone. This was not shown with desogestrel as in Cerazette™.

7.43 What are the effects on carbohydrate metabolism?

Once again a consensus view is that the effects are minimal. However, some studies have shown a slight deterioration in glucose tolerance and a tendency to hyperinsulinism, particularly in users of the levonorgestrel POPs. Some studies cannot exclude the possibility that adverse metabolic findings are the result of selection of the POP by users who have arterial disease risk factors, so that use of the POP is coincidental not causal.

7.44 Can the POP be used by frank diabetics?

Certainly – after the diaphragm or sheath the POP can be the method of choice. Workers in Edinburgh have found that with POPs containing 350 µg norethisterone no increase in insulin dosage appeared necessary, and there was no change in the incidence and severity of retinopathy. They consider the POP to be an ideal choice from the metabolic point of view. In addition, only one pregnancy occurred among 50 women during the period of observation (1050 woman-months) and the woman concerned omitted a number of pills.

Generally, diabetics have exceptionally good compliance because they take their pill with each evening dose of insulin. But for younger and more fertile diabetics the extra efficacy plus still no EE content of Cerazette™ would make it even more attractive.

7.45 Would you use current POPs in a diabetic with definite evidence of tissue damage, especially arteriopathy?

Yes. In my view the uncertainty about metabolic effects, especially on lipids, makes this WHO 3 for old-type POPs and WHO 2 for Cerazette™ (i.e. certainly usable); but other options like an IUD or IUS might be even better.

7.46 Have any other metabolic effects been described?

1   When progestogens are administered alone they have little if any effect on hepatic secretion of plasma proteins – compare this with the COC (see Q 5.98).
2   Thyroid and pituitary–adrenal function also appear to be unaffected.
3   Progestogens beneficially affect the biochemistry and physiology of cervical mucus (see Q 7.17), thereby probably protecting the user against pelvic infection. They also appear to improve aspects of erythrocyte metabolism in sickle cell anaemia (see Q 8.15).

7.47 So, does the POP affect the risk of circulatory disease?

We lack much data. In the Oxford/FPA study there were just two cases of venous thromboembolism and two of stroke in 3303 woman-years of study. Considering the women were in the older age group and in general more likely to have other risk factors for circulatory disease, this seems a highly acceptable incidence. The more recent WHO study was also reassuring, but again based on small numbers.

7.48 Does the POP affect BP?

Reassuringly, apparently not. Studies have shown neither the slight rise in systolic and diastolic pressure that occurs in almost all individuals given oestrogen-containing preparations and nor (and this includes Cerazette™) do they appear to increase the risk of frank hypertension risk. COC-induced hypertension usually reverts to normal on the POP.

The same appears to apply to DMPA and other oestrogen-free methods in this chapter. Though the data come from mostly small studies, progestogens seem to have an adverse effect on BP only if oestrogens are also administered.

SELECTION OF USERS AND OF FORMULATIONS

7.49 For whom is the POP method particularly indicated?

Lactation (see (8), below) has hitherto been the main indication, although the working rule has been:

Wherever there are contraindications to or side-effects with the COC, and an oral hormonal method is preferred? Try the POP.

Previously there was the obstacle of reduced efficacy in making this choice, but that disappears with the advent of Cerazette™:

1 *Women above 35 who smoke* cigarettes. On present information it is acceptable to continue use of the POP even in a smoker on her say-so until beyond the average age of the menopause (i.e. about 51 years) (*see Qs 7.62–7.64* about establishing menopausal infertility).

2 *Oestrogen-linked contraindications* or side-effects on the COC. Some of those listed on the left of *Table 6.1* (*Q 6.22*) might improve. The POP should not be chosen preferentially for conditions such as endometriosis because it does not reliably suppress endogenous oestrogen (though Cerazette™ might be tried for maintenance therapy).

But importantly this category of indications for the COC includes:

3 *History of or any predisposition to thromboembolism*, including known prothrombotic coagulation factor changes: since adverse effects on clotting mechanisms have not been demonstrated (*see Qs 7.40 and 7.41*).

It follows, accordingly:

4 *Chronic systemic diseases* in which oestrogen is the hormone that might exacerbate the condition (e.g. SLE) or where there is an extra thrombosis risk (e.g. complicated structural heart disease (*see Q 7.52*), severe cases of Crohn's disease or ulcerative colitis (*see Q 5.145*) and, again, SLE (*see*

Q 5.146). Sickle-cell disease is another example. But (*see* Q 8.15), for this indication DMPA might be an even better option.

5 Patients with *diabetes or obesity*. Diabetics do particularly well on the POP, especially with regard to compliance (*see* Q 7.44). There are efficacy considerations for the obese (*see* Qs 7.14–7.16).

6 Patients with *hypertension*, either related to the COC or other varieties if well controlled by treatment.

7 Patients with *migraine* (including, with appropriate caution and advice, young women with migraines which are severe or with aura) (*see* Qs 5.151–5.168).

8 During *lactation* (*see* Qs 7.54 and 7.55). This is a well-established indication in which the method has the highest efficacy.

9 At the *woman's choice*: such as a reliable pill taker who prefers a hormonal method yet wishes to use the least possible amount of exogenous hormone.

7.50 What are the contraindications to the POP?

As we have seen, a long list of conditions contraindicating use of POPs can be found in the manufacturers' SPC sheets, but most are there for medicolegal reasons, with no epidemiological basis. In general, and with the exceptions suggested below, the absolute contraindications to the COC (WHO 4) are only relative contraindications (of varying importance, most commonly WHO 2) for the POP.

As before, any list of contraindications must be to some extent a matter of personal judgement (*see* Q 5.135) and, with the POP, involve some informed guesswork – given the dearth of good data.

7.51 What then are the absolute contraindications to the POP, in your view?

Here (as in the next questions) the WHO categorization is used (WHO 4 in this section):

1 *Any serious side-effect occurring on the COC and not clearly due only to oestrogen* – or associated with past progestogen-only use. Liver adenoma or cancer, and severe past sex-steroid-associated cholestatic jaundice would come here, because it is not clear with which of the two hormones in the COC they are primarily linked.

2 *Current breast cancer* – for fear of worsening the prognosis. This is WHO 4 pending more data, but can be WHO 3 after the woman has shown no evidence of current disease for 5 years, according to the WHO (*see* Q 7.52).

3 *Recent trophoblastic disease* (*see* Q 5.77) but only while the hCG is elevated.

4 *Acute porphyria*, past history of an actual attack (*see* Q 6.42). See below if latent, with no history of past attack.

So it is a very short list although, as for all medical methods, we must add:

5   Severe *allergy* to a constituent.
6   *Undiagnosed abnormal genital tract bleeding*, because the POP will confuse diagnosis.
7   Actual or possible *pregnancy*.
8   *The woman's own continuing uncertainty* about POP safety, even after full counselling.

7.52   In your view, what are only relative contraindications to the POP (i.e. when can it be used but with some added caution)?

There is much obvious overlap with *Q 7.49*. The WHO 2 'broadly usable' category (which mainly applies) makes the POP an excellent second choice when the first choice is a pill but the COC is now 'out' for some reason:

1   *Risk factors for arterial disease (WHO 2, or 3 if severe or multiple)*:
    (a)   established hypertension once it has been diagnosed and controlled
    (b)   the presence of more than one risk factor can be tolerated more readily than with the COC. Prothrombotic coagulation factor abnormalities are rightly included above as 'indications', since they should not be worsened at all by the POP
    (c)   likewise, there is not the oestrogen-related concern about thrombotic stroke in migraine, including migraine with focal aura – though the headaches may be still be affected by the POP hormone.
    (d)   Significant lipid abnormalities might be slightly worsened by the POP, but probably less so with Cerazette™. If the disorder has a good prognosis with lipid-lowering treatment by diet and drugs it would be no more than WHO 3 for all POPs. Take the laboratory consultant's advice and continue monitoring of blood levels.
2   *Significant structural heart disease, including where there is an added risk of arrhythmia (especially atrial fibrillation) and systemic embolism*: Cerazette™ is the particularly relevant choice (WHO 1 in fact) among POPs here for young, highly fertile women, many of whom come into the 'grown-up congenital heart disease' category (*see Q 5.134*).
3   *Past subarachnoid haemorrhage*: if there has been good recovery and definitive treatment such that the neurologists are confident recurrence is unlikely, this is WHO 2. But COC can also be usable (*see Q 5.144*).
4   *Sex-steroid-dependent cancer (WHO 3)*: in general, discuss this with the oncologist looking after your patient, particularly for *breast cancer*. According to WHO, once this has been in remission (they say for

5 years but I have been prepared to define this as after 2 years for my own patients) the POP is cautiously useable (WHO 3).

5 *Current liver disorders (e.g. jaundice, cirrhosis) with persistent biochemical changes (WHO 2 unless severe changes)*: focal nodular hyperplasia is WHO 3 (*see Q 5.134*).

6 *Acute porphyria, latent without a past attack* WHO 3: needs caution, and full counselling regarding risk of a future attack (*see Q 6.42*).

7 *Relevant interacting drugs*: WHO 3 the dose can be increased in selected cases (*see Q 7.28*).

8 *Chronic systemic diseases (see also Q 7.49)*: the same fundamental approach as in *Q 5.138* for the COC applies here. The POP (not Cerazette™) has the slight disadvantage of lesser efficacy, especially if pregnancy is made more dangerous by the particular disease. But this is balanced by the likelihood that if hormones were one day shown to worsen the prognosis, the tiny dose in the POP ought to have less effect than the COC.

9 *Functional ovarian cysts (FOCs)*: these are definitely associated with the POP (*see Qs 7.34 and 7.53*) and still occur in Cerazette™ users (*see Q 7.35*). A past history of hospitalization for severe pain resulting in this diagnosis would be WHO 3. However, some women might prefer to continue using the method, as most episodes of FOC formation will be asymptomatic.

10 *Unacceptability of irregular menstrual bleeding*: this remains a problem with all progestogen-only methods, certainly including Cerazette™.

11 *Previous ectopic pregnancy (see Q 7.33)*: is WHO 2 according to the WHO, but I classify this as WHO 3 for a nullipara. She is at risk of recurrence, plus a future second ectopic could endanger her future fertility as well as her life. Her remaining tube (or tubes) deserves maximum protection, which an anovulant method like the COC or DMPA or Cerazette™/Implanon™ could provide.

12 *Where complete protection against pregnancy is vital*: especially if the woman is likely to be at all erratic as a pill-taker. In my view, only Cerazette™ – and not the older POPs – is appropriate on efficacy grounds for teenagers in general.

7.53 What are the clinical implications of an increased rate of functional ovarian cysts (FOCs)?

1 Ultrasound studies suggest that most FOCs are asymptomatic (*see Q 7.34*).

2 It is likely that irregular oestrogen production by functional cysts can explain some of the menstrual irregularity.

3 The main risks of FOCs are those of unnecessary surgery, especially laparoscopy, and rarely also necessary surgery for acute events such as

ovarian torsion. This is why the past history of symptomatic FOCs, either before use of the POP or while taking it, should now be considered WHO 3.

In my experience, however, some women so much prefer this method to the alternatives that they are prepared to take the risk of recurrences. They should be advised to take prompt medical advice as indicated. Given the problem of distinguishing this syndrome from ectopic pregnancy, pelvic ultrasound and ultrasensitive pregnancy tests should be utilized to minimize the need for diagnostic laparoscopy.

USE OF THE POP IN LACTATION

See Q 7.23 for the enhanced efficacy implications of the POP during breastfeeding. This is in fact the most common context in which POPs are used.

7.54 What are the effects of the POP on lactation?

The COC can reduce the volume and alter the constitution of milk. Some of the artificial steroids are transferred to the infant. By contrast, the POPs (including Cerazette™ but *see Q 7.16*) are suitable choices for lactating women. Indeed, progestogens, when administered alone by any of the means discussed in this chapter, appear to reduce neither the volume of milk nor the duration of lactation, and some reports suggest that both are increased. Careful studies on norethisterone-, levonorgestrel- and desogestrel-containing POPs show that the amount transferred to the milk is minute and most unlikely to present any hazard. Studies of the blood of suckling infants have been unable to demonstrate any progestogen because the concentration is below the limits of the sensitivity of present assays.

Last, but not least, the contraceptive combination of lactation plus old-type POP is for practical purposes 100% effective. (*See Qs 7.16, 7.23*).

7.55 What are the implications for prescribing the POP during lactation?

1 First and foremost, the above findings need discussion. The prospective user might be interested to learn that, according to Scandinavian studies of 30-μg levonorgestrel POPs, after 2 years of lactation with regular POP taking the infant will have received at most the equivalent of one tablet! If this is not sufficiently reassuring, of course, another method should be adopted.

2 Another advantage is that the main symptom with the POP – irregular bleeding – is unlikely during lactational amenorrhoea, except when it is first commenced postpartum (*see Q 7.56*).

7.56 When should the POP be commenced after delivery?

1 As, unlike the COC, the POP does not affect lactation nor the risk of venous thrombosis, it is medically safe to start it in the immediate postpartum period. WHO calls such early use WHO 3, because of the concern that the neonate might be at some risk if exposure is in the first 6 weeks after delivery.

2 Studies have shown a greater likelihood of spotting and bleeding problems with starting early in the puerperium. So unless there are special reasons to start earlier, initiating the POP a little later – at around day 21 – is recommended by the FPA (see *Table 7.4*), as with the COC. Of course, even a 6-week time of starting would be fully effective when combined with full breastfeeding (*see Q 2.36*).

7.57 How should weaning be managed in POP users?

Some women simply continue using the POP long term. However, I well remember a clinic in which two consecutive women described how they had unwantedly conceived another pregnancy through not being warned that the margin for error of their POP method would plummet once they weaned their child! That was before the days of Cerazette™, of course.

Therefore if greater efficacy is desired, the woman who is beginning to wean her infant should either switch to Cerazette™ or be prescribed in advance a suitable COC to follow her old-type POP. She should be instructed to start taking the COC when breastfeeding frequency halves, or once solid food is being given or at the first bleed: whichever comes first. Remember that the first fertile ovulation is more likely to happen without a first warning bleed, if it is more than 6 months since delivery.

The increased dose of hormones in the breast milk is not believed to have any relevance to the health of the baby, but the COC might very well hasten the end of lactation.

7.58 With or without lactation, which POP should be chosen?

After consideration of the contraindications (*see Qs 7.51 and 7.52*), there are few guidelines:

1 Neogest™ is not a very logical choice because it gives an added unnecessary dose of non-contraceptive dextro-norgestrel.

2 During lactation, on theoretical grounds Norgeston™ is possibly preferable to the other old-type POPs because such a negligible amount reaches the breast milk (*see Q 7.55*) – due to particularly strong binding to SHBG in the blood.

3 No study has shown statistically different rates of effectiveness between the levonorgestrel POPs (Norgeston™, Neogest™) and the

norethisterone group (Micronor™, Noriday™ and Femulen™). Cerazette™ is in a different league (although old-type POPs are nearly 100% themselves, when combined with breastfeeding or other states of relative infertility such as perimenopausally).

4 A 'best buy' can also not be stated for menstrual disturbance.

The initial choice of POP for cycling women therefore depends on the degree of efficacy desired. One would have to predict that Cerazette™ will corner the POP market for most highly fertile young women and those who are above 70 kg in weight (*see Q 7.16*); but old-type POPs would be equally suitable during lactation and other states of reduced fertility.

INITIAL MANAGEMENT AND FOLLOW-UP ARRANGEMENTS

7.59 What are the main aspects to convey during counselling?

The truth of the phrase 'forewarned is forearmed' is never so clear as in counselling about the unpredictable bleeding pattern of the POP (as indeed for all the oestrogen-free methods in this chapter). The good efficacy, second only to Cerazette™, the combined pill and injectables, of old-type POPs (especially in older women), should also be stressed – provided always that the rules for successful pill taking are followed (*see Qs 7.20–7.28*).

As for other methods, a supplementary leaflet (e.g. that produced by the FPA) should always be supplied along with the PIL.

7.60 How should POP use be monitored?

1 A baseline BP and weight are valuable.
2 Routine cervical smear examinations are good screening practice, although (as before) not believed to have any special relevance to the contraceptive method.
3 The woman should be seen 3 months after starting the POP and normally after 6 months – but all checks can then be extended to annually, and performed by a family-planning trained nurse with recourse to a doctor only if problems arise, such as pelvic pain.
4 Routine examinations should be kept to a minimum.
5 BP need only be measured annually.
6 Body weight is of no relevance to monitoring.

7.61 For how long can POP use be continued?

At present the answer is 'indefinitely' as long as contraception is required, into the late 50s – in the absence of contraindications, multiple-risk factors, or the occurrence of important complications.

7.62   How can the menopause be diagnosed in older POP users?

If an old-type POP user develops prolonged amenorrhoea, yet was previously observing bleeding episodes, it can be difficult to distinguish between amenorrhoea secondary to the POP and the arrival of the menopause. Symptoms, especially hot flushes, can be a useful guide.

There is also evidence that the finding of a high level of FSH can have some relevance at the menopause despite continued POP-taking. Low levels, on the other hand, suggest that the woman is in group 4 of Q 7.5, still potentially fertile, and should certainly continue to use this or some alternative contraceptive method.

7.63   How do you act if the FSH is high in an older POP user? Is there a practical protocol?

If the FSH is found to be high (at menopause levels for the laboratory), my practice above age 51 is to suggest that the woman discontinues the POP and transfers to a simple barrier method. The FSH is then repeated at 4–6 weeks, on two occasions if there is any doubt.

If the woman is still amenorrhoeic, has vasomotor symptoms and menopausal FSH results are again obtained, she can be advised that her chances of conception are low enough to discontinue alternative contraception – whether or not she now transfers to taking hormone replacement therapy (HRT).

No guarantee of total infertility can be given, however, and she is warned to return for advice should she develop any subsequent (non-HRT-related) bleeding. And women who want more complete reassurance should continue a simple method of birth control until 1 year after the last spontaneous bleed.

7.64   What if FSH measurements are still low?

If she is amenorrhoeic, the POP can simply be continued into the 50s with periodic FSH checks. But if she remains symptom free there is usually no pressure actually to establish final ovarian failure.

7.65   What about Cerazette™ use perimenopausally?

It is even more likely than with old-type POPs that a user of this pill will be amenorrhoeic at this age, but even when the ovaries are non-functional FSH levels might be maintained low, because of strong suppression of the hypothalamus/pituitary. There is medically no rush to get her off this very safe product, unlike with the COC at this age but it is a bit of a 'contraceptive overkill' – why not use a cheaper POP?

So a good option is to transfer to an old-type POP and proceed as above (see Qs 7.63 and 7.64). Or, if she develops unacceptable vasomotor symptoms, like any POP-user she could move to the excellent LNG-IUS plus HRT combination mentioned in Q 9.102 and 9.155; or more controversially (we badly need good studies on this) be given HRT while continuing on Cerazette™ (always if so on the 'named patient' prescribing basis discussed in *Appendix A*).

7.66 Should I be concerned about hypo-oestrogenism in any POP-user who develops prolonged amenorrhoea, especially with Cerazette™?

This is a difficult one: as in the similar situation applying to DMPA, there are insufficient data. But here there is actually reassuring data from the premarketing studies about average estradiol levels, with both Implanon™ and Cerazette™. Yet both suppress the ovaries more than old-type POPs, so it is believed that there is enough follicular activity through some ongoing FSH secretion and hence adequate oestrogen production with all these progestogen-only methods – regardless of whether or not they bleed.

Pending more data therefore, my current view – and this is a change from the last edition – is that, unlike with DMPA (*see Qs 8.23–8.27*) there need be no particular concern about hypo-oestrogenism, osteoporosis or arterial disease in long-term users of any kind of POP.

If an individual user develops significant vasomotor symptoms she should either switch to another method or perhaps try the combination of Cerazette™ with HRT proposed in *Qs 7.64 and 7.67*.

7.67 If add-back oestrogen is taken by a POP user won't this make her more likely to conceive?

Not when she starts off in group 4 of Q 7.5, which means she is not ovulating. She is not relying on the mucus effect for contraceptive efficacy anyway, so it cannot enhance her fertility if the mucus is improved by the added oestrogen.

However now we have Cerazette™, I would normally recommend eliminating that concern (whatever ovarian function group a POP user might be in) by using only that anovulant POP when HRT is also desired (as always, on a 'named patient' basis, see *Appendix A*).

A stronger evidence-base for the advice given in the last six questions is high on my personal wish-list!

MANAGEMENT OF SIDE-EFFECTS OR COMPLICATIONS

7.68 What should be the second choice of POP if bleeding problems develop and cannot be tolerated?

1   First, examine the patient for a coincidental gynaecological cause (see *Table 5.15* and Q 5.168).

2 An understanding of the spectrum of individual reactions to the POP is of some help (*see Qs 7.5 and 7.6*). It would appear that the bleeding problems are concentrated in groups 2 and 3. Group 1 cycles are generally the most acceptable. With good counselling, women in group 4 can also accept their long episodes of amenorrhoea. Careful assessment of the bleeding pattern therefore aids decision making.

3 If it appears that a reduction in dose might transfer a woman from group 2 or 3 to group 1, one could, for example, switch from Femulen™ to Micronor™/Noriday™.

4 The reverse could be tried if reaching group 4 seemed likely to be achieved thereby, i.e. a trial of Femulen™ (the strongest old-type POP available) or Cerazette™. But the bleeding irregularity might get worse, if amenorrhoea does not result.

7.69 What minor non-bleeding side-effects have been described in POP takers?

The short answer is that POP-users report almost all of the minor side-effects reported by COC-takers but in general less frequently. In the Oxford/FPA comparative study, headaches, psychological disturbance (including depression) and hypertension were particularly associated with COCs as causes of discontinuation of the method. However, menstrual disturbance and, interestingly, breast discomfort, were reported more commonly among POP users. Mildly androgenic effects such as acne also occur, with no difference noted in the premarketing studies between the old-type LNG POP (4.2%) and Cerazette™ (4.1%).

7.70 Which second choice of POP should follow if non-bleeding minor side-effects develop?

The decision to change to a different POP has again to be empirical. For example, if headaches occur on a levonorgestrel POP it might be worth transferring to one of the norethisterone group – or the newest desogestrel product. With support and reassurance, however, the subjective symptoms often disappear after a few months of continuing to take the same POP.

7.71 What action should be taken if a POP user complains of low abdominal pain?

As usual, causes unrelated to contraception should be excluded. Two important possibilities must be borne in mind, although the first has a reduced likelihood with Cerazette™. Importantly, both cause menstrual irregularity and perhaps a unilateral mass as well as pain:

1 ectopic pregnancy.

2 pain due to the formation/torsion or rupture of a functional ovarian cyst: referral for ultrasound and (rarely) laparoscopy may be required (*see Q 7.53*).

7.72 Which symptoms should lead a POP user to take urgent medical advice? Should she transfer to another method at once?

Abdominal pain is probably the only acute symptom requiring urgent advice. But neither for this nor for any of the symptoms in the 'stop COC' list in *Q 6.13* (which are mostly irrelevant because they relate to oestrogen), must the woman discontinue the POP instantly. Continuing to take the POP for a few more days can do no significant harm – whereas an unplanned pregnancy might.

7.73 What should be done if a POP user is immobilized after an accident or requires emergency (or elective) major surgery?

There is no reason for a woman using any oestrogen-free preparation to discontinue the method in either of these clinical contexts.

7.74 What are the risks if a woman should become pregnant while taking the POP?

1 If she has conceived, although the old-type POP does not cause ectopics, a higher proportion of conceptions than usual prove to be extrauterine: so it would be clinically important to exclude the condition (*see Q 7.33*).

2 The available findings concerning teratogenesis are extremely reassuring. No cases of congenital abnormality have been reported, although there have been no good large studies. In the Oxford/FPA study there were 30 accidental pregnancies in continuing POP users. Of these, seven were terminated, 15 ended in live births without malformations, one was ectopic and seven ended in spontaneous miscarriage (*see also Q 6.46*). Given its small dose of only one hormone, the usual 'armchair thinking' about the POP would lead one to expect an even lower rate of fetal abnormalities in breakthrough POP pregnancies than with the COC. The rate for the latter (which is more firmly documented) is itself already remarkably low.

There is certainly no need to advise switching from the POP to another method for any arbitrary time before a planned conception (indeed this is unimportant even for the COC, *see Q 6.48*).

7.75 Are there any known special risks or benefits for ex-takers of the old-type POP?

There are no data to support or refute any such ex-use effects. If they exist at all they are likely to be clinically insignificant. Because of the known advantages of long-term anovulation, several of the ex-use benefits of the COC must be expected for ex-Cerazette™ users, but its arrival on the scene is too recent for any of these yet to be demonstrable.

PATIENT QUESTIONS

QUESTIONS ASKED BY USERS ABOUT THE POP

The general public does not ask many questions about the POP because few know of its existence as a separate method. Much confusion, particularly that these 'mini-pills' are not low-dose combined pills, has to be cleared up. The following short list can be instructive.

7.76 Does the POP ever cause an abortion?

No. Although not its usual method of action, one possible way the old-type POP operates on some occasions is by stopping implantation: the process by which a dividing fertilized egg becomes embedded in the lining of the womb. Stopping this is not now felt by most people to be causing an abortion, for the reasons explained in *Qs 10.3 and 10.4*. But the POP is thought to use this mechanism very rarely anyway and *never* when combined with full breastfeeding (*see Q 7.23*). If this is of concern to you, the newest product – Cerazette™ – does not appear to require to operate this way, when correctly taken even outside of breastfeeding.

Reading the question a different way, deliberately taking any or even a large number of POPs (or combined pills for that matter) is not a recognized abortifacient method: it is most unlikely to stop a fully established implanted pregnancy (even though they do work as emergency contraceptives prior to implantation, see *Chapter 10*).

7.77 If the old-type POP is not so effective as the combined pill, why are some women recommended to use it?

This method is only a little less effective than the combined pill, especially in the older age group. Indeed, above the age of 40 or when combined with breastfeeding it is as effective as the COC would be for a 25-year-old.

7.78 My period is overdue on the old-type POP or Cerazette™. What does this mean?

First, we might need to exclude the possibility that the method has let you down. Once that has been done, the most likely explanation is that the pill is preventing egg release. So, paradoxically, you will be more effectively protected from pregnancy than a girlfriend who is being reassured by seeing regular periods (*see Q 7.7*).

7.79   I know that COC users do not see proper periods – is that also true of the bleeds I get on the POP?

On the old-type POP, some episodes of bleeding are caused like normal periods. In these the special structure in your ovary known as a corpus luteum stops producing the two hormones that stimulate growth of the uterine lining, and this leads to it coming away, and hence a period. However, many POP users and users of Cerazette™ who bleed at all, have other bleeding or spotting episodes as well. These are either shorter or longer than a normal period and can be lighter or heavier. They are caused by irregular shedding of the womb lining, in turn caused by combined effects from the artificial hormone of the POP and the oestrogen and progesterone produced by your ovary (*see Qs 7.4–7.6 and Fig. 7.1*).

7.80   I am breastfeeding my baby and have been given the POP – won't this harm my baby?

Although a very tiny amount of the hormone does get into the breast milk, it has not been possible to show any changes in milk quantity or in quality, with either the old-type POP or with the newer product Cerazette™.

   There cannot be absolute proof that the POP hormone in the milk would be completely harmless: so if you are unhappy it would be important to discuss another method with your family doctor or a local clinic. However, the amount taken by the baby is very small; for example with Norgeston™ your baby will take only the equivalent of one tablet if you continue to breastfeed for 2 years! It is extremely improbable that such a minute dose would affect your baby at all (*see Qs 7.54 and 7.55*).

Injectables and implants

8

SELECTION OF USERS AND OF FORMULATIONS

INITIAL MANAGEMENT AND FOLLOW-UP ARRANGEMENTS

BACKGROUND AND MECHANISMS

8.1 What are injectables?

The two available in the UK are progestogenic steroids given on a regular basis by deep intramuscular injection for contraception. Experience with them dates back to the early 1960s. According to WHO (2003), DMPA is currently used by about 13 million women worldwide.

8.2 What injectables are available in the UK?

1   *Depot medroxyprogesterone acetate (DMPA)*: this is available in aqueous microcrystalline suspension and is normally given in a dose of 150 mg every 12 weeks. Other regimens have also been tried and proved effective.
2   *Norethisterone oenanthate (NET EN: Noristerat™, Norigest™)*: this is available in a vehicle of benzyl benzoate and castor oil, the dose being 200 mg every 8 weeks. Other regimens are not now recommended.

DMPA is an example of a pregnane progestogen, which is more closely related to natural progesterone than either oestrane progestogens such as norethisterone or gonanes such as levonorgestrel – all derived from 19-nortestosterone.

8.3 What is the status and availability of injectables worldwide and in the UK?

DMPA has been repeatedly endorsed by the WHO, the International Planned Parenthood Federation (IPPF) and virtually every other relevant authority. It is currently available for long-term contraceptive use in more than 130 countries. It is, in fact, the first-choice reversible method in South Africa and was approved for similar licensing in the US at end of 1992. In 1984, the UK Minister of Health agreed to the recommendation by the CSM that the method could be used long-term for contraception by selected women after full counselling about its long-term (and slow-to-reverse) nature. It now has the status of a first-line option in the UK. Yet it is still chosen currently by a very small minority – less than 2% of women use reversible contraception in the UK. This low usage is largely provider led: the option is offered so infrequently. But most of those who do use it are very satisfied customers!

NET EN is used, chiefly in Germany and a number of developing countries, even less widely. It is also available in the UK, a product licence for antifertility use having been granted. Although it is only officially for short-term use at present, longer-term use is acceptable in selected patients after counselling. But the oily injection is more painful than DMPA and its duration of action is only 8 weeks.

8.4 What is the mode of action of injectables?

The primary action of the progestogen dose given by both injectables is, like the COC, to prevent ovulation. As with other hormonal methods, this is supplemented chiefly by contraceptive actions at the endometrial and mucus level (*see Q 7.4* and *Table 7.2*).

8.5 Do injectables provide a steady dose?

No – see *Fig. 8.1*. Although the levels fluctuate far less than any oral method (COC or POP), there is a much higher level initially, declining exponentially thereafter. The release of hormone at a relatively constant or so-called zero-order rate is one of the advantages sought in newer injectables, and also rings and implants.

8.6 What is known about individual variation in blood levels?

This exists, as for the oral methods. However, the interindividual variation is rather less marked because variable absorption from the gut and variable first-pass metabolism (*see Q 5.33*) are not involved. Blood levels seem to

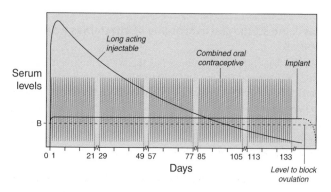

▲

Fig. 8.1 Blood levels of progestogen hormone in users of three delivery systems. Q 8.5. This is a schematic representation for DMPA. After an injection there is a relatively high level (B indicates the level to block ovulation), then a decline as time passes. Oral contraceptives (the POP would be similar, without a 7-day break) show wide fluctuations – a sawtooth pattern. Implants result in remarkably constant blood levels (adapted from Population reports K2, May 1983. Population information program. Johns Hopkins University, Figure 1).

decline more rapidly in thin women (*see Q 8.9*). NET EN has a shorter duration of action than DMPA.

8.7   What effects do injectables have on ovarian function?

As ovulation is generally inhibited, the 'spectrum effect' described in *Q 7.5* for the POP is not observed with these agents. However, minimal follicular activity occurs, especially towards the end of the injection period and more in some women than others. Importantly, this follicular estradiol keeps serum concentrations in the range normally found in the early to middle follicular phase (90–290 pmol/L). This prevents clinical hypo-oestrogenism (whether as symptoms or signs), probably in the majority of users. However, there is some concern about a few who in long-term use are found to have abnormally low estradiol levels (*see Qs 8.19 and 8.23*).

EFFECTIVENESS

8.8   What is the overall effectiveness of injectables?

Among available reversible contraceptives the use-effectiveness of these methods is greater than the COC because the factor of the user's memory is almost eliminated. The range of efficacy quoted for DMPA is 0(0.3 according to WHO)–1/100 woman-years, and for NET EN 0.4–2/100 woman-years.

8.9   What factors influence the effectiveness of injectables?

As usual, the rate of failure is marginally higher in younger, more fertile women. With either compound, but especially NET EN, it is essential not to massage the injection site (*see Q 8.44*) because this shortens the duration of action, increasing the failure rate in early studies. Local infection of the injection site can also be a factor (*see Q 8.16(11)*). It is important to insert the complete dose without spillage and ensure it is truly intramuscular even in an obese woman.

For the ticklish problem of overdue injections, see *Q 8.53ff*.

8.10   What are the recommended starting routines for injectables?

1   In menstruating women the first injection should normally be given before day 7 of the cycle (according to IPPF and WHO and it can certainly be even later if there has been 'believable abstinence or the equivalent' up to that date). With either drug before day 7 WHO does not advise added precautions. Yet, because of the analogy with the COC (see *Table 5.4*, p. 134), and conceptions in my service (one was ectopic), I advise extra precautions for 7 days whenever the first dose is later than day 2.

2   If a woman is on the POP or COC, and definitely not pregnant if
    amenorrhoeic on the former (see footnote to *Table 5.4*, *Qs 5.49 and*
    11.22), the injection can be given any time, and with no added
    precautions. The medical suitability of this 'overlap' of the two methods
    can be useful, for example in a combined pill-taker over the time of
    elective major surgery (*Q 6.17*).
3   Postpartum (whether or not the woman is breastfeeding): it
    recommends that the first injection should preferably be postponed until
    5–6 weeks after the delivery. Earlier administration increases the
    likelihood of heavy and prolonged bleeding. However, this is not
    inevitable and DMPA can also be given early even in the first week
    postpartum, exercising clinical judgement, if there is doubt whether the
    woman will return at the right time for her first dose. She must then be
    forewarned about the increased bleeding risk. Lactation is not inhibited.
4   After miscarriage or termination of pregnancy (first trimester): the
    injection is normally given within 7 days of the procedure and no extra
    precautions are required (*see also Qs 5.77 and 8.36 re* trophoblastic
    disease).

8.11 Do interactions with other drugs pose any problem with injectables?

There is certainly no problem with non-enzyme-inducing antibiotics
because the drug is not recycled from the gut.

Drugs inducing liver enzymes (*see Q 5.36*) pose a theoretical problem.
However, there has been a change in the clinical advice about this since the
last edition of this book because data that was already on file with the
Pharmacia company has been made available, and this supports *not*
shortening the injection interval or increasing the dose – even when the
most potent enzyme inducers (rifampicin or rifabutin) are used with
DMPA. The reason is that in studies the hepatic clearance of DMPA is
found to equate to hepatic blood flow. In other words, the liver is normally
eliminating all the medroxyprogesterone acetate (MPA) hormone in each
unit volume of blood that flows through it, and an incease in enzyme
activity in the hepatocytes cannot make the liver do better than 100%!

8.12 Might injectables affect the action of other drugs?

Due to possible and variable interference with warfarin metabolism, in
patients also using DMPA the INR needs to be checked additionally – as
with the COC and following emergency contraception. But because of the
increased risk of haematoma after each injection it would be far more usual
now to advise another method (e.g. Implanon™, *see Qs 8.58ff*). No other
interactions of this type have impacted on clinical practice with DMPA.

ADVANTAGES AND BENEFITS

8.13 What are the beneficial effects of injectables?

CONTRACEPTIVE BENEFITS

1   *High effectiveness*: definitely greater than the COC. Moreover, uniquely, its efficacy remains unaffected by enzyme-inducing drugs (*see Q 8.11*).
2   *Minimizes 'forgetability'*: a problem that exists with all pill methods.
3   *Highly convenient, non-intercourse-related.*
4   *Fully reversible*: although with some delay.

NON-CONTRACEPTIVE BENEFITS

Most of those in *Q 5.56* are believed to apply.

5   In many women there is a reduction in the disorders of the menstrual cycle:
  (a) less heavy bleeding, often culminating in amenorrhoea (which can be a health benefit in reducing the risk of gynaecological disorders as listed in *Q 5.57* – but with the caveats in *Qs 8.23–8.27*)
  (b) less anaemia, indeed the haemoglobin has been noted to rise regardless of the bleeding pattern, suggesting a direct haemopoietic effect as well as less quantity of loss
  (c) less dysmenorrhoea
  (d) fewer symptoms of premenstrual tension (not invariably – in some women similar symptoms (*see Q 8.16(10)*) occur early in each injection interval)
  (e) no ovulation pain.

Given the common side-effects of frequent or prolonged bleeding (*see Q 8.16*) none of the above improvements can be reliably predicted for the individual woman.

6   Less pelvic inflammatory disease (PID): like other progestogen-containing contraceptives. Confirmed by a WHO study (1985).
7   Fewer extrauterine pregnancies because ovulation is inhibited.
8   Possibly fewer FOCs overall for the same reason (*see Q 5.60*), but this has not been well studied.
9   Reduction in the growth of fibroids but, once again, only if oligo- or amenorrhoea is achieved.
10 A possible reduction in the rate of endometriosis, which indeed can be treated by high-dose oral MPA or by DMPA (unless they fail to produce amenorrhoea).
11 Overdose extremely unlikely and would not be fatal.
12 Beneficial social effects, especially because the method is under a woman's control.
13 Protection against endometrial cancer (*see Q 8.31*).

It is not known how many of the other benefits described for the COC (*see* Q 5.56) apply also to injectables (namely, a reduction in risk of benign breast disease, thyroid disease, rheumatoid arthritis, TSS, trichomonal vaginitis and, above all, ovarian cancer). On theoretical grounds most are likely benefits, only waiting to be firmly established.

BENEFITS NOT (NECESSARILY) SHARED WITH THE COC

14 Definite beneficial effects on frank sickle-cell disease (*see* Q 8.15).

15 Aggression, mood swings and epileptic attacks: especially in patients with severe learning disabilities, DMPA is reported as very beneficial if the timing of these problems is regularly premenstrual or menstrual. 'Tricycling' of the COC or using Cerazette™ or Implanon™ can be a way of obtaining a similar benefit, providing amenorrhoea is achieved (*see* Q 5.31).

16 Lactation is not suppressed and might even be enhanced due to increased production of prolactin – but the POP is lower-dose and equally effective (*see* Q 8.40).

17 Complete freedom from side-effects due to oestrogen. Its mortality rate approaches very close to zero.

> These improvements are variable, and dependent on the bleeding pattern experienced by individual women.

8.14 In view of the above advantages, why has there been so much adverse publicity over the years about injectables?

Mainly because of:

1 Unfounded excessive anxiety about cancer as a result of irrelevant studies on different species (e.g. dogs). The balance of the evidence is actually favourable (*see* Q 8.31).

2 The possibility of abuse (by providers, 'pushing' the method on women or, worse, giving it without their knowledge or consent). This is a potential problem with any injection but one that is not best solved by banning a good product.

3 The impossibility of removing the injection if side-effects occur.

Yet, overall, safety is clearly greater than the COC, which itself is amazingly safe. Wherever injectables have been made available as a realistic choice, continuation rates are better than for most other methods.

8.15 What is the effect of DMPA on homozygous sickle-cell disease?

A careful trial in the West Indies demonstrated a highly significant improvement in the haematological picture, and a reduction in the number of painful crises, in patients treated with 3-monthly injections of DMPA. It is suggested that this could be the method of choice both in sickle syndrome and sickle-cell disease.

There are theoretical reasons for believing that all progestogen-containing contraceptives would be similarly beneficial, including the POP, Cerazette™ implants (*see Q 8.59*) and even perhaps the COC – although with the last the artificial oestrogen content has its own potential disadvantages (*see Q 5.143*).

MAIN PROBLEMS AND DISADVANTAGES

8.16 What are the main disadvantages of injectables?

1 First and foremost, the fact that the *injection cannot be removed* once given. This must always be mentioned to the potential user: the method is irreversible for at least 2–3 months (depending on the injectable used) and early side-effects would therefore have to be tolerated for a long time.

2 *Disturbance of menstruation* when it occurs can be so marked and variable over time that it has been called 'menstrual chaos'. With reassuring counselling amenorrhoea is usually very acceptable (*see Q 8.43*).

3 Possible, as yet unconfirmed, *risks of long-term hypo-oestrogenism* (*see Q 8.23*).

4 *Delay in the return, but no loss of, fertility* (*see Q 8.39*).

5 *Weight gain*: with most other contraceptives the method is often blamed unfairly, but not so with this one. Most women gain weight – up to 2 kg (4.5 lb) in the first year – and a few do so very rapidly after the very first dose. This possibility must always be discussed with users in advance. The increase is not associated with fluid retention and diuretics are useless.

6 Possible *adverse effects on the fetus* (*see Q 8.56*).

7 *Galactorrhoea* can occur, with a raised prolactin (usually within the normal range).

8 *Mildly androgenic effects* such as acne can happen but are surprisingly uncommon.

9 *Enuresis* has rarely been reported as recurring in women who were enuretic at adolescence. If the link is causal it might attributable to a relaxing effect of the progestogens on smooth muscle.

10 *Subjective 'minor' side-effects*. These are many and varied, as with all hormonal methods. Some can be truly attributable to the method and in some cases they might be placebo reactions. The following have been reported:

   (a) loss of libido, vaginal dryness (relatively rare, but biologically plausible, *see Qs 8.23 and 8.27*)

(b) lassitude
(c) depression (*see Q 8.50*) and other mood changes
(d) bloatedness
(e) dizziness
(f) breast symptoms (increase or decrease in size and tenderness)
(g) leg cramps
(h) headaches
(i) acne – rare, because MPA is a progesterone-based molecule.
11 Local complications:
   (a) haematoma of the injection site (particularly in patients using anticoagulants, which are therefore a strong WHO 3 contraindication to the method, especially as the needle of an obvious alternative, Implanon™, is inserted far more superficially)
   (b) infection of the injection site. I am aware of a legal action alleging that an abscess caused failure of the method. Therefore if this rare event occurs that particular injection should be deemed to be ineffective.

8.17 What are the effects of injectables on metabolism?

Although many studies have been reported (particularly on DMPA) they tend to be cross-sectional and poorly controlled, especially for cigarette smoking, and might not be standardized for the time since the last injection was given, individual variation, the presence or absence of ovarian activity, and so on. Too often the studies tell us more about the users than about DMPA.

8.18 What are the effects on blood coagulation and fibrinolysis?

To summarize much research, there is no proven effect of any significance on either of these. In the WHO Collaborative Study (1998) there was a small and non-significant increase in the odds ratio for venous thromboembolism. This could have been related to selective use of the methods by women at greater risk, and to diagnostic bias.

For the present, it remains good practice to use either DMPA or NET EN where there is a past history of venous thromboembolism (WHO 2).

8.19 What are the effects on blood lipids, especially HDL-C?

Available data about blood lipids are scanty and difficult to interpret. Most researchers have reassuringly found no effect or even a decrease in triglycerides or total cholesterol with both injectables. A few DMPA studies show a less encouraging increase in LDL and decrease (of up to 15%) in HDL-C levels with DMPA. In a prospective study of NET EN, HDL-C declined more markedly, by about 25% after the first injection, but did not change further with up to 4 years of use.

These results are hard to interpret because so many DMPA users smoke, but they could also be at least partly related to the lower endogenous estradiol production in users of injectables. Their relation to amenorrhoea and the overall clinical significance for arterial disease are not clear (*see Q 8.23* and, with regard to contraindications, *Qs 8.36 and 8.38*).

8.20 What are the effects on carbohydrate metabolism?

Some reports find an increase in insulin levels with both these injectables, which would cause some theoretical concerns, but most report no change. The development of overt diabetes in women using DMPA for contraception has not been reported, and WHO does not consider this a contraindication to the method.

8.21 Do any other surrogate tests suggest a risk of arterial wall disease?

Yes, a small study by Sorensen et al 2002 (*Circulation* 106:1646–1651), of 12 DMPA users and 9 controls used magnetic resonance imaging (MRI) to evaluate arterial function in the brachial artery. The results (after 1 year) suggested that endothelial function might be slightly impaired in the DMPA users, in a manner that has been proposed as a possible surrogate marker for risk of arterial disease. The recency of this technique and its non-clinical end-point makes us wary of drawing conclusions or changing practice through this study alone (*but see Q 8.23ff*).

8.22 Are there any other metabolic effects?

In general, only minimal effects have been shown. Because all progestogens appear capable of causing attacks of acute porphyria, and injectables cannot be rapidly reversed, they are absolutely contraindicated, even in latent acute porphyria (WHO 4, *see Qs 6.42 and 8.36*).

Injectables do not appear adversely to affect liver function. They are metabolized by the liver but can be used safely by women with a history of jaundice or hepatitis B carrier states (WHO 2). If there is chronic cirrhosis with mild liver function test abnormality this would be WHO 3. But injectables should not be used at all if liver function tests are currently grossly abnormal (WHO 4) – if any hormonal method were suitable the POP (WHO 3) would be preferred.

8.23 What is the present information on hypo-oestrogenism and progestogen-only injectables?

For DMPA the evidence is still too scanty to give any confident answer, and data are all-but absent for NET EN. The discussion below relates to DMPA only. There is some cause for concern, in my view, as follows:

1   It has been known since the 1970s that DMPA is a powerful suppressant of FSH as well as LH levels, so that estradiol levels in long-term DMPA users are always on the low side, as in the follicular phase of the cycle; although after 5 years of use most are above those of postmenopausal women and do not suggest true functional insufficiency. However, very low levels are found in some individuals – well under 100 pmol/L (compare this with 150–200 pmol/L as the target bone-sparing threshold level in low-dose oestrogen replacement after the menopause). Recent work shows that estradiol levels can be very low whether women are seeing bleeds (bleeds from the endometrium in DMPA users not being 'periods' anyway) or have complete amenorrhoea. Contrariwise, some other long-term users even with complete amenorrhoea do have enough ovarian follicular activity for perfectly adequate estradiol levels – up to over 300 pmol/L – to be measurable (*see Q 8.27*, *Box 8.1* (4)).

2   It is also well established that premature menopause (idiopathic or after bilateral oophorectomy) increases the risk of AMI and osteoporosis thereafter, unless the missing oestrogen is replaced.

So the big question is: does hypo-oestrogenism in a proportion of DMPA users signify similar long-term risks to having a premature menopause?

8.24 What do we know, then, about the osteoporosis risk in long-term DMPA users?

Results from a study by Cundy et al, working in New Zealand, were published in the *British Medical Journal* in 1991. In brief, 30 current users of DMPA, with a minimum 5 years' previous use and all with continuous amenorrhoea, were compared in a cross-sectional study with 30 premenopausal volunteers and 30 postmenopausal controls. The bone density values in the DMPA users were lower by about 7% than those in the premenopausal women. This is too small a reduction for any fracture risk and, moreover, the values were higher than in the postmenopausal women, whose mean duration of relative oestrogen deficiency was similar (about 10 years).

There are many problems with this study. The laboratory and technical work might be good but numbers were small and the researchers were let down by the basic design (there was no knowledge of the bone status of the DMPA-users prior to starting the method). Also, the attempted matching process could not correct for gross disparity between the studied groups. Four times as many DMPA users were smokers (40%) as the premenopausal controls, although the DMPA-related difference persisted when the (only) 21 women who were concordant for smoking habits were compared.

However, a later study by Cundy was larger and confirmatory (Cundy et al 1998 *Obstetrics and Gynecology* 92:569–573) and, reassuringly, documented recovery of bone density, with the restoration of more normal estradiol levels, when DMPA users were monitored before and after stopping DMPA. The effect might prove comparable to prolonged lactation, where bone density loss is reversed after cessation. And a study of postmenopausal former DMPA users showed very similar bone densities to never-users.

Other studies in the world literature are mostly (although not all) reassuring about osteoporosis. Another finding, like for bleeding pattern, is that there is no significant correlation between bone density in DMPA users and serum estradiol levels (Gbolade et al 2002 *Journal of Family Planning and Reproductive Healthcare* 28:7–11). But this might be because of the many confounding variables affecting the data, which are mostly cross-sectional and which could be telling us much more about the women who select or are selected for DMPA than about effects of DMPA itself!

In short, the jury is still out as to whether there is, in reality, a minor adverse effect on bones in long-term users and how completely reversible this might be: especially in smokers, the very underweight, in adolescents under 18 who are still building their peak bone mass post menarche and among women above age 45. In their eligibility monograph, WHO put the latter two groups in category WHO 2 on this account.

8.25 But are the bones the main concern? What do we know about the risk of heart attacks and other arterial diseases in long-term DMPA users?

My chief concern is not with the bones at all. My concern is far more about whether the analogy with premature menopause means that long-term DMPA users will resemble women with (premature) menopause for subsequent risk of arterial disease, especially in smokers. Some of the metabolic (lipid) changes (described many years ago) in long-term users are not very reassuring (*see* Q 8.19), nor is the MRI study discussed in Q 8.21, nor the 1998 WHO study of BP and injectables (Q 8.29).

The 1998 WHO Collaborative study (*Contraception* 57:315–324) is encouraging about all arterial disease including AMI in current injectable users. However, WHO admits that the study has a 'major limitation':

… the potential for false negative findings … resulting from the small numbers of cases and control subjects.

I would add that a clinically important real difference in AMI risk might only be detectable in ex-users, and many years later, because women (fortunately) have so low a risk of AMI in the childbearing years.

8.26 We all want to practise evidence-based medicine, so what does this add up to?

Given some metabolic 'surrogate markers' of possible risk, and the uncertain picture from so-far inconclusive clinical/epidemiological studies, we all face a dilemma. I summarize it in the following completely true statements:

1   There is insufficient evidence that long-term hypo-oestrogenism in DMPA-users *does* increase the risk of a later heart attack or other arterial event (or of osteoporosis).

2   There is insufficient evidence that long-term hypo-oestrogenism in DMPA-users *does not* increase the risk of a later heart attack or other arterial event (or of osteoporosis).

Both statements cannot be refuted. It becomes a matter of clinical Judgement, with a capital 'J'!

I prefer to act on the precautionary principle. One day the evidence will be incontrovertible. I will find it easier to look my patients in the eye if it then emerges that I have over the years unnecessarily changed some women to using another method (even if this led to some unwanted pregnancies) or given them 'add-back' oestrogen; than if it turns out they have been exposed for years to a real and possibly long-term increased risk of AMI, or indeed of osteoporosis (although this is a far less fatal condition).

There is no simple answer. *Box 8.1 (see Q 8.27)* outlines the protocol I currently recommend. But I have to report that many other UK and international authorities (and staff-members in my former service!) consider this, as they are perfectly entitled to do, an over-reaction. They would not proactively raise the issues of arterial disease or bone density loss with any long-term user and they would rarely – and only on the basis of concern about these two issues – consider a change of method or add-back oestrogen. In this they are being reassured by statement (1) above and they are well supported by all recent publications of WHO and IPPF, which in general simply do not discuss the arterial issue!

8.27 But how do you personally feel long-term users of DMPA should be managed, pending more data?

Given the uncertainty, I start from the view that DMPA is a very useful contraceptive but that it would be best to consider it, as a general rule, as being normally time-limited to 5 years use (*Box 8.1*). Thereafter, given several new choices among 'forgettable' contraceptives (e.g. Implanon™, newer IUDs and the IUS), it should normally be possible to switch at about that time to a satisfactory alternative.

Box 8.1 admittedly describes a rigmarole but I feel myself pushed into it by the conflicting data. *Hence my strong preference, especially now we have excellent new choices, for generally short-circuiting it by simply recommending a change of method in most women after about 5 years.*

BOX 8.1 A protocol for DMPA management

1. Contraindications

Pay careful attention to contraindications (*see Qs 11.36, 11.38*): with special reference to risk factors for:

(i) *arterial disease* (WHO 4 if multiple or severe, down to WHO 3 if an older smoker, or WHO 2 if a young smoker, see *Table 5.11*, p. 190)

(ii) *osteoporosis* (WHO 3, meaning usually avoid the method, if these are marked such as corticosteroid treatment, anorexia nervosa, bulimia; and WHO 2 for under 18s and over 45s as actually advised by WHO).

Should either type of risk factor apply then the potential user should be informed of the unproven additional adverse effect of DMPA on their particular risk.

2. Review at 5 years

Generally, only after 5 years use should the issue be reviewed with the woman herself, but at any time earlier if she has actual symptoms suggestive of hypo-oestrogenism (notably dryness of the vagina, hot flushes).

3. The consultation

This will have three main outcomes:

(i) *Does she want to change her method?* Most commonly, once this concern is addressed, the woman chooses to change her method anyway. This will regularly increase her mean oestrogen levels, either exogenously (the COC) or endogenously from her own ovaries (as after vasectomy, IUD or IUS insertion and all the lower-dose progestogen-only methods including Implanon™ and Cerazette™).

(ii) *Does she want simply to continue DMPA* without either investigations or supplements? A woman in this group decides differently from (i), given the genuine scientific uncertainty about what an estradiol in the low follicular-phase range means for health, and all the other risks she takes in life anyway (especially relevant thinking for a smoker!). Such a woman often says she would always choose to continue with DMPA on the balance of risks, including those of pregnancy. If so, this discussion should simply be recorded meticulously, she should be advised about diet and exercise, and the question readdressed with her periodically, at least at 5-yearly review visits or when new research data are published. Remember, in a moderately overweight individual, oestrogen levels are more likely to be higher anyway, due to peripheral conversion of androgenic precursors to oestrogens.

(iii) *She thinks she might want to continue and wants investigation before deciding* to change the method or maybe take added oestrogen (see 4, below).

4. Testing – whether and what to test?

(i) There is no point in doing FSH levels because these will always be low in DMPA users as a result of pituitary suppression.

(ii) There is also not much point in doing expensive bone scans or blood lipid assays, although they could be appropriate on specific clinical grounds (e.g. a bone scan for a thin teenage athlete or on the emergence of an anorexia history, lipids because of a relevant family history of AMI).

(iii) *Serum estradiol?* Although it does not correlate with bone density in the available studies (but these have so many potential confounding variables, *see Q 5.103*), it is nevertheless in my view the proximate determinant of the issue of concern here, which is that very low levels for a long time of this quintessentially female hormone might not be good for health, particularly of the arteries. So, in my view, in a symptom-free user of DMPA for 5 years, if any test is done (testing should be rare given that Group 3(iii) ought to be a small residual group after counselling) to aid the decision whether to continue for longer, this is it:

   (a) it is not expensive, but the laboratory will stress that results are not accurate at this low end of the sensitivity range – they are only '± 25 pmol/L' anyway. This does not matter because we are only looking for results significantly below 100 pmol/L.

   (b) estradiol should be measured in the week before the day of her next injection, to get a measure of its level well after the peak of the MPA levels and thus when minimum suppression would be expected (*see Fig. 8.1 and Q 8.6*).

5. Actioning the results

(i) Sometimes the *first result is good*, well above 100 pmol/L, implying (according to present knowledge) ovarian follicular activity that might well be sufficient both for arterial and bone health. If so, and the woman is happy with the injectable, it can continue to be used (long term), plus the usual diet and exercise advice and a periodical review at 5 years or when new data emerge.

(ii) *First estradiol is definitely less than 100 pmol/L.* Alternatively: consider if there might be an added clinical indication for a bone scan and, if so, arrange, manage according to the result obtained.

(iii) Will the DMPA user *now* accept a change of method? This would be ideal, see above.

(iv) *Or* (and after working through this protocol there should now be only a tiny minority of the original population of 5-year DMPA-users): *does she want to continue the DMPA method?* This is entirely in her gift. If so, does she want oestrogen add-back?

    (a) *No*: in which case (although it would really have been better she never got herself tested!) follow the management and careful record-keeping at 3(ii), above.

    (b) *Yes*, if and only if she is interested in that option, I would prefer to repeat the test (see above regarding timing), to provide support for a somewhat controversial decision (Gbolade 2002) with long-term implications. If two oestrogen results less than 100 pmol/L are obtained, I would then be prepared, pending more data, to supply natural oestrogen by any chosen route and usually continuously.

It must be fully explained and recorded (as in Appendix A), that this add-back concept is not licensed. Nor is it fully evidence-based that this combination will reverse the arterial disease or osteoporosis risks; nor that MPA by this route will fully protect the uterus from the effects of added oestrogen. Stress the need for good future follow-up. But do not retest estradiol levels at any later time while the woman is taking the added oestrogen; this would be somewhat meaningless.

6. Clinical grounds

There is one other option, which is to use clinical grounds alone, without measuring estradiol at all, to provide the add-back oestrogen by any chosen route (always on a 'named patient' basis; see Appendix A). One example might be a very committed/enthusiastic DMPA user aged 45-plus with vasomotor symptoms that are such a problem to her that (combined with reaching the 'HRT age') one would wish to treat anyway. But then I would have encouraged her to switch away from DMPA (perhaps to an old-type POP) by age 45 anyway!

8.28 **What protocol would you follow for NET EN users? And for long-term oligo- or amenorrhoeic users of any POP (including Cerazette™), of Implanon™ or of the LNG-IUS?**

With DMPA the problem seems to be long-term suppression of FSH and, as we have seen, the occurrence of some bleeding is no guide to oestrogen levels. But with all the other methods mentioned in the question there seems generally to be sufficient FSH release to maintain enough follicular activity and supply adequate oestrogen for (presumed) arterial and (measured) bone health. And with the LNG-IUS, after the first year 85% of users are cycling normally (*see Q 9.145ff*) – almost all are oligo- or amenorrhoeic but this is due to local effects of the LNG at the end-organ, the endometrium.

All these proposals (*see Qs 8.23–8.28*) are tentative, for the time being, and until we have better data.

8.29 What effects do injectables have on BP?

Studies show no consistent and certainly no significant change in either systolic or diastolic BP in women using either injectable. But limited WHO evidence (1998) suggests that women with hypertension may have an increased risk of cardiovascular events if they use DMPA.

Interestingly, neither WHO nor IPPF in their latest guidelines recommend regular BP measurements, aside from the first visit to assess pre-existing hypertension. In the UK it is usual to check BP at least every 6 months. Yet would not annual checks be more than adequate after the first year, and surely doing it at every 12-week visit for an injection is over the top?!

8.30 Do injectables affect neoplasia in animals?

Given enormous doses of DMPA, beagle bitches (which are by nature prone to breast lumps) can develop malignant tumours of the breast. Two out of 12 rhesus monkeys given 50 times the human contraceptive dose in a 10-year trial developed endometrial carcinoma. No cases were observed in monkeys treated with the human dose or 10 times the human dose.

The animal models (beagle bitches or rhesus monkeys) are believed by most authorities to be manifesting species-specific reactions that are not applicable to the human, and the doses used have been irrelevantly high.

8.31 What are the latest data about DMPA and cancer in the human?

The 1991 publications by WHO from good hospital-based, case–control studies in developing countries (including *International Journal of Cancer* 49:182–195) still provide the best data to date. The findings were:

1 *Endometrial cancer*: a protective effect, in fact a five-fold reduction in risk. There was also an ex-use protective effect detectable for at least 8 years after cessation of DMPA use. It seems the reduction in risk is as great for DMPA as for the COC.

2 *Epithelial ovarian cancer*: protective effect as with the COC was (surprisingly) not demonstrated but there is certainly no increase in risk

either. It might be that protection would be shown only in a population of DMPA users at high risk of ovarian cancer (not so far studied).

3 *Primary liver cancer*: no increased risk, and this was in countries (Thailand and Kenya) where hepatitis B is endemic.

4 *Cervical cancer*: no increased risk. This is the finding of a larger and better WHO study than the earlier one reported in 1984, which showed a small association with DMPA use. It confirms the suspicion at the earlier time that the association was due to confounding by factors such as sexual activity and smoking.

5 *Breast cancer: see Q 8.32.*

Overall, these results are very favourable to this much-maligned method.

8.32 Does DMPA increase the risk of breast cancer?

In the large WHO (1991) hospital-based, case–control study from five centres, reported in *The Lancet* (338:833–838), there was no link with breast cancer in the total population (869 cases, 11 890 controls), nor any increased risk with increased duration of use. The only statistically increased risk was for use in the first 4 years after initial exposure, mainly in women under 35. There was no increase in risk among women who started DMPA more than 5 years previously.

On the one hand, DMPA might – perhaps – be bringing forward the appearance of cancers that would have become manifest later. On the other hand, it is possible that the association in the WHO study is entirely caused by detection bias; recent users (who would necessarily be younger) or their physicians being more likely to discover breast lumps in the first 4 years of DMPA use.

The 1996 CGHFBC study differs slightly, giving similar results for DMPA to those for the COC (*see Q 5.83*), i.e. a possible but *non-significant* increased risk in current users, which diminishes reassuringly by to nil after 10 years in ex-users. More data are needed and the jury is still out.

8.33 Can DMPA be used in cases of trophoblastic disease?

In the UK it is recommended that DMPA, like all contraceptive steroids, should be avoided until hCG is undetectable (*see Q 5.77*). Thereafter there is no objection to this method, which can be a very suitable means of preventing pregnancy for the 2 years of designated follow-up.

8.34 Is there any evidence that injectables affect the development or growth of benign tumours?

The growth of uterine fibroids is usually inhibited, presumably because of hypo-oestrogenism. Other benign tumours appear to be unaffected.

SELECTION OF USERS AND OF FORMULATIONS

8.35 For whom are injectables particularly indicated?

1 First and foremost, if a systemic, non-intercourse-related method is chosen by the woman and *other options* (particularly those containing oestrogen) are *contraindicated, or disliked*. This includes the categories:

(a) postvenous thromboembolism or known prothrombotic abnormality of coagulation (WHO 2). A good example of the latter is severe SLE (*see Q 5.146*)

(b) to cover relevant elective surgery (*see Q 6.17*)

(c) forgetful pill-takers.

2 Women wanting hormonal contraception and on long term enzyme-inducers, since they affect the efficacy of DMPA (*Q 8.11*).

3 Women in whom *long-term progestogens are indicated anyway*, e.g. sickle-cell disease (*see Q 8.15*) and some with fibroids and endometriosis.

4 Past history of a *tubal ectopic pregnancy*: because like the COC it is an anovulant and will prevent pregnancy in any location (*see Q 8.31*).

5 *Epilepsy*: the frequency of seizures can sometimes be reduced.

6 At the *woman's choice*.

8.36 What are the absolute contraindications (WHO 4) to injectables?

These are identical to the first six relating to the POP (*see Q 7.51*), with the need for a little more caution (as also in *Q 8.38* with respect to relative contraindications) because:

1 The dose is larger, blood oestrogen levels are lower (*see Qs 8.23ff*) and lipid changes greater.

2 There is the aforementioned reversibility problem after any given injection is given.

ABSOLUTE CONTRAINDICATIONS

1 Past *severe arterial disease*, or current exceptionally high risk of the same. Pending further information I would not prescribe an injectable to a woman known to have current ischaemic heart disease (including angina) or to have already suffered a thrombotic stroke; nor to women with marked and multiple risk factors (e.g. a 45-year-old heavy-smoking hypertensive diabetic!) – or if so one would certainly only use the method as a WHO 3 short-term expedient (*see Qs 8.19 and 5.102*). Severe hypertension (*see Q 8.29*) and hereditary lipid abnormalities with a poor prognosis come into this category WHO 4. However, the injectable might be prescribed with extra counselling and supervision in the presence of milder abnormalities with a good prognosis (WHO 3 or even 2).

2   *Any serious side-effect occurring on the COC and not clearly due only to oestrogen* – or associated with past progestogen-only use.

3   *Liver adenoma* and severe past steroid-associated *cholestatic jaundice*, also any current *severe liver impairment* with grossly abnormal liver function tests.

4   *Recent trophoblastic disease* (*see* Q 5.77), until hCG is undetectable.

5   *Acute porphyria*, WHO 4 even if only the latent condition, without a past attack history (*see* Q 6.42).

As for all medical methods, we must also add:

1   *Severe allergy* to a constituent (particularly the methyl parabens excipient)

2   *Undiagnosed abnormal genital tract bleeding* since the injectable will confuse diagnosis

3   Actual or possible *pregnancy*

4   *The woman's own continuing uncertainty* about the safety of DMPA or NET EN, even after full counselling.

8.37   Why is past ectopic pregnancy an indication rather than a contraindication to injectables, whereas the POP would not be a preferred method?

Because, like the COC, injectables almost always block ovulation and hence virtually eliminate the risk of an ectopic. The woman with damaged tubes is, of course, still at risk of getting her ectopic later, when the anovulant treatment cases.

8.38   What are the relative contraindications to injectables?

See Q 5.135 – here is my list, but as usual the judgements of different authorities such as WHO differ to some extent. The category is WHO 2 unless otherwise stated:

1   *Risk factors for arterial disease (WHO 3)*: this category includes hypertension once it has been diagnosed and controlled and also migraine with focal aura (*see* Q 5.151). The presence of more than one risk factor can be tolerated more readily than with the COC – but there are limits. Prothrombotic coagulation factor abnormalities are actually included above as 'indications' because they should not be worsened at all by an injectable. Likewise, there is not the oestrogen-related concern about thrombotic stroke in migraine although it might be affected as a symptom. Lipid abnormalities might perhaps be worsened by the injectables. Any of the POPs or Implanon™, having fewer metabolic effects, would therefore normally be a better choice (*see* Qs 7.52, 7.66 and 8.73ff).

2 *Significant risk factors for osteoporosis (see Qs 8.23–8.27 and Box 8.1, p. 331)*: Corticosteroid treatment, anorexia nervosa, and athletes with amenorrhoea and bulimia would be WHO 3; also women aged under 18 or over 45 are WHO 2 states, as advised in WHO's *Eligibility criteria* monograph. If any of these risk factors apply then the potential user should be informed of the possible additional adverse effect of DMPA, with careful review after 5 years.

3 *Sex steroid-dependent cancer (WHO 3)*: the POP is preferred as lower dose and more readily reversible (*see Q 7.52*). But seek the advice of the oncologist looking after your patient. The WHO *Eligibility* monograph permits DMPA on a WHO 3 basis for women with breast cancer in remission for 5 years.

4 *Active liver disease, with moderately abnormal liver function tests*: caution is required (WHO 3). Focal nodular hyperplasia (FNH) is also WHO 3 for DMPA (*see Qs 5.96 and 5.134*).

5 *Other chronic systemic diseases*: the comments in *Q 5.138* for the COC apply. The great effectiveness as a contraceptive often helps to outweigh the continuing uncertainty as to what effect (either way) an injectable might have on the disease. With that proviso, and given the reversibility problem, DMPA might be a possible choice (WHO 3) for the conditions listed as absolute (*see Q 5.134*) or relative (*see Q 5.136*) contraindications to the COC – including severe SLE or diabetes with tissue damage.

6 *Unacceptability of menstrual irregularities*: especially cultural/religious taboos (e.g. Islam and Orthodox Judaism) associated with bleeding – or amenorrhoea.

7 *Obesity*: although further weight gain is not inevitable (*see Q 5.123*) and there is a possible oestrogen advantage, see Box 8.1, p. 331).

8 *Past severe endogenous depression*: above-average support is needed.

9 *Planning a pregnancy in the near future (Q 8.39)*: this contraindication would become 'absolute' if she wished to conceive within 6–9 months of the proposed injection.

10 *In the years leading up to the menopause*: there are five concerns:
   (a) the effect on HDL-C (*see Q 8.19*), particularly if the woman is a smoker
   (b) the possibility of hypo-oestrogenism and its uncertain implications (*see Q 8.23*).
   Objections (a) and (b) might, in a few selected cases, be overcome by 'add-back' oestrogen replacement (see *Box 8.1*, p. 331).
   (c) irregular bleeding might necessitate endometrial sampling
   (d) the menopause will be masked (*see Q 8.47*)
   (e) the method is perhaps too strong, a 'contraceptive overkill' (*see Qs 11.32 and 11.49*).

These concerns add up to WHO 3 in my view so, in practice, at around age 45 it would nearly always be better to switch, e.g. to the POP.

8.39 What effects do injectables have on future fertility?

Return of fertility is slow, especially with DMPA, but complete. In the largest study (*Fig. 8.2*) of parous women in Thailand, the mean time to conception was 9 months after the last injection. Now the last injection has a significant antifertility effect for about 15 weeks (the 12-week injection frequency being set to prevent, not the average, but the most DMPA-resistant woman from conceiving). So the true delay after stopping the method is a median of only 5.5 months, comparing very favourably with discontinuation of the COC (mean delay 3 months, *Fig. 8.2*). Underweight women regained their fertility faster.

The same study showed that 91% of DMPA-users had conceived by 2 years from discontinuation, as just defined, compared with 95% of former COC users – not a statistically significant difference and confirming the lack of any permanent fertility loss.

Secondary amenorrhoea does persist in a minority and should be investigated and treated if it lasts for more than 9 months after the last injection (*see Qs 5.62–5.67*). This is extremely treatable by standard ovulation induction methods.

Cumulative conception rates for women discontinuing DMPA, COCs and copper IUDs to become pregnant

Fig. 8.2 Cumulative conception rates for women discontinuing DMPA, COCs and copper IUDs to become pregnant. Q 8.39. *Note*: Researchers assumed that users 'discontinued' DMPA 15 weeks after their last injection (source: Pardthaisong 1984 *Journal of Biosocial Science* 16:23–34).

8.40 What are the effects of injectables on lactation?

1 Both injectables appear to increase the volume of breast milk.
2 Most studies suggest no important change in its composition.
3 The amount of hormone transmitted to the infant in breast milk is very small, less than 0.5% of the maternal dose.

Although no long-term effects on infant growth and development have been reported, the amount of exposure to an artificial hormone is obviously greater than with the POP. In view of this minimal uncertainty, in my view it would be preferable for most lactating women in the UK to use the POP, transferring to the injectable as one option when the child is weaned. (The combination of POP plus full lactation is already almost 100% effective contraception.)

If DMPA or NET EN *are* used in lactation, they should ideally be given 5–6 weeks after delivery, this delay being helpful to minimize bleeding problems. But it is sometimes right to give an injectable much earlier than this.

8.41 Which injectable should be chosen?

1 The natural first choice is DMPA, because its effects are better known and it is marginally more effective. The injection is less uncomfortable and only needs to be given four times a year. Moreover NET EN is still not licensed for long term use.
2 Possible reasons for selecting NET EN include:
   (a) more bleeds, reduced likelihood of complete amenorrhoea if that state is rejected by the prospective user
   (b) shorter time until spontaneous reversal of the effect, if unacceptable side-effects were to develop after the first injection
   (c) more rapid return of fertility after the last injection
   (d) less risk of marked weight gain
   (e) if DMPA proves unsatisfactory, as an empirical second choice.

INITIAL MANAGEMENT AND FOLLOW-UP ARRANGEMENTS

8.42 What should be done at the first visit prior to giving an injectable?

1 A good medical history should be taken with special reference to the absolute and relative contraindications, especially those related to arterial disease and osteoporosis (*see Qs 8.36 and 8.38*).
2 Record the weight. This is more important than with other hormonal methods.
3 Record the BP. The evidence suggests it is not especially relevant to the method (*see Q 8.29*) but it is desirable as a baseline.

4   Discuss breast self-examination/awareness with a good leaflet – not leading to a nerve-racking ritual. Offer to examine the breasts if she has any concern, and with a lower threshold in women above age 40 (as a baseline).

5   Carry out a pelvic examination only if there are clinical grounds – i.e. rarely – and take a cervical smear only if due. A bimanual examination might be clinically indicated after childbirth to exclude the possibility of retained products.

8.43 What is the minimum information that should be conveyed at counselling?

Failure to counsel adequately has been the main cause of adverse publicity in the UK. The following should be discussed:

1   *Impossibility of rapid reversal if any side-effect was unacceptable.*

2   *Amenorrhoea*: as Dr Wilson of Glasgow has declared, reassurance that a 'monthly clean-out' of the 'bad blood' is not necessary for good health might make all the difference between happy acceptance and chronic anxiety and dissatisfaction.

3   *The possibility of frequent irregular bleeding*: Reassure the woman that medical advice is available if this should occur (*see Q 8.48*).

4   *Weight gain*: this is not inevitable. If potential users are forewarned in a very positive way, experience shows they can sometimes succeed in resisting the DMPA-caused weight increase by lifestyle change, including taking more exercise.

5   *Delay in fertility return*: women should be told on average it might take 9 months from the time of the last injection to conceive (*see Q 8.39*) but even longer is possible.

6   *Theoretical long-term risks*: the cancer balance seems on present evidence to be rather favourable to the method (*see Q 8.31*). The issues of arterial disease and osteoporosis, especially if there were to be prolonged amenorrhoea, are still not fully resolved. In my view they should be routinely raised at this stage only if there are relevant risk factors (*see Qs 8.23, 8.27 and 8.36–8.38*). It could be mentioned that this is 'a great method for at least 5 years'. How much else is told must depend on the doctor's judgement of the patient's understanding and background but an opportunity for questions must be given and they must be frankly answered.

7   *Supply the FPA's leaflet*: in addition to the licensed product information leaflet in the pack.

8.44 How are the injectables given?

By deep intramuscular injection. In the UK this is usually from the preloaded syringe into the upper outer quadrant of the buttock, outer thigh or (less often, because there is less muscle there) into the deltoid. Avoid major nerves and aspirate with care before injection of the dose. Warfarin treatment is WHO 3 because no amount of care can completely eliminate the haematoma risk.

The DMPA ampoule should be very thoroughly shaken to remove any sediment. NET EN should be warmed to body temperature. The site of either injection should not be massaged.

See also Q 8.9. If any of the dose is spilled, the amount lost should be carefully (over-) estimated and replaced by another injection.

8.45 What are the requirements for successful monitoring and follow-up?

1 Careful planning of the date for the next dose when each is given. Try to avoid the complexities of *Qs 8.53 and 8.54* by explaining that if a planned date proves inconvenient, it is far better to ask for the next dose a week or two early than to be late.
2 Equally important is the ready access between injections to medical advice by telephone or in person, to deal with any anxieties arising.
3 BP needs checking at most annually (*see Q 8.29*) and weight at each visit in the first year; but thereafter, if stable, mainly at the patient's request.
4 Cervical screening is performed according to local policies.

8.46 For how long, and to what age, can use of injectables be continued?

There are no known reasons for arbitrarily restricting the duration of use in younger women with adequate endogenous ovarian activity. The implications and management of prolonged use is discussed in *Qs 8.23–8.27*.

At around age 45 a review is appropriate (earlier for those with significant arterial cardiovascular symptoms or osteoporosis risk factors): transferring to another method should, in my view, be routinely considered then.

8.47 How can the menopause be diagnosed?

With difficulty – the scheme for the POP in *Q 7.63* is not appropriate for injectables. The method has to be discontinued and alternative contraception practised, e.g. most usefully an old-type POP in fact, then following the *Q 7.62 and 7.63* protocol, which simplifies diagnosis of ovarian failure at the menopause.

Injectables are by way of being a 'contraceptive overkill' around the climacteric (*see Q 11.50*). Transfer to another method before age 45 is therefore normally preferable as just suggested.

MANAGEMENT OF SIDE-EFFECTS AND PRACTICAL PROBLEMS

8.48 How should non-acceptable, prolonged or much too frequent bleeding be managed?

The patient should be examined to exclude an unrelated cause: notably retained products of conception, polyps, *Chlamydia* or carcinoma. An ultrasound scan might be required. If the uterus is firm and non-tender, with a normal closed cervical os, it is unlikely that the bleeding has any cause other than as a side-effect of the injectable.

Drugs: enquiry should be made but, by rights no interacting drug should cause bleeding (*see Q 8.11*).

POSSIBLE TREATMENTS

1   Best option: give oestrogen (if not contraindicated). Simply giving two or more packets of any convenient 30 μg COC (e.g. Microgynon-30™) can be of benefit. The extra progestogen matters not at all, so this source of oestrogen is often convenient. Giving it cyclically rather than continuously (to produce hopefully a couple of 'physiological curettages') works best in my experience. If the COC is contraindicated, use any convenient source of natural (HRT) oestrogen. Forewarn the DMPA user that if there is benefit, the bleeding pattern might not continue as well as when her oestrogen course runs out, but it 'might be more live-with-able'. Repeat as necessary if unacceptable irregularity follows the final withdrawal bleed. But WHO points out that add-back oestrogen 'is likely to be of short term or no benefit.'

2   Other options are more rarely successful:
    (a) Give the next dose early but no earlier than 4 weeks since the last.
    (b) Haemostatics such as prostaglandin synthetase inhibitors (PGSIs), tranexamic acid and ethamsylate have been tried. They rarely work and their risks would therefore usually outweigh the benefits for this indication.

Iron treatment is very rarely indicated to correct anaemia (*see Q 8.13(4)*). The actual amount lost over many days is usually not great.

It might be possible to help a woman through initial difficulties, particularly by the use of one, or sometimes more, courses of oestrogen. But irregular bleeding remains the most common reason for discontinuing the method. The problem is most pronounced postpartum, often helped by delaying the first dose to 5–6 weeks.

8.49 How should amenorrhoea be managed?

1   Pregnancy should be eliminated as the (very rare) cause.

2   The woman should be counselled as in *Q 8.43(1)*. I find it helpful to say 'there's no blood coming away because there is no blood to come away'.

The establishment of prolonged amenorrhoea can often be the best solution for women with bleeding problems.

3 One cycle or even just 7 days of the COC (or a natural oestrogen) will cause a withdrawal 'period' and can sometimes be helpful as an adjunct to reassurance.

8.50 What about other minor side-effects?

Management can only be empirical, for example, switching to the other injectable or another method. Weight gain is the most common complaint: dieting is possible but difficult. Diuretics are useless. Pyridoxine treatment can be tried if depression is reported (*see Q 6.23*) but there have been no good studies – moreover, the depression is not uncommonly related more to factors within the user herself than to her contraceptive.

8.51 What symptoms should lead an injectable-user to take urgent medical advice?

There are none known that are specifically related to the method. There are sporadic reports of massive uterine 'flooding', not necessarily causally related.

8.52 Are prolonged immobilization or major surgery contraindications to injectables?

There is no need to discontinue either DMPA or NET EN before any kind of surgery. Indeed, an injectable can be a very satisfactory option instead of the combined pill for women at high risk of pregnancy while on the waiting list for major surgery (*see Q 6.17* for the practical management).

8.53 How should one handle the problem of overdue injections? How can one maintain contraception without avoidably risking fetal exposure to the drug?

This is a very difficult practical problem. Even if the woman is not amenorrhoeic, any bleeds she has give no information about when she may ovulate. Waiting 'till the next period' risks the woman conceiving during a potentially very long wait (Q 8.39)!

According to WHO there is a full 2 weeks of leeway for late injections with both injectables, so the late dose might simply be given at 14 weeks. In the UK, the manufacturer of DMPA is *much* more cautious (see note to *Box 8.2*). My own current advice is a working compromise between them.

Using other anovulants as a model, the likelihood of conception when up to 7 days overdue is acceptably low, so I now recommend the following protocol (*Box 8.2*) for this common problem (subtract 4 weeks or 28 days from all numbers if the injectable is NET EN not DMPA).

BOX 8.2 Overdue injections

Assuming regular intercourse has been continuing:

1   Up to 13 weeks (91 days): give the due dose, advising also added precautions for 7 days. Beyond that the chances of a blastocyst being in the genital tract increase. Assuming intercourse has been continuing:

2   If the due dose is late by a further 3 days (up to 94 days): do a sensitive pregnancy test and hormonal postcoital contraception can be given plus an immediate DMPA injection – plus 7 days added precautions.

3   Up to 96 days: if the earliest ovulation is assumed to be at 13 weeks, the intervention is still before implantation 5 days later. Hence after a negative pregnancy test an emergency copper IUD insertion can be carried out in good faith, with the usual *Chlamydia* test and antibiotic cover (*see* Q 10.24), plus an immediate injection plus later removal of the IUD – or neither of the latter, if the woman chooses to switch to the IUD as her future method. Up to 96 days it would also be legitimate to offer postcoital levonorgestrel such as Levonelle™. This is not contraindicated though unlicensed beyond 72 h. How much efficacy will be reduced when required to work as an anti-implantation method 5 days after ovulation is not yet quantified (*see* Q 10.9) and certainly not as good as the IUD method. But the ethical/legal situation is, surely, the same, 5 days after the earliest postulated ovulation, as with the copper IUD option.

In all these cases added precautions for a further 7 days are advised, plus 100% follow-up with exclusion of pregnancy 3–4 weeks later. Counselling must include discussion of the (very low) potential of harm to any fetus. It should be recorded that no promise has been made that she will not conceive, nor that any fetus would be born normal.

Note: There are other 'rules' around! Given that the manufacturer states (in sharp contrast to the WHO!) that the safety margin of DMPA is only up to 89 days after the last dose, i.e. only 5 days late, some authorities cautiously recommend reducing the total durations at (1), (2) and (3) by 4 days in each case.

8.54 What if the injection is more than 5 days beyond the 1 week assumed safety margin for the first possible ovulation?

According to the protocol in Q 8.53, this means beyond 96 days, with DMPA. In a currently sexually active user one would have to follow the policy described in Q 11.22.

In brief, insist that she agrees to avoid all risk of conception – by abstinence, combinations of methods, whatever – for a total of at least 12 days since the last intercourse. She then returns with an early morning urine.

If this gives a negative result by one of the ultrasensitive pregnancy tests now available for primary care use (with a minimum sensitivity of at least 25 mIU/L, e.g. Clear-view™), this can be interpreted as no fertilization up to 12 days (14 days with a less sensitive test) previously, since when she had additionally agreed to be 'safe'.

After discussion, recorded as in the italicized section of *Box 8.2*, the next due injection can be given. For extra security the couple should use the condom for a further 7 days and, again, there must be a follow-up visit to exclude pregnancy after 3–4 weeks.

The above protocol is surely preferable to the medical paranoia that has led to conceptions through refusal to give the late DMPA dose at all…

8.55 Beyond 14 weeks, what about the option of just giving the next dose, along with due warnings to the woman?

In very rare cases, if a continuing sexually active woman at high risk of conception without her DMPA absolutely refuses to follow the policy just described (*see Q 8.54*), it might sometimes be acceptable (given a negative ultrasensitive pregnancy test at the time) to give the next dose anyway, plus a supply of condoms for the next 7 days. There should certainly be recorded warnings of the (low) risk of fetal harm along with 100% follow-up. Beyond 14 weeks this would normally be *without* giving postcoital levonorgestrel.

8.56 What are the risks if a fetus is exposed to injectables?

1   There is no evidence of an increase in ectopic or miscarriage rates.
2   There is some concern that offspring of women exposed to DMPA during pregnancy, especially in the 4 weeks after an injection, are at increased risk of low birth weight and subsequent infant mortality. But it has been suggested this could be due to confounding, e.g. by social class.
3   Masculinization of the female fetus, particularly transient enlargement of the clitoris, and a possible increase in the incidence of hypospadias in males exposed to MPA and similar hormones, have been reported. But no serious fetal malformation risks have been established with the very low doses used for contraception in DMPA and NET EN. Meaningful conclusions about what must be very low potential teratogenic risks are unlikely ever to be reached because proceeding to term after exposure to injectables is such a rare event.

Every effort must of course continue to be made to prevent fetal exposure (*see Qs 8.54 and 8.55*).

8.57 Are there any known risks or benefits for ex-users of injectables?

There are no established teratogenic effects on pregnancies among recent ex-users of injectables. The only known problem is prolonged amenorrhoea and delayed return of fertility (*see* Q 8.39). There is a definite ex-use protective effect against carcinoma of the endometrium.

SUB-DERMAL IMPLANTS

8.58 Subdermal implants – what's new? Is this route of contraception still worth offering, since Norplant™?

It is sadly true of Norplant™ that the media, combined with legal action, destroyed public and professional confidence in what, since 1993, had been a very satisfactory option for many women. But the implant route is not defunct; it has – and is – being used by 11 million women worldwide (according to WHO estimates).

Implants contain a progestogen in a slow-release carrier, made either of dimethylsiloxane (as in Norplant™ with six implants and the very similar two-rod Norplant II, now called Jadelle™) or EVA, ethylene vinyl acetate (Implanon™). After an initial phase of several weeks giving higher blood levels they deliver almost constant low daily levels of the hormone (in the case of Implanon™ 60–70 μg falling in a few weeks to a steady 30–40 μg of etonogestrel – as shown in *Fig. 8.1*.

Implanon™ is now the only marketed implant in the UK. Its main features are summarized in *Table 7.2*, p. 282. It works primarily by ovulation inhibition, supplemented by the usual mucus and endometrial effects.

8.59 What is Implanon™? How effective is it?

1 It is a single 40-mm rod, just 2 mm in diameter, inserted far more simply than Norplant™ (*Fig. 8.3*). The implant contains 68 mg of etonogestrel – the new name for 3-keto-desogestrel. This is dispersed in an EVA matrix and covered by a 0.06-mm rate-limiting EVA membrane.

2 Its duration of use is for 3 years, with the unique distinction of a zero failure rate in the trials up to the launch date in 1999 – although the 95% confidence interval ranges up to 7 in 10 000. The latest (2003) manufacturer's estimate of true failures is 14 worldwide, with about 1 million units sold. Most 'failures' are pre-insertion conceptions or failures to insert (by the clinician).

3 Because, in the international studies, serum levels do tend to be lower in heavier women, contraceptive efficacy might be lower in the grossly obese, especially in the third year, when it might rely more on the cervical mucus effect for its efficacy. Noting what Kovacs found (*see* Q 7.17) for another progestogen-only method, and assuming the reduced effect relates to dilution, in a greater total body water of

Fig. 8.3 Implanon™. Q 8.59. Note picture (c) taken from *above* the patient.

distribution (*see Q 7.15*), I would consider action only in young presumed highly fertile women weighing more than 100 kg – as opposed to any level of BMI. This action could either be advising additional contraception (perhaps with a daily added Cerazette™ tablet, see Appendix A) or reimplanting sooner than 3 years.

4   If enzyme inducer treatment is necessary, the manufacturer – primarily because of having almost no data either way – recommends 'additional contraceptive precautions'. A second implant is not advised: one short-term option might be to add in a daily Cerazette™ tablet (but see Appendix A). But e.g. the LNG-IUS would usually be preferable long-term.

8.60 How is Implanon™ inserted, and when?

Although not difficult, specific training is essential. A few tips: the upper non-dominant arm is the best site (*Fig. 8.3*), under local anaesthetic (LA); implants at other sites can migrate. Insertion is direct from a dedicated sterile preloaded applicator with a cleverly shaped wide-bore needle, with similar dimensions to those used for blood transfusion. Positioning immediately subdermally by an injection/withdrawal technique is helped by the smooth bevel behind the sharp needle-tip. *Always check correct insertion by immediate palpation.*

Having had to perform a difficult removal (under ultrasound control) when a too-deep Implanon™ was partially imbedded in the neurovascular bundle, I prefer an insertion site slightly anterior to the manufacturer's recommended site, midway between biceps and triceps, which is directly over it. Beware also the thin woman with muscular arms in whom inadvertent insertion into muscle is now a well-recognised problem.

TIMING OF IMPLANON™ INSERTION

1   Day 1 to 5 of the woman's natural cycle. If any later than day 2, at the Margaret Pyke Centre we would recommend additional contraception for 7 days. We would only accept insertion later than day 7 if there has been believable abstinence ever since the LMP; or if, as preferred, since the counselling visit another highly effective method has been in use (see (5)). Cerazette™ can be ideal here as a trial of what is a bit like 'oral Implanon' (*Q 7.11*).

2   Following first-trimester abortion: immediate insertion is best.

3   Following delivery or second-trimester abortion: Implanon™ insertion on day 21 is recommended and, if later, with additional contraception for 7 days. If still amenorrhoeic pregnancy risk should be excluded (*see Q 11.22*).

4   During breast feeding, the manufacturer is now less cautious. Although uncertainty about possible effects of the tiny amount of etonogestrel

reaching the breast milk must be discussed (as for the POP, *see Qs 7.54 and 7.55*), it is – like Cerazette™ (*see Q7.56*) – very usable. A study from Thailand demonstrated that even during the earliest time after insertion, when the mean release rate was highest at 67 μg of etonogestrel per day, the amount ingested by the suckling infant would never be greater than a negligible 10–20 ng/kg/day. WHO classifies breastfeeding for this, like all progestogen-only methods, after 6 weeks as WHO 1; but says initiation after 6 weeks is preferable (because of slight concerns about the immaturity of the neonate and extra risk of irregular bleeding).

5 Changing from any combined hormonal or any (other) progestogen-only or intrauterine method: Implanon™ can be injected on any convenient day. Condoms should then be used, or the preceding method continued, for 7 further days.

8.61 What are the advantages and benefits of Implanon™?

1 Above all, efficacy and convenience, if the bleeding pattern suits it has that great feature of 'forgetability' as a contraceptive.

2 Long action with one treatment (3 years), plus very high continuation rates.

3 Absence of the initial peak dose given orally to the liver.

4 Blood levels are steady rather than fluctuating (as the POP) or initially too high (as injectables). This minimizes metabolic changes: HDL/LDL lipid ratios remained essentially unchanged and there were no important changes in clotting factors – as for Norplant™.

5 Oestrogen-free, therefore usable if past VTE (this is WHO 2, in my opinion). An excellent choice for many diabetics (*see Q 5.147*).

6 Median systolic and diastolic blood pressures were unchanged in trials for up to 4 years.

7 Being an anovulant, special indications can include past ectopic pregnancy (*see Q 8.35(5)*), and otherwise as for Cerazette™ (*see Q 7.11*) commonly after an initial trial of the latter.

8 The implant is rapidly reversible. After removal, serum etonogestrel levels were undetectable within 1 week. Within 3 weeks 44 out of 47 women were ovulating normally.

8.62 What are its problems and disadvantages?

1 *Altered bleeding pattern*: in the premarketing randomized comparative trial of Implanon™ with Norplant™, the bleeding patterns – analyzed in 90-day reference periods – were very similar, with one main difference. As expected for an anovulant method, amenorrhoea was significantly more common (20.8% versus 4.4%). The infrequent bleeding and spotting rate was 26.1%. Normal cycling was reported by 35%. But the combined rates for the more annoying 'frequent bleeding and spotting'

and 'prolonged bleeding and spotting' totalled 18% (actually more than the 12% for Norplant™).

2 *Treatment of irregular bleeding*: the best short-term treatment is cyclical COC therapy – logically with Marvelon™ or with natural oestrogen patches – after which the bleeding pattern, although not necessarily still as good, might (or might not) become acceptable.

3 *'Minor' general side-effects*: reported in frequency order these were: acne, headache, abdominal pain, breast pain, 'dizziness', mood changes (depression, emotional lability, usually improving after the first 3 months), libido decrease, hair loss. The frequencies were amazingly similar to Norplant™ and, as usual, forewarning plus encouragement over the initial weeks yields dividends.

4 *Body weight*: in a non-randomized comparative study the mean weight increase over 2 years was 2.6% with Implanon™ and 2.9% with Norplant, but in users of an IUD the weight increase was 2.4%! Although this implies a normal increase over time, by 24 months 35% had put on more than 3 kg. As with DMPA, forewarning is essential: some individuals do put on an unacceptable amount of weight.

5 *Possible hypo-oestrogenism*: because Implanon™ suppresses ovulation and does not supply any oestrogen, the same long-term concerns arise as with DMPA (*see Q 8.23*). However, as for Cerazette™, follicular activity is more evident than in DMPA users because FSH is minimally inhibited. Moreover, in the comparative study just mentioned, after 2 years use of either Implanon™ or a copper IUD the findings on mean oestrogen levels and bone density were almost identical.

6 *Local adverse effects*: discomfort, at insertion and removal, can be minimized by good training. Expulsion, infection of the site, migration, deep insertion (which is the main cause difficult removal) and scarring should all be very infrequent in a good programme.

8.63 Who might choose this method?

Indications for use follow from *Q 8.61*, especially for women wanting effectiveness without the finality of sterilization.

ABSOLUTE CONTRAINDICATIONS (WHO 4) – A VERY SHORT LIST!

1 *Progestogen-dependent tumours* (including active trophoblastic disease, liver adenoma). Also *current breast cancer* – Implanon™ useable (WHO 3) after remission for 5 years (WHO advice).

2 *Current severe hepatic disease* with markedly abnormal liver function.

3 Known or suspected *pregnancy*.

4 *Undiagnosed vaginal bleeding*.

5 *Severe hypersensitivity to any component*.

6 *Acute porphyria* (*see Q 6.42*).

The manufacturer adds 'active venous thromboembolic disorder', but in my view this history (past or present) would be WHO 2. There is no evidence that Implanon™ would increase the risk.

RELATIVE CONTRAINDICATIONS

In my view, these are as for Cerazette™ (*see Q 7.52*), i.e. the same as for old-type POPs but without any concerns about lower efficacy, including against ectopics. They are all no more than WHO 2. Liver disease like cirrhosis is WHO 3 unless very severe. Breastfeeding is now WHO 1 for Implanon™, like all progestogen-only methods.

8.64 What about follow-up? And removal of Implanon™?

No treatment-specific follow-up is necessary, including no BP checks. In the UK context it is usually helpful to schedule one 3-month visit, for encouragement and management of any bleeding or non-bleeding side-effects. Much more important is a genuine 'open house' policy, at any time, without any provider pressure to persevere if the woman really wants the implant out.

8.65 How is Implanon™ removed?

Removal is usually easy, with training. In the comparative study the mean insertion time was 1.1 min and the mean removal time 2.6 min (range 0.2–20 min). This was approximately four times faster for both procedures than for Norplant™.

Implanon™ is radiotranslucent. If an implant cannot be palpated it should be removed under ultrasound control: indeed all difficult cases are best discussed with the manufacturer's medical department, to arrange referral to a specialist centre.

FUTURE DEVELOPMENTS

8.66 Will the transdermal route be used for contraception?

Yes (*see Q 6.80* regarding the combined oestrogen and progestogen patch marketed as EVRA™). At the moment I know of no plans however for a progestogen-only patch for contraception

8.67 What are other theoretical routes?

For completeness, one should mention the rectal, transnasal and sublingual routes, all of which are in current use for other drugs. There are no known plans at present for routine contraception by those routes.

8.68 What further implants can be expected?

Perhaps implants that slowly biodegrade and would never need removing: but they should remain removable if desired.

A much improved estradiol implant, releasing steady levels for 1–3 years (rather than, as currently, with declining levels over 6 months) is in the pipeline. We can anticipate combined implants of progestogen with this oestrogen, also that other contraceptive compounds will be delivered by this route, such as gonadotrophin-releasing hormone antagonists – and methods for the male.

8.69 What are vaginal rings?

Like implants, current versions use a silastic or EVA carrier, which is in the shape of a ring between 4 and 6 cm in diameter and 4–10 mm thick. There are two main designs. In core-rings all the hormone is in a central core. In the shell design the inner core is hormone free but encircled by a narrow, hormone-filled band. Both types are then covered by tubing, giving controlled (zero-order) release to the vaginal mucosa.

Research into progestogen-releasing vaginal contraceptive rings generally received a set-back during a study of a levonorgestrel-releasing ring at the Margaret Pyke Centre during 1991–92. Asymptomatic erythematous patches were discovered, apparently associated with the areas of contact of the rings with the vaginal fornices. It is still not clear whether these were caused by physical pressure or a chemical effect. The long-term effects on the vagina and cervix of all future rings will certainly need careful monitoring.

8.70 What is currently the most promising type of ring?

The combined type (the NuvaRing™ version of this was discussed in Q 6.82).

8.71 What is the natural progesterone ring?

This is a WHO ring designed especially for lactating women. Over 3 months, it releases 5–10 mg/day of progesterone, thereby minimizing concerns about the composition of breast milk. With this method I would foresee (as with the POP) the need for great care to transfer to a more effective method during weaning: if unwanted conceptions are to be avoided when the progesterone is no longer supplemented by the contraceptive effect of full lactation.

PATIENT QUESTIONS

QUESTIONS ASKED BY USERS

Most questions asked are about DMPA, or Depo-Provera™, as it is best known by the general public.

8.72 What are in practice the most effective purely hormonal contraceptives currently available?

Implants and injectables. The COC fails far more often – through human error.

8.73 Do injectables cause cancer in women?

This currently seems very unlikely and one cancer (of the lining of the womb) is less frequent (*see Qs. 8.30–8.33*).

8.74 But is it safe? How does the safety (freedom from health risk) of Depo-Provera™ compare with 'the pill'?

Overall, because it doesn't contain oestrogen, its safety is believed to be greater than that of the combined pill. No deaths have ever been clearly blamed upon it (*see Q 8.14*).

8.75 Why are some people so opposed to Depo-Provera™?

Mainly because of its potential for abuse and the fact that if side-effects occur – and there are fewer overall than with the pill – the drug's action cannot be reversed once given. You have to wait for the last injection to wear off (*see Q 8.16*).

8.76 So is it a 'last resort' method?

No! In the UK its licence used to require it to be used only after discussion of all the alternatives and after very special counselling along with the special package leaflet. But it is now approved as a 'first-line' option.

8.77 Can I be too young to be given Depo-Provera™?

Some doctors are reluctant to give it to very young teenagers who are just beginning their normal menstrual cycle. Up to age 18 it is used a bit cautiously (WHO 2; see *Box 8.1*, p. 331). Injectables or the implant Implanon™ would normally be preferable to insertion of an IUD for a teenager, if that was the alternative choice.

8.78 Won't I put on a lot of weight?

Depo-Provera™ unfortunately does seem to increase people's appetites. But forewarned is forearmed! Experience shows that if you are on the look-out it is possible to avoid gaining much weight, especially if you also start taking more exercise.

8.79 Can I be too old to be given Depo-Provera™?

Over the age of 45 injectables are stronger contraceptives than are really required and there is an increasing risk of disease of the arteries. Many other good choices are now available, so other methods are usually preferable, especially in smokers (*see Qs 8.19 and 6.49*).

8.80 Where (on the body) is the injection given?

Usually into the upper outer region of the buttocks, on either side, but it can sometimes be given into the shoulder or thigh muscles.

8.81 Why can't the injection be given right after having my baby?

If given too soon it tends to cause more bleeding problems in the weeks after childbirth. These are less if it is given at about 5–6 weeks but because it does not have any thrombosis risks it can sometimes be given much earlier, if you are prepared to accept some extra irregular bleeding.

8.82 How long does the injection last?

Officially for 12 weeks, and each injection should be on time. If you are overdue a dose, abstain from sex or use condoms, although if you forget, up to 14 weeks something can still be done about it (see *Box 8.2*, p. 345). Although some women can become pregnant if they are just a few days overdue, others (and we do not know who they are in advance) go on being affected for much longer (*see Q 8.83*).

8.83 How far ahead should I discontinue injections if planning another baby?

You should plan for about 1 year after the last injection because it is quite usual (and nothing to worry about) for conception to be delayed that long.

8.84 Excess bleeding – will it harm me in any way if I can live with it?

The short answer is 'no'. You ought to be examined to eliminate any cause not related to the Depo-Provera™. A blood test is sometimes done to check that you are not anaemic. Some treatments can be tried to stop the bleeding (*see Q 8.48*). Otherwise if you can live with an unpredictable bleeding pattern it will do you no harm. If you choose to have intercourse during bleeding that too is medically harmless.

Intrauterine devices

9

PAIN AND BLEEDING

PATIENT INFORMATION AND FOLLOW-UP ARRANGEMENTS

QUESTIONS ASKED BY CURRENT USERS

BACKGROUND AND MECHANISMS

9.1 How would you define an intrauterine device?

This is any solid object that is wholly retained within the uterine cavity for the purpose of preventing pregnancy. Such devices are usually inserted via the cervical canal and might have marker thread(s) attached, which are visible at the external os. There are three main types with frames: inert, copper-bearing and hormone-releasing (often called 'systems'). There are now also two frameless (implantable) varieties: copper-bearing (GyneFIX™ being the sole representative thus far) and hormone-releasing.

9.2 Should they be abbreviated IUD or IUCD?

Underlying this question is the possibility of confusion of 'intrauterine device' with 'intrauterine death' of a fetus. Hence many gynaecologists prefer IUCD, for **i**ntra**u**terine **c**ontraceptive **d**evice. But this leads to problems in translation and moreover IUD is now well established in the world literature. An amusing compromise adopted by an expert committee of the World Health Organization (WHO) in the 1970s was the following: to use IUD (without full stops) for intrauterine device, and I.U.D. for intrauterine death! This agreed notation will be used here.

9.3 What is the history of IUDs?

An oft-quoted but poorly substantiated story describes the first IUD as a stone or stones placed in the uterus of camels in North Africa to prevent pregnancies during long caravan journeys. One version of the story, however, suggests that the stones were actually put in the vagina, making the method more akin to a chastity belt than an IUD! Over 2500 years ago, Hippocrates is credited with using a hollow lead tube to insert pessaries or other objects into human uteri. (The translations differ as to whether this was for contraception or other purposes.) Casanova recommended a gold ball; and as recently as 1950 one woman apparently used her wedding ring as a do-it-yourself IUD!

Cervicouterine stem pessaries were used from the late nineteenth century. They were made from material as exotic as ivory, glass, ebony and diamond-studded platinum, and were used for many purposes – including contraception. Some were shaped like collar-studs or had V-shaped flexible wings inserted into the lower uterine cavity. When the devices fractured, as they sometimes did, leaving just the intrauterine part in position, it was learnt that the latter (rather than the surface cap covering the external os) was the contraceptive. The first completely intrauterine device was a ring made of silkworm gut, described by Dr Richter of Braslaw. Later, silver wire was wound around the silkworm gut by Grafenberg and it is of interest that later versions were made of German silver, an alloy that contains copper.

Now made of coiled stainless steel, the design is still one of the most widely used in the world (because it is so popular in China).

Many of the early devices were used as abortifacients as well as contraceptives, and the resultant haemorrhage and pelvic infection led to widespread condemnation by the medical profession. This retarded acceptance of the method, which was only really achieved in 1962 at the first International Conference on IUDs in New York City. The Lippes loop was presented to this conference by its inventor, and became the standard inert device (*Fig. 9.1*) against which many newer devices were compared: many now being bioactive, bearing copper or releasing hormones. The lay terms 'loop' and 'coil' are out-of-date and best not used.

The intrauterine method received a body blow in the mid-1970s with severe illnesses and even deaths linked to the now infamous Dalkon Shield™ device: this was the biggest single factor in the IUD's subsequent undeserved reputation – that of causing severe pelvic inflammatory disease (PID) and later tubal factor infertility. This still prevents many potential users in the UK, and even more in the US, from giving the intrauterine approach a fair hearing when it is proposed – it has too much 'baggage' with it from the past. Yet the latest IUDs are much improved and very different from those of 30 years ago; and as for the LNG-IUS (*see Q 9.145ff*), I see no reason to retract a statement of mine in the 1990s that it is 'the greatest advance in the contraceptive field since the combined pill'.

9.4 How prevalent is use of the IUD?

It is estimated by WHO that about 156 million IUDs are in use worldwide, around 60 million of them in one country – China. In the UK, IUDs are fitted in a mere 4% of women in the childbearing years (see *Table 1.3*). This is far fewer than might be predicted from the method's advantages (*see Q 9.19*). So, as it is as has been well said, it is long past 'time to forgive the IUD'.

9.5 What are the effects of IUD insertion on the genital tract?

Many cellular and biochemical changes have been described but it is now clear that any IUD in situ long term acts chiefly by interfering with gametes and fertilization (*see Q 7.7*).

1 All types of IUD lead to a marked increase in the number of leukocytes, both in the endometrium and in the uterine and tubal fluid. All the different types of white cell involved in a typical foreign body reaction are represented.
2 Inert and copper devices lead to elevated levels of many prostaglandins.
3 Copper enhances the foreign body reaction and leads to a range of biochemical changes in the endometrium, affecting enzyme systems and hormone receptors.

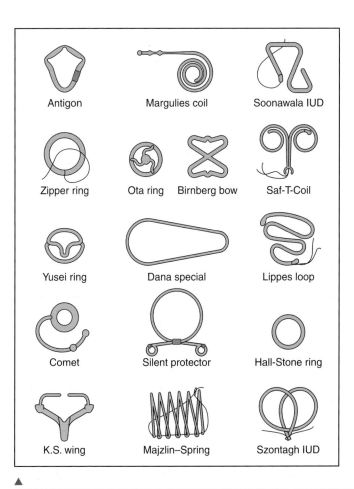

▲

Fig. 9.1 Past inert IUDs. Q 9.3. See Figs 9.9, 9.12 and 9.13 for bioactive IUDs.

4   Copper ions are also toxic to sperm and blastocyst.

5   Progestogen-releasing IUDs alter endometrial histology with a decidual reaction and glandular atrophy, and block oestrogen and progesterone receptors. They also markedly reduce the sperm penetrability of uterine fluid and cervical mucus to sperm. In the first year of use they do also inhibit ovulation in a significant minority of cycles.

9.6 Are there any known systemic effects of IUDs (outside the genital tract)?

An increase in some circulating immunoglobulins has been reported but neither this nor the minute amount of copper entering the systemic circulation in users of copper IUDs is thought to be of clinical significance (except in Wilson's disease, *see Q 9.86*). Absorption of hormones or any other chemicals that are carried by bioactive devices must always be presumed but systemic effects even of the progestogen-releasing IUDs are small (and depend on the release rate).

Inert and copper IUDs have no effect on the pituitary or ovary. However, uterine shedding starts 2–3 days before circulating levels of oestrogen and progesterone have reached the levels usual at the start of the menses in non-IUD users.

9.7 So what is the main mode of action of IUDs?

The main effect is now believed to be by the blocking of fertilization. The inflammatory cells of the fluid in the whole genital tract (including the tubes) appear with all IUDs to impede sperm transport and fertilization. Actual phagocytosis of the sperm has been reported. Copper is also directly toxic to the sperm and ova. In various studies of long-term IUD users, viable sperm have very rarely been found in the uterine cavity, the tubes or in aspirates of the pouch of Douglas, in clear contrast with the findings in sexually active controls.

However, an implantation-blocking effect is a back-up contraceptive mechanism. The remarkable effectiveness of copper IUDs when inserted postcoitally, up to 5 days after ovulation, indicates that they can still be exceptionally effective when the action cannot be by blocking fertilization. To work by this mechanism IUDs seem only to require to be present in the uterus for the last 9 days of each cycle. This implies the need for caution whenever IUDs are removed (*see Qs 9.13 and 9.14*).

The progesterone or progestogen-releasing IUDs (*see Qs 9.145–9.151*) markedly impair the sperm penetrability of cervical–uterine fluid, as well as sometimes stopping fertile ovulation. But they also have an anti-implantation effect: one that builds up too slowly for the LNG-IUS to be a reliable postcoital contraceptive (*see Qs 9.148, 10.5, 10.34*).

9.8 So how do IUDs mainly act when they are in situ long term?

They mainly act before fertilization; the post-fertilization effects are potential but rarely utilized by in situ IUDs or IUSs. However, a prospective long-term user cannot be guaranteed that her IUD or IUS will never in an occasional cycle block the implantation of a blastocyst. If she has ethical problems about that possibility she should perhaps only use anovulant, barrier or natural methods (or sterilization) (*see Q 10.2*).

9.9 Why are inert devices now no longer used in the UK?

Their market was taken by the copper IUDs. As the surface area of inert devices is reduced, so the bleeding and pain side-effects are minimized but the failure rate increases. By virtue of its additional contraceptive actions (*see Q 9.5*), copper enables smaller devices to be used without loss of efficacy. The major advantage of inert devices (long-term use through to the menopause) is disappearing with the steady increase in permissible duration of use of copper IUDs, now at least 10 years for the *banded* devices.

From this point until *Q 9.145*, the LNG-IUS section, unless otherwise stated, I shall deal only with modern copper IUDs.

EFFECTIVENESS

9.10 What is the overall failure rate?

For all current devices this is low, in the range of 0.2–2.0/100 woman-years, including pregnancies that are due to unrecognized expulsions (estimated at about one-third of the total) – in the first year.

Three IUD designs stand out as the most effective currently available. These are the T-Safe Cu 380A™ and its clones (now marketed in the UK as T-Safe Cu 380A™), GyneFIX™, which like T-Safe Cu 380™, utilizes copper bands, and the levonorgestrel-releasing (LNG)-IUS discussed later (*see Q 9.144*). Based on no less than 16 000 woman-years of use in multicentre WHO and Population Council studies, the first of these is now the 'gold standard' among copper devices. At 7 years of use the cumulative failure rate was 1.4/100 women, putting it in the same league as female sterilization! The LNG-IUS is equally effective but all other IUD designs, being unbanded, appear to be less so. The former market-leader, the Nova T (200)™, had a much higher failure rate (*Fig. 9.2*) and its distribution ceased in October 2001. It has been replaced by the confusingly named Nova-T 380™, with more copper wire but still not apparently quite as effective as the 'gold standard' (*see Qs 6.95, 9.94*) and the user has to have more reinsertions (*Q 9.11*).

9.11 What factors influence failure rates (and other problems) of IUDs?

1   By far the most important is the competence of the doctor or other professional inserting the device into the correct high fundal position. The few appropriate comparative studies that have been done show that the difference between doctors, for all the problems (summarized in *Q 9.21*), is greater than the difference between devices. Therefore also long-lived (i.e. banded) copper IUDs are better, though requiring fewer reinsertions.

Fig. 9.2 Five-year cumulative gross intrauterine and ectopic pregnancy rates per 100 women: for 1124 women using the LNG-IUS versus 1121 using the CuT 380 Ag (a clone of T-Safe Cu 380 A™) on the left and another 1821 women using the LNG-IUS versus 937 using old-style Nova T. Data from two separate RCTs: Sivin et al. 1990 *Contraception* 42:361–78 & Andersson et al. 1994 *Contraception* 49:56–72.

2   The second most important factor in comparative studies is the age and hence relative fertility of the population. Above 35, the first-year failure rate (of 0.1–0.5/100 woman-years with any device) is so good that IUDs become the method of choice for many older women (*see Qs 9.20 and 9.22*).

3   Duration of use (*see Q 9.134*).

9.12 Are the various aspects of device design almost irrelevant then?

No. Attention to the shape and size of a device and of its introducer, and the insertion technique, can all influence efficacy. The ideal design would maximize delivery of any bioactive agent such as copper to the most important (high fundal) zone, and minimize the:

1   likelihood of malposition (especially too low in the cavity)
2   likelihood of expulsion
3   liability to and seriousness of translocation and perforation (*see Qs 9.43 and 9.45*).

Also, if possible:

4   the severity and duration of bleeding and pain (*see Q 9.77*)
5   any liability to exacerbate pelvic infection (*see Q 9.62*).

The implantable GyneFIX™ (*see Q 9.141*) approach looks promising, particularly in regard to expulsion, malposition and device-related pain – always provided it is implanted by a good operator.

9.13 How can insufficient caution when removing an IUD cause iatrogenic pregnancy?

The answer follows from Q 9.7. If one of the major actions of IUDs is to block implantation, removal at any time before the last 9 days of the cycle can enable the blastocyst to arrive at a non-IUD-bearing uterus. Pregnancy could therefore result even if a woman were being sterilized at the time of removal, and this has in fact been reported. A more serious risk would be a clip-induced ectopic, due to trapping the blastocyst in the tube. These events are rare because of the strong prefertilization effects of in situ IUDs (*see Q 9.5*) but they are entirely preventable (*see below and Q 11.16*).

9.14 How can such pregnancies be avoided?

Either by removal during a period or, more usually, by following a '7-day rule', i.e. advice in advance to abstain or use a barrier method for 7 days before any IUD is removed; 7 days is believed to allow sufficient time – namely that between ejaculation and the latest likely implantation – for the IUD to have its antinidatory effects in that cycle. The 7-day rule is particularly important before sterilization, for fear of that iatrogenic tubal ectopic. It is also wise before any attempted replacement of an IUD.

Occasionally an IUD needs to be removed midcycle although it has been recently relied upon (*see Q 9.67*). Postcoital hormone treatment should be considered in such cases (see *Chapter 10*).

9.15 How can excessive caution about the time of insertion of IUDS cause iatrogenic pregnancies?

By slavish adherence to the myth that it is best to insert only during or just after the menses! If women are told to wait until after their next period, not a few return pregnant. Several US-based studies have shown that IUDs can be inserted with relative safety on the day they are requested, provided the woman's history indicates she will not have an implanted pregnancy. For many women this 'quick start' approach is even more appropriate than for the COC (*see Q 6.17*).

Especially relevant was a US study that showed a statistically significant doubling of the rate of expulsion if copper-T IUDs were inserted on days 1–5 of the cycle as compared with days 11–17. Because the patients were unaware of the expulsion (usually partial) in nearly 40% of the cases, extra pregnancies are possible if IUDs are inserted only during the menses.

Finally, of course, deliberate postcoital IUD insertion up to day 19 of a 28-day cycle (adjusted for cycle length) is very effective (see *Chapter 10*).

9.16 What is the likely explanation for a high expulsion rate when IUDs are inserted very early in the cycle? And what might be done about it?

The main increase in expulsion rate occurs when IUDs are inserted during the menstrual flow, and is probably linked with extra myometrial activity at that time due to prostaglandins. The intraluminal pressure can rise above 100 mmHg and the fundal cavity is also narrower than that at midcycle.

Sometimes there is no practical alternative to fitting an IUD or IUS menstrually or just premenstrually. In particular, if there is a history of dysmenorrhoea I now suggest that the prostaglandin inhibitor treatment routinely given as a premed for the insertion (a prostaglandin synthetase inhibitor (PGSI) such as mefenamic acid or ibuprofen) is continued – until and during that next period.

9.17 So when are IUDs best inserted?

The answer is not during heavy days of the menses but at any time from their ending phase through until about midcycle. At the Margaret Pyke Centre we target days 4–12 of a normal cycle. Beyond that, if intercourse has been continuing, postcoital insertion in good faith is still permissible up to 5 days after the calculated ovulation day (*see Q 10.15*) but with caution and counselling, appropriate screening, consideration of antibiotics, good records and follow-up.

9.18 Should adjunctive contraceptive measures be recommended to IUD users following insertion?

Many women select this method precisely because they desire a non-intercourse-related method. However, there are three arguments in favour of added use of a male or female condom:

1 Very short term, in the first 3–4 days following insertion or reinsertion of any IUD or IUS (although abstinence would be preferable). This is a personal recommendation of mine, because insertion is the time when there is interference with the protective barrier to upper genital infection provided by the cervix (*see Q 9.56*). Moreover, sperm seem able to act as bio-vectors of STIs.

2 To provide some protection in the event of unrecognized expulsion, which is common especially in early months and might be unnoticed in the menstrual flow.

3 To provide protection longer term against both sexually transmitted and non-specific pelvic infection (*see Qs 9.49 and 9.50*), particularly if there is a partner change *or* in the not uncommon scenario that a monogamous woman doubts the monogamy of her partner.

ADVANTAGES AND BENEFITS

9.19 What are the advantages of IUDs?

1 Effective:
   (a) highly, comparable to female sterilization, indeed better than some methods of the latter
   (b) postcoitally (not the LNG-IUS)
   (c) postabortally.

2 Safe:
   (a) mortality 1:500 000
   (b) no known, unwanted systemic effects (not LNG–IUS).

3 Independent of intercourse.

4 Does not require any day-to-day actions, such as taking a pill.

5 Motivation is chiefly required around the time of insertion and never subsequently if side-effects are acceptable – it then being truly a 'default' method, for over 10 years duration of use in the case of T-Safe Cu 380A™.

6 Relatively cheap and easy to distribute.

7 Does not influence milk volume or composition.

8 With sympathetic providers the method is under a woman's control and (a point of occasional relevance) if the threads are removed, can be undetectable by her partner.

9 Continuation rates high.

10 Reversible (*see Q 9.139*).

What a remarkable list of advantages, amounting to transcervical sterilization without a general anaesthetic or hospital visit! Add to them a hint – unproven so far – from five out of six case–control studies that copper IUDs might actually be protective against endometrial cancer (see Grimes 2000 *The Lancet* 356:1013–1019) and, although it has been around too short a time to prove the point, there is much more reason to expect a reduction of this risk in users of the LNG-IUS, through its endometrial suppressive action.

It makes one wonder why we do not at least offer this choice, as a routine, to all parous young women and also to many more who, although nulliparous, are in mutually faithful relationships. See below!

9.20 For whom are IUDs indicated?

The answer is: upon request for contraception, unless the absolute contraindications apply (*see Qs 9.85 and 9.86*) or if the relative contraindications are unacceptable to the woman herself after discussion in the light of alternatives. More specifically, in view of the threats to fertility to be discussed (which are not due to the intrauterine method but to prevalence of STIs in most societies), and the fact that these are not only more serious when there is no family but also more probable in the very young: IUDs are still not first-choice methods for most young women until they have had children. But nulliparity in monogamous relationships is no more than WHO 2 and often a good choice for older women above 35 – especially any with the view that their career will be likely to take precedence over ever having a child.

Modern intrauterine contraception can substitute well for female sterilization (*see Q 11.56ff*). Unless the man volunteers for vasectomy, which does add (10-fold) greater efficacy, the IUD (or IUS) might be so acceptable that it remains in use until final removal 1 year after the menopause.

MAIN PROBLEMS AND DISADVANTAGES

9.21 In summary, what are the main problems and disadvantages of intrauterine contraception using copper?

These can be listed briefly as in Box 9.1 (please read this box in conjunction with Q 9.22). *Note: these are **not** in order of frequency and are far more related to the skill or otherwise of the inserting clinician than any problems with the method itself.*

BOX 9.1 Problems that may occur during intrauterine contraception using copper

1 *Intrauterine pregnancy*: increased risk of miscarriage, hence of infection.
2 *Extrauterine pregnancy* (but no increase in overall population risk, *see Q 9.30*).
3 *Expulsion or partial expulsion*, with risks of pregnancy (see (1)).
4 *Malposition* of the device, which could cause items (1), (3), (7) and (8) in this list, as well as being one cause of 'lost threads'.
5 *Perforation* with risks of pregnancy, also risk of IUD penetration of bowel/bladder and adhesion formation – and the resultant risks of surgery.
6 *Pelvic infection/salpingitis*: although IUDs are definitely **not** the initiating cause (*see Q 9.49*).
7 *Pain*.
8 *Abnormal bleeding*: this can be increased in amount, duration, and/or frequency.

All available data are reassuring concerning carcinogenesis, whether of endometrium or cervix. Rare problems are considered at *Qs 9.73, 9.88, 9.113, 9.127*

9.22 Are the problems in *Box 9.1* (Q 9.21) interconnected? Please give examples.

Very much so, and it is instructive to see how:

■ *Insertion*: first and foremost is capable (either directly or indirectly) of causing any one of problems (1) to (8). The importance of this factor cannot be over-emphasized: its impact must be minimized by skill: through good training and maintained experience.

■ *Pain*: can be a symptom of (1) to (6) in Box 9.1. Hence these should first be excluded before terming it a side-effect (i.e. something that the woman might or might not be able to live with). Beware the stoical woman or the one who tries too hard to avoid troubling the doctor!

■ *Bleeding*: might sometimes mean directly or indirectly numbers (1), (2), (3), or (4) and even (6) (chlamydial endometritis can cause bleeding). So this too is not necessarily just a side-effect.

■ *Fertility*: can be impaired (indirectly or directly) by any of (1) to (6) (*see* Qs 9.24, 9.32, 9.49). Hence the general view that young nulliparae should think twice before using this method.

■ *'Lost threads'*: can signify any of (1), (3), (4) and (5) (see Q 9.33).

■ Malposition of the device: can cause numbers (1), (3), (7) and (8) in Box 9.1, as well as 'lost threads'.

■ *Increasing age*: has been found to increase the risk of (2) (ectopics), possibly because more years' of sexual activity means more chance of an initial or recurrent infection to damage a tube, and of (8) (heavy periods). These risks are regardless of whether there is also an IUD present. But age definitely reduces the risk of (1), (3) and (6) (*see* Qs 9.11, 9.38 and 9.53).

■ *Duration of use*: reduces most problems, i.e. (1), (3), (6), (7) and (8) (*see* Qs 9.134 and 9.135).

INTRAUTERINE PREGNANCY (IUD IN SITU)

9.23 Does intrauterine pregnancy pose problems for IUD users? Is there an increased risk of teratogenesis?

There is absolutely no evidence for an increased risk of any of the more common fetal abnormalities, whether the device is present at the time of conception or during organogenesis – at least for the inert and copper-containing types. Proof of this is (as usual) impossible, especially as 2% of all babies have an abnormality, and most particularly for the rarer disorders.

There are as yet no adequate data concerning any possible effects of a high local dose of progestogen on a continuing pregnancy (*see* Q 9.147).

9.24 Should the device be removed and, if so, surely this will increase the risk of miscarriage?

Counterintuitively, the 'obvious' course of action – which is to leave the device alone so as to avoid disturbing the pregnancy – has been shown to result in a high rate of miscarriage (above 50%). Moreover, more often than expected this occurs in the second trimester with dangerous complications, particularly haemorrhage and sepsis; septic second-trimester abortions were 26 times more frequent in one study. There is also evidence that the risks of antepartum haemorrhage, of preterm delivery and of stillbirth are increased if the IUD remains present.

Such problems are not restricted to the Dalkon Shield™, although first reported for that device. Tatum (the inventor of the first T-device) produced good evidence that removal of a copper device in the early part of pregnancy reduced the spontaneous abortion rate from 54% to 20%. So the slogan is: if an IUD fails and a woman wishes to proceed to full-term delivery, do not leave the device in situ.

9.25 How should removal of the device be managed?

1 Begin by counselling the woman and warning her that she is at increased risk of miscarriage whatever is done, but that the risk can usually be reduced considerably by gentle removal of the device.

2 Arrange an ultrasound scan. Occasionally the device can be identified above the pregnancy sac and it might be judged that removal would cause excessive trauma/rupture of the membranes. But far more commonly the device is below the sac (displacement having been the probable cause of the method failure, in fact).

3 Removal should then be performed, at the earliest possible stage in pregnancy, whenever the threads of the device are still accessible. In rare cases of heavy bleeding or leakage of liquor thereafter, the woman might need immediate admission. However, she can usually continue as an outpatient, with appropriate advice about the subsequent occurrence of any pain or more bleeding than the slight show to be expected at IUD removal. If the threads are (already) missing, consider the possibility of perforation, not only of expulsion; and in all cases categorize/supervise the pregnancy as 'high risk' (*see Q 9.24*).

See also *Q 9.28*: the vital importance after delivery of establishing where the IUD is …

9.26 What if the outcome after counselling is to be a legal abortion?

Clearly the removal of the device is then best performed at the time of termination. In my view there should be routine *Chlamydia* testing and antibiotic cover for all such procedures. The latter is essential:

1   If the woman is first seen with an IUD-associated incomplete abortion.
2   If medical induction of the termination is planned with mifepristone and/or prostaglandins (PGs). This is because of anecdotes especially in the second trimester of severe infections, implying that the presence of the foreign body increases the sepsis risk. Indeed, the IUD should be removed at the outset of treatment, whether by mifepristone or PG pessary, and not left to come away with the products of conception.

9.27 Should an ultrasound scan be done after all failures of an IUD or IUS, even if the woman does not go on to full term?

In my opinion, yes, because the pregnancy might have resulted from the device being malpositioned or even placed in one horn of a bicornute uterus.

9.28 What if the original IUD is never found following spontaneous or induced abortion? Or at full term?

It is unbelievable how often the original presence of an IUD is forgotten, especially after delivery. There should be a thorough search for it in the placenta and membranes, and its presence or otherwise recorded. Otherwise a women might find herself, at a later stage, with two intrauterine IUDs or with one in her uterus and one still at large – free in the abdomen (thus explaining how the original conception occurred). Many legal cases have resulted, and they are indefensible. One can nearly always exclude either an embedded or perforated device with plain abdominal X-rays as a supplement to ultrasound scanning (*see* Q 9.35).

EXTRAUTERINE PREGNANCY

9.29 What is the risk of extrauterine pregnancy when an IUD user becomes pregnant, and is the rate really increased?

No! to the second question. First and foremost, since the last edition of this book it is now clearly established that copper IUDs do *not* increase the overall risk of ectopics in a population, as compared with suitable non-IUD-using controls.

The rate of ectopics is fundamentally dependent on the rate of pelvic infection (*see* Q 9.50) in that community. Because in situ copper IUDs drastically reduce fertilization rates (*see* Q 9.7), even women with damaged tubes (who will be at definite risk of an ectopic when they come to try for a pregnancy) might well escape this while using an IUD.

The risk among current users of the Progestosert™ (progesterone-containing) IUD appears to have been truly higher; but the more potent LNG-IUS seems to block fertilization so well that in the Population

Council study (1990, see *Fig. 9.2*) no ectopics at all occurred during a massive 3371 woman-years of use! However, they do very rarely occur even with the IUS.

9.30 But surely ectopics are more common among IUD conceptions?

Precisely, but this does not invalidate the above answer. As a working rule, the ratio increases roughly 10-fold. Thus, approximately 1 in 10–20 IUD-associated pregnancies will be extrauterine if the background rate is 1 in 100–200 pregnancies among non-IUD users. My assessment of the literature is as follows: IUDs do not prevent extrauterine pregnancy (through the antifertilization effect) quite as well as they prevent intrauterine pregnancy (with the added anti-implantation effect). Hence there will be such a great reduction in the denominator of uterine pregnancies as to lead to an increased rate, even though the numerator of ectopic pregnancies is also reduced (but not by so much). It might help to use real numbers (*Table 9.1*, which, for simplicity, assumes an unreal population having 100 percent fertility by the end of 1 year).

Thus although 1 in 10 among the IUD conceptions is ectopic, this is actually a tenfold reduction in the expected number in the population. The numerator of the first ratio is truly lower, instead of ten so it is myth that IUDs cause ectopics; but the denominator of total conceptions is so massively reduced (by 990) as to allow there to be relatively more ectopics among the few conceptions.

The ectopic problem is caused by pre-existing tubal damage and should not be blamed on the IUD. Very probably, even the one woman who has an ectopic while using the IUD was due to get one (along with the other nine women) in the future, anyway, when trying to conceive.

TABLE 9.1 Ectopic pregnancy risk with IUDs

	Annual conceptions (no.)	Ectopics (no.)	Ratio
Ordinarily, in a society, let the ectopic rate be 1 in 100 pregnancies.			
Assuming zero infertility, if 1000 women use no contraception:	1000	10	1:100
If the same 1000 women use a copper IUD with a 1st-year failure rate of 1/100 woman-years:	10	1	1:10
Reduction:	990	9	

A similar explanation holds for the apparently increased rate of ectopics among conceptions with the POP, which nevertheless also protects against ectopics overall as compared with non-contracepting controls.

9.31 What are the implications for management?

The main point is that, even if only by the above selection mechanism (more ectopics being allowed to happen relative to the intrauterine pregnancies), once an IUD user is pregnant she could well have an ectopic. So the clinical slogan is:

Every IUD user with menstrual irregularity and pelvic discomfort has an ectopic pregnancy till proved otherwise.

In practice, every IUD user in whom pregnancy is suspected, with or without a positive pregnancy test, should have a pelvic examination to detect adnexal tenderness; and each IUD user should be warned prospectively, backed by a leaflet, that any marked pelvic pain should always receive prompt medical attention, particularly if her period is late.

Beware also of the IUD user who has just been sterilized. She could have a clip-induced ectopic if she was not advised appropriately (*see Qs 9.13 and 9.14*), i.e. not to rely on the IUD for 7 days before surgery (although actually this risk would be even higher if she was operated on late in the cycle while using no effective contraception at all).

9.32 Is past tubal pregnancy a contraindication to the modern banded copper IUD, or to the LNG-IUS?

In my view this is a relative contraindication (WHO 2), and even stronger (WHO 3) in young nulliparous than parous women. Although the method definitely reduces the overall risk of ectopics in a population it does, as we have seen, sometimes selectively fail to prevent them. The woman concerned should ideally use a method that will provide maximal protection to her one remaining tube. This is why I differ from WHO, which classifies past ectopic as WHO 1 for the IUD and IUS.

A poor choice would therefore be the old-type progestogen-only pill (*see Q 7.33*). Good choices would be the combined pill, Cerazette™, an injectable or Implanon™ (*see Q 8.61*). The common factor is that all these are anovulants and therefore equally good at stopping ectopics and intrauterine conceptions.

If a copper device is nevertheless chosen, as the WHO 2 category permits, the T-Safe Cu 380A™ or the GyneFIX™ should be used, because ectopics (like all conceptions) are much less frequent with these banded products. The LNG-IUS would be another option with this history: an ectopic was more than 10 times less likely in the randomized European trial (Andersson et al, see *Fig. 9.2*, p. 372) than among users of the old Nova T 200™.

9.33 What is the differential diagnosis of 'lost threads' with IUDs?

The first possibility is that the threads are in fact present but not being palpated by the user. This could be because of her inexperience or because the threads have retreated to just within the external os. If the threads are truly absent then the differential diagnosis is as shown in *Table 9.2*.

9.34 What are the 'do's and don'ts' of the management of 'lost threads'?

The first message from *Table 9.2* is another IUD 'slogan', namely that:

IUD users with lost threads are either already pregnant or at increased risk of becoming pregnant.

This is hardly surprising: the device is just as bad at preventing pregnancy – just as absent from the uterine cavity – after perforation (under the liver …?) as after expulsion (in the toilet …?). And if the IUD was only malpositioned this might still leave part of the cavity unprotected and increase the conception risk:

1 All such women therefore need to be advised to use an alternative contraceptive method until the protective presence of an IUD has been established.
2 Consider also the possible need for postcoital contraception, especially if recent expulsion is diagnosed (*see Q 10.23*).
3 In general, X-rays and any form of intrauterine manipulation should be arranged in the follicular phase of the menstrual cycle, for fear of disturbing a pregnancy.
4 Above all, women with this problem need full explanations and supportive counselling throughout the management, which is described below (*see Q 9.35*).

9.35 What is the recommended protocol for the management of 'lost threads'?

I recommend the very practical scheme in *Fig. 9.3*, amplified below. Diagnosis and treatment are simultaneous in most cases, with minimum use of hospital facilities. Exclude implanted pregnancy. Take a careful menstrual history, do a bimanual examination and if indicated perform the most sensitive pregnancy test available. If the woman is pregnant, the management is primarily that of the pregnancy itself. Note, however, that if an IUD is not recovered in the products of conception or, much later, at full term in the placenta, an X-ray should be taken before assuming expulsion (as opposed to perforation or malposition).

TABLE 9.2 Differential diagnosis of 'lost threads' with IUDs

Main diagnoses A: Not pregnant	Clinical clues	B: Pregnant	Clinical clues
(1) **Device in uterus** Threads cut too short, or caught up around device during original insertion or avulsed at a previous removal attempt; or device itself malpositioned	(a) Periods likely to be those characteristic of IUD in situ (b) Uterus normal size	(4) **Device in situ + pregnancy**	(a) Amenorrhoea (b) Pregnancy test likely to be positive, with clinically enlarged uterus (sufficient to pull up thread)
(2) **Unrecognized expulsion**	(a) Recent periods as woman's normal pattern (b) Uterus normal size	(5) **Unrecognized expulsion + pregnancy**	(a) Amenorrhoea, following one or more apparently normal periods (i.e. unmodified by IUD) (b) Signs of pregnancy variably present (may be too early on first presentation) or pregnancy test positive
(3) **Perforation of uterus**	As (2) plus (rarely) mass or actual IUD palpated on bimanual examination	(6) **Perforation of uterus + pregnancy**	As (5) plus (rarely) mass or actual IUD identified on bimanual examination

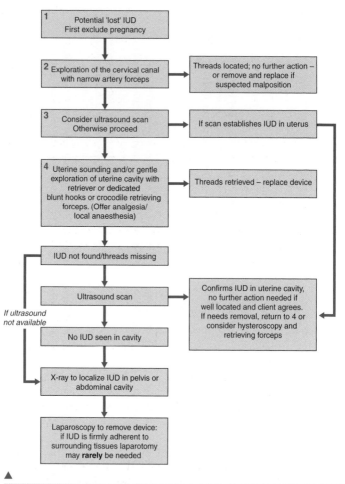

Fig. 9.3 Management of 'lost' IUD threads. Q 9.35.

In the absence of pregnancy, proceed as follows:

1   First, insert and open the jaws of *long-handled narrow artery forceps* (Spencer-Wells or equivalent) within the endocervical canal – without reaching the level of the internal cervical os. In a (1992) study of 400 women with 'lost threads', the Margaret Pyke Centre found that almost 50% of the IUDs were identified/retrieved this way, meaning that the

woman had had a wasted trip because this could so easily have been done by the referring doctor.

2 If the threads are readily located without having being pulled and the IUD judged to be correctly located, no further action need be taken; but disappearance of the threads might be a sign of malposition. So it is often advisable (after discussion with the woman) to remove and replace the device. An ultrasound scan is very helpful here but, if not available on site (as it increasingly is), this can be deferred until later in the sequence because it might be unnecessary if the device is removed successfully.

3 *Try the use of thread-retrievers.* The most established of these in the UK is the Emmett retriever, which is available presterilized and disposable. It has a handle to which is attached a thin plastic strip with multiple notches designed to trap the threads, when the edge is used like a curette against each surface of the fundus. The MI-Mark Helix™ was found to be significantly less effective than either this or the (no longer available) Retrievette™, in the Margaret Pyke Centre study above.

   What about analgesia? Ideally (and this is policy at the Margaret Pyke Centre) a prostaglandin inhibitor such as mefenamic acid should be routinely given about 30–60 min before any intrauterine manipulations – as for all IUD insertions. A few women, especially nulliparae, require a paracervical block with local anaesthetic (*see Q 9.111*). If the cervix is stenosed, pretreatment with EE (30 mg daily for 5 days) can soften and dilate the canal. Misoprostol 200 mg vaginally as a single dose the night before has been tried (unlicensed use) but was not particularly helpful in my own small series.

4 Next, try *small, blunt IUD-removal hooks* (Grafenberg pattern). In skilled hands these metal devices can be used to hook down either a thread or part of the device itself, but they can also cause trauma at the internal os. Blind traction on a partially perforated device can be dangerous (*see Q 9.48*).

5 *Various resterilizable IUD retrieving forceps* (e.g. the Patterson alligator forceps), with short jaws opening wholly in the uterine cavity, can next be tried with success. Otherwise, and usually after imaging (if not already done), try suction using a Karman curette, and hysteroscopy. All require good analgesia but local anaesthesia is nearly always sufficient. General anaesthesia should very rarely be required for any device that is in utero.

6 Arrange *appropriate imaging.* An ultrasound scan can be arranged at this point, if it has not already been done. In fact, the scan should have been done earlier if the device was not readily located by sound or retriever at (3), so as to avoid unnecessary discomfort. Confirmation of correct intrauterine location within a non-pregnant uterus can be helpful for a woman who wishes to continue using the same device but if there is any suspicion that it is malpositioned (e.g. too low or rotated), appropriate

steps should be taken for its removal as above. If the scan shows unequivocally that the uterus is empty, an X-ray is then required to differentiate between expulsion and perforation (*see Qs 9.38–9.48*). If the latter is confirmed, refer to an expert (2) laparoscopist (see *Fig. 9.3*).

9.36 What if ultrasound facilities are not available?

It might then be useful to arrange an X-ray with a uterine marker. The most practical marker is another IUD, preferably of a different pattern from that originally fitted. There are three possible X-ray findings:

1 *Only the newly inserted device visible*: this implies unrecognized expulsion of the first device.
2 *IUDs shown on the abdominal radiograph in close proximity*: if a lateral view also shows that the IUDs are contiguous this means that the first device is actually in utero. This should be a rare finding if the X-ray is arranged only after stages (1) to (5) above. However, it is well worth removing the second IUD, as this might bring down part of the original device.
3 *The IUDs might be clearly separated on the X-ray*: this establishes the diagnosis of complete perforation (translocation) (*see Qs 9.43–9.48*).

9.37 Some IUDs, especially the Chinese steel spring one, do not have threads anyway, how are they removed?

After excluding pregnancy (i.e. usually by a normal LMP), and at minimum giving a PGSI premed (but considering a full paracervical block if dilatation will be required, *see Q 9.111*), blunt hooks nearly always work. Patterson forceps should be available as back-up. *See Qs 9.105 and 9.126* for a discussion on oestrogen pretreatment if the woman is hypo-oestrogenic (e.g. postmenopausally).

EXPULSION

9.38 What influences the frequency of partial or complete expulsion?

In most large studies of framed IUDs the rate ranges widely, from about 3 to 15/100 women at 1 year. The rates are influenced by:

1 Characteristics of the woman (age, parity and uterine shape) – also the wrong timing of insertion in relation to the menses (*see Qs 9.15–9.17*, sometimes indicating a course of PGSIs (*see Q 9.16*))
2 The size and nature of the device: the implantable GyneFIX™ has it is claimed the lowest rate (0.4% in the first year)
3 *Above all*, the skill of the person performing the insertion (*see Q 9.22*).

9.39 When do expulsions most commonly occur?

During the menses, most particularly the first or second menstruation after insertion. About one-third of first-year pregnancies among IUD users occur after unnoticed expulsion. This should not happen if women are taught to check for the presence of the threads (and the absence of any part of a partially expelled device), after each period and prior to relying on the device for that cycle. Among users for more than 3 years, the expulsion rate with most devices approaches nil (*see Qs 9.34 and 10.23*).

9.40 What effect do age and parity have on the expulsion rate?

Young nulliparous women have higher expulsion rates for all devices than parous women. After the first child there is a negligible effect of increasing parity on the expulsion rate. However, IUD expulsion rates seem to decline in a fairly linear fashion with increasing age. In studies either of parous or of nulliparous women, the rates of expulsion are about half over the age of 30 than in women below that age.

9.41 What is the effect of the size and shape of the uterus?

If the cavity of the uterus is significantly distorted, either congenitally or by fibroids, there will be an increase in uterine activity (and cramps) after insertion and an increased likelihood of both malposition and expulsion. Ideally, therefore, such women should avoid framed IUDs, although the GyneFIX™ is often usable. Careful sounding, as described in *Q 9.113*, during the insertion might lead to a change of plan but in practice quite gross distortions of the uterine cavity can be difficult to identify clinically (see *Fig. 9.10* (p. 420) and *Q 9.92*). If in doubt, a good preinsertion ultrasound scan of the contours of the uterine cavity is invaluable, and this should always be done if fibroids are identified.

9.42 What is the effect of the size and shape of the device itself?

Different expulsion rates between devices certainly exist. For example, the rate for the now obsolete Copper 7™ (particularly for partial expulsions) was considerably higher than that for the T-shaped IUDs, even after controlling for other variables. In an RCT, the Flexi-T 300™ had a higher expulsion rate than the T-Safe Cu 380A™.

Aside from insertion skill, expulsion rates are probably most correlated with the precise fit of any framed device within the uterus of different women.

The GyneFIX™ solves the problem of fitting different sizes and even shapes of uterus comfortably in a unique way (*see Q 9.141*) and so, always provided it is fitted optimally initially, it can have a particularly low expulsion rate.

PERFORATION

9.43 What problems are associated with uterine perforation?

1 *Pregnancy*: most perforations first present as a pregnancy with 'lost threads'.
2 *Adhesions or penetration*: if the device is bioactive (copper or progestogen-containing) it leads to adhesion formation or might penetrate the wall of bowel or bladder. 'Closed' devices (e.g. rings) are particularly associated with bowel strangulation.

Yet the uterus always heals so completely that any IUD or IUS may be used in future if requested (WHO 2).

9.44 Should perforated devices be removed? Should it be considered an emergency?

In countries with developed medical services the benefits of removal always outweigh the risks. There are usually no specific symptoms so removal can be elective but prompt after diagnosis (*see Q 9.35*).

While waiting for hospital admission the patient should be warned to use alternative contraception, and that any abdominal pain, particularly if there is associated diarrhoea, must be reported promptly. Serious complications involving the bowel have been reported (including one death from peritonitis in a Copper 7™ user).

9.45 What is the frequency of uterine perforation following IUD insertion?

The true incidence is difficult to establish but is commonly quoted as around 1 per 1000 insertions. It is probably even lower for T-shaped IUDs that are positioned by a 'withdrawal' technique. Only one perforation in 1815 insertions of such devices was reported by Chi in 1987 (*see also Q 11.24*).

9.46 What factors affect the perforation rate?

The rate is affected by the usual three kinds of variable:

1 *Features of the woman*: the main factor here is recent pregnancy, puerperal insertions having a higher rate (*see Q 11.24*).
2 *Features of the device*: linear devices, such as the Lippes loop, that were inserted by a 'push' technique (rather than the 'withdrawal' techniques now more commonly used) were more likely to perforate. An important safety factor is to avoid loading any IUD into its inserter too far ahead of the insertion, so that the plastic loses its 'memory' (*see Q 9.115*).
3 *Features of the inserting clinician*: this is again by far and away the most important factor. As Lippes himself observed: 'IUDs do not perforate. For this to happen we need a practitioner'. Almost all perforations are

produced at insertion even though the diagnosis might be long delayed (and frequently emerges only when the empty uterus permits a pregnancy). Perforations are more common:
(a) when the operator is inexperienced
(b) when the position of the uterus is misdiagnosed (especially unrecognized retroversion) and probably:
(c) when a holding forceps or tenaculum is not used (*see* Q 9.113).

9.47 What is the best way to remove perforated devices?

This can sometimes be done with minimal trauma by simple colpotomy (when the device is palpable in the pouch of Douglas) or, more commonly, at laparoscopy. Even if there are adhesions, the device can usually be grasped at one end or the other and pulled through its own 'tunnel'. However, great care is necessary because devices can sometimes be adherent to the actual wall of bowel or bladder. Laparotomy might be required, but very rarely these days. If operative laparoscopic removal is not successful I would arrange more detailed imaging and referral to an expert in minimal access surgery, not now proceeding to a laparotomy under the same anaesthetic.

9.48 Are there any special points about embedding and partial perforation?

If part of a partially translocated device can be grasped within the uterus it might be possible to remove it transcervically. However, this should be done with great gentleness. It is possible for the part of the device which is through the uterine wall to be adherent to bowel or bladder. Removal at hysteroscopy under ultrasound or laparoscopic control is much safer in such cases (*see also* Q 9.125 and *Fig. 9.11*, p. 427).

PELVIC INFECTION

9.49 Do IUDs cause pelvic inflammatory disease (PID)?

 The evidence-based answer to this question now is No! (see Q 9.51). Although studies have repeatedly shown an increased risk of such infections in IUD users as compared with controls, the controls are protected (*see* Q 9.50). When they occur, in some studies, attacks appear to be of greater severity than in cases without the associated foreign body.

According to Westrom, one severe attack of laparoscopically diagnosed PID of any type carries a 1 in 8 risk of infertility due to tubal occlusion; two attacks, a 1 in 3 risk; and three attacks a 1 in 2 risk. So this infection risk has rightly become the greatest single anxiety about the IUD method, particularly for use by nulliparae especially since the Dalkon shield disaster of the 1970s (Q 9.63).

> PID is primarily caused by people, not by devices; and the people are most often MEN, bringing the infection into what the woman believed to be a monogamous relationship.

9.50 What is the actual frequency of PID among IUD users?

The absolute risk varies enormously according to the background rate of (sexually transmitted) PID in the population studied. The problem is that in most comparative studies the controls have been themselves protected against infection, either by using barrier methods or the combined pill. Progestogen-containing (i.e. mucus-altering) contraception generally about halves the risk of PID (*see Q 5.40*).

Westrom (1980) studied all women aged 20–29 in the town of Lund, Sweden, and found the incidence of PID per 1000 woman-years to be 52 for IUD users, compared with 34 for sexually active users of no contraception, 14 for barrier method users and 9 for pill users. This study usefully shows that the lion's share of the six-fold difference at that time (early 1970s) when IUDs were compared with pills was caused by the protective effect of the latter: four-fold compared with users of nothing.

9.51 As shown by that Westrom study, a doubling of the risk of PID through use of the IUD would surely still be important?

Definitely, but even that is a huge exaggeration. Factors like diagnostic bias are operative: PID is more likely to be thought about/diagnosed when pelvic symptoms occur in IUD users. Several studies have shown low or absent risk in women claiming only one sexual partner – and that's even without good information about what their partner is up to!

More convincingly, in the massive WHO study (*see Q 9.55*) there was not one single case of PID reported among 4301 women fitted with IUDs in China in the 1980s: a country where true (two-sided) monogamy was then a reality, and at that point, virtually an STI-free zone (not so now). Two other Chinese trials referenced in an excellent review by David Grimes (2000 *The Lancet* 356:1013–1019) and totalling 3300 women, also reported no cases of PID at all. If 7600-plus IUDs can be fitted (anywhere) with no PID during follow-up, is it not a bit unfair to blame the IUD per se for causing the condition?!

9.52 So what factors have been suggested as affecting the rate of PID in IUD users?

In summary, and in order of clinical importance, the factors are:

1   the woman's risk of acquiring PID from a partner
2   the insertion process, combined with point (1) (*see Q 9.54ff*)

3 features of the IUD:
   (a) foreign body effect – unlikely (*see* Q 9.62)
   (b) the cervical tail(s) – very unlikely if they are monofilament
        (*see* Q 9.63).

9.53 What features of the woman can influence the PID rate?

Age, acting as a marker for the risk of sexually transmitted infections. The
risk is highest in young women under 20 and declines in a linear fashion as
age increases (*Fig. 9.4*). In a study at the Margaret Pyke Centre, the
incidence of infection was 10 times greater below the age of 20 than it was
above 30 – although the 871 women were all nulliparous, had received the
same type of IUD (Copper 7™), at the same centre and all in the first 10
days of the cycle.

There is no evidence that the uterus becomes more resistant to infection
with age and, because the isolation of specific cervical pathogens and rates
of PID in non-IUD users show a decline with age and correlates with sexual
lifestyle, this again is indirect evidence that the vast majority of cases of PID
in IUD users are primarily sexually acquired.

It needs to be stressed again that the infection is often transmitted to a
woman:

■ who is practising monogamy (serial monogamy, anyway) by her
  partner who is not
■ at the time of partner change.

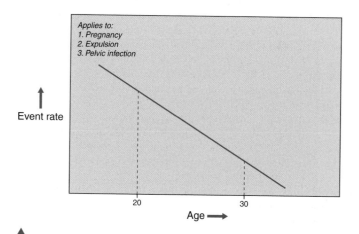

Applies to:
1. Pregnancy
2. Expulsion
3. Pelvic infection

Event rate

20   30

Age ⟶

Fig. 9.4 Effect of age on IUD performance. Q 9.53. See also Qs 9.11 and 9.40.

Very often, if the right questions are asked, the attack of PID comes after a recent partner change. After the age of 30 it is an observed fact that partner change becomes less frequent.

9.54 So how should we question and counsel women who wish to use the IUD method?

Verbal screening concerning lifestyle of self/partner and recent partner change(s) is of great relevance but unlikely to be sufficient: in study during the mid-1980s by the Margaret Pyke Centre, the background rate of *Chlamydia* carriage was 2.4% in the general clinic population but higher – 8.2% – in the pre-IUD group who had first been sensitively questioned about their likely exposure!

Thus, in most metropolitan areas of the UK today, I consider it suboptimal to fit copper or progestogen-releasing devices without microbiological screening: the money for preinsertion *Chlamydia* testing must just be found. This argument is greatly strengthened by the WHO study depicted in *Fig. 9.5* and the discussion that follows.

9.55 What light is thrown on this PID problem by the thorough database review of international WHO studies published in 1992 (Farley et al *The Lancet* 339:785–788)?

One of 10 types of IUD had been inserted in 13 trials (12 of them RCTs). There were 22 908 IUD users (almost all parous) from five continents, fitted

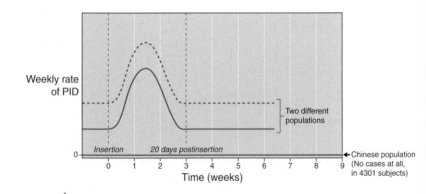

Fig. 9.5 Graphic representation of PID rates post-IUD insertion. Q 9.54 (from Farley et al 1992 Lancet 339:785–788).

and followed up to a common protocol from 1975 to about 1990, and there were no less than 51 399 years of follow-up. Of the users, 9% were using the inert Lippes Loop, copper IUDs were used by the majority – 17 019 women – and hormone-releasing devices (the Alza progesterone T™ and the LNG-IUS) were used by the remainder (16%).

The overall rate of PID among the women recruited was low, 1.6/1000 woman-years of use (contrast with Q 9.50!), and lower still in the late 1990s – suggesting that later in the trials in all centres there was greater care in user selection, because there was no prescreening or antibiotic prophylaxis. The most important findings were:

1   PID risk was more than six times higher during the first 20 days after insertion than later; the risk was constant and relatively low thereafter for up to 8 years with no evidence that it was then any higher than the local background rate (see *Fig. 9.5*).
2   PID rates varied by geographical area. They were highest in Africa and nil in China, and were inversely associated with age. This mirrors exactly the background risk of sexually transmitted diseases (STIs).
3   Whether considered individually or grouped by type, the PID rates for copper-bearing, hormonal and inert IUDs were statistically indistinguishable. For all these devices this makes a specific IUD factor in the attacks very improbable, especially as previous studies were readily able to show that one device, the Dalkon Shield™, did specifically increase PID risk (*see* Q 9.63).
4   In China, 4301 IUDs were inserted and not a single case of PID was reported either in the critical first 3 weeks or later!

9.56 It looks, then, as though insertion time is the main danger time for IUDs, but why?

The postinsertion infection 'bulge' of *Fig. 9.5* is most unlikely to be because of bad insertion technique (i.e. the doctors introducing new organisms) occurring only among the doctors outside China. Westergaard et al (1982 *Obstetrics in Gynecology* 60:322–325) showed that carrying out a termination of pregnancy in the presence of *Chlamydia* or gonococcal infection of the cervix increased the risk of postabortal infection about three-fold.

IUD insertion is another procedure that can temporarily impair (at a cervical level) the protective mechanisms that protect the upper genital tract from organisms. This was shown by Mishell et al (1966 *American Journal of Obstetrics and Gynecology* 96:119–126). Although the doctors in all the centres were searching for monogamous women, they might well have been successful in this search only in China. In mainland China, through the 1970s and 1980s (it would not be true now), monogamy was the norm, and it was also two-sided, with a consequential very low incidence of STIs of all kinds.

As there was no systematic prescreening, in the other countries PID-causing organisms (especially *Chlamydia trachomatis*) are presumed to have been present in a proportion of the women.

In a later study from California (Walsh et al 1998 *The Lancet* 351:1005–1008) when there *was* effective prescreening (verbal plus microbiological), the postinsertion 'bulge' of PID was – unsurprisingly – not detected even when antibiotics were not given. The screening of clients was so good that few if any pathogens would have been in the lower genital tracts of the subjects, and the incidence of PID was minimal (1:1000 in early months of use regardless of antibiotic treatment).

So in the WHO studies without prescreening the process of insertion would enable clinically silent infection to spread from the lower genital tract, where it had been, into the upper genital tract, including the fallopian tubes, becoming symptomatic. Everywhere except in China. In summary:

1 The greatest risk of PID is in the first 20 days, believed to be caused by pre-existing carriage in the lower genital tract of that woman of sexually transmitted pathogens (STI organisms).
2 PID rates thereafter, like preinsertion, relate to the background rate of STIs.
3 Insertions should ideally only be through what I light-heartedly call a 'Chinese cervix', minimizing the IUD-related postinsertion 'bulge' of PID (see *Fig. 9.5*).

9.57 So what is a 'Chinese cervix', as you use the term?!

Quite simply, it is a pathogen-free cervix! *Either* because the woman comes from a society/culture where, quite simply, there are no such pathogens (an almost unique feature of the Chinese mainland in the 1970s and most of the 1980s) *or* because she has been so effectively screened by a combination of verbal screening and assessment *and* – except when assessed as personally at very low risk – at least by an accurate *Chlamydia* test.

9.58 In summary, what are the practical implications for arrangements at IUD insertion in a society with a moderate or high prevalence of STIs?

Defining 'moderate prevalence' arbitrarily as over 3% *Chlamydia* carriage, it is my view that:

1 All prospective IUD users should be questioned closely about their own STI risk, which means a proper sexual history (*see Q 1.14*), including the ticklish issue of how likely it might that a pathogen might have been transmitted from a sole current partner and then:
2 Ideally this verbal screening (including the background factors of age and parity) should be supplemented by microbiological screening at least for *Chlamydia*, prior to all IUD insertions or reinsertions.

3 Evidence of recent exposure to an STI or a purulent discharge from the cervix indicates more detailed investigation at a genitourinary medicine (GUM) clinic anyway.

4 If *Chlamydia* is detected, an urgent GUM appointment should follow. Unless there is clinical PID (requiring more vigorous treatment), treatment is usually by doxycycline 100 mg bd for 7 days, or azithromycin 1 g stat, *after* other STIs have been looked for. Contact tracing should be arranged and the IUD insertion postponed – maybe indefinitely. There should certainly be a serious reappraisal of the implications of her (and her partner's) lifestyle for use of this method – most particularly, as usual, if she is nulliparous.

5 If the *Chlamydia* result is negative this, now highly likely to be a pathogen-free 'Chinese cervix', should be very thoroughly physically cleansed before the device is inserted – following the manufacturer's instructions with minimum trauma.

9.59 What if the (copper) IUD needs to be inserted when *Chlamydia* screening is not available, or before the results of the recommended *Chlamydia* screening are known – which is the norm in emergency contraception cases? Could one not eliminate the postinsertion 'hump' of infection shown in *Fig. 9.5* by simply routinely prescribing the appropriate antibiotics?

Because attenders for EC are known to be at high risk of *Chlamydia* (Faculty of FPRHC Guidance 2003 *Emergency Contraception* 29:9–16), in my view full antibiotic treatment (as detailed in *Q 9.58(4)*) should normally be given, with 100% follow-up to enable contact tracing if the *Chlamydia* test does return positive.

But some will dispute this because a Cochrane Review (Grimes et al 2002 Cochrane Library, Issue 4, Oxford: Update Software) was not able to demonstrate that prophylactic antibiotic use prior to *routine* IUD insertion conferred any benefit, aside from a significant reduction in unscheduled return visits to the provider clinic in one Kenyan study. Aside from the fact that evidence is lacking for similar treatment at the time of *emergency* IUD insertion, in my opinion the four main RCTs in the excellent review by Grimes could not detect an advantage. This would be either because, through excellent screening, the women studied were at too low a risk without prophylaxis (Walsh's California study, *see Q 9.56*, and probably the study from Turkey) or perhaps because the studies in Kenya and Nigeria gave inadequate treatment (a single 200-mg dose of doxycycline preinsertion).

Even within the Cochrane Review there is the statement:

In populations with a high prevalence of sexually transmitted diseases, such as Kenya [Sinei 1990] prophylaxis may offer modest protection against both pelvic inflammatory disease and unscheduled visits to the clinic.

Now, according to the Faculty guidance mentioned above, EC requesters in the UK are indeed such a population with respect to *Chlamydia*. Moreover, absence of proof of benefit is certainly not proof of absence of benefit. Pending more data, therefore, I would withhold a proper course of prophylactic antibiotics from a prospective IUD user in these particular circumstances only if verbal screening of the particular individual was very convincing that she was *at low risk*. I would also then arrange her first IUD follow-up visit at 7 days (*see Q. 9.60*).

Note that if the high risk circumstances of the individual do justify that antibiotic, they would usually justify *also* doing a *Chlamydia* test, if available, to have the option of contact tracing and to minimize the woman's risk of later infection by her partner.

9.60 What are the implications of *Fig. 9.5* for follow-up?

At the Margaret Pyke Centre, our initial reaction to the 1992 WHO publication was to arrange a (new) first postinsertion visit after 7 days (additional to the routine 6-week follow-up): designed to pick up any women with postinsertion infection (during the 'hump' of *Fig. 9.5*). I would still recommend this if no microbiological screening was done.

However, now that effective *Chlamydia* screening by a highly sensitive DNA test is available, we find it is sufficient to give screen-negative women a hand-out, at the insertion visit, with a list of the symptoms suggestive of PID:

■ low abdominal or pelvic pain, especially if any postinsertion symptoms had initially improved
■ dyspareunia
■ abnormal vaginal discharge
■ a temperature above 38.3°C, especially if preceded by rigors.

She is instructed to telephone our Advice Sister should she be in the slightest doubt. As a minimum in general practice, a similar handout could be used and it might be advisable for the woman to be asked routinely to 'touch base' by telephoning the practice nurse about a week postinsertion.

9.61 How do you manage those who report problems?

If examination reveals cervical excitation tenderness and/or adnexal tenderness then an urgent GUM appointment is indicated. If frank PID is confirmed, sometimes laparoscopically (*see Q 9.66*), metronidazole is usually added to a full 2 weeks of doxycycline.

9.62 What features of the device itself might increase risk of PID, and how might they be changed?

As we have seen, PID is primarily a 'self- or partner-inflicted wound'. Because IUDs are foreign bodies they have the *potential* suggested in early studies such as Vessey et al. 1981 (*BMJ* 282:855–57) to facilitate sexually transmitted infections or to promote secondary invaders and the severity of attacks. However, studies summarized in David Grimes' 2000 Review quoted in Q *9.51* do not support this: more evidence is needed.

If the foreign body effect of IUDs were a factor in worsening (sexually acquired) PID, it cannot – by definition – be eliminated. However it is *theoretically* reducible by:

1 avoiding embedding of part of the device in the myometrium
2 elimination of the plastic carrier, as in the GyneFIX™ (*see Q 9.141*)
3 release of progestogens into the cervical/uterine fluid, which might hinder transfer of pathogens to the upper genital tract with the LNG-IUS, although whether this truly lowers PID risk is not proven (*see Q 9.146*)
4 similar release of antiseptic substances – attempted in small experiments, never taken further.

9.63 What could be the effect of the threads traversing the cervical canal?

The thread of the now defunct Dalkon Shield™ was multifilament in design and this was shown to act as a 'wick'. This was disastrous and, because a very few Dalkon Shields™ might still be in situ, they should always be removed on suspicion of their presence.

9.64 So should we go back to using threadless IUDs, like the old Birnberg Bow?

No. The RCTs quoted in Q *9.51* have shown no difference in PID rates between thread-bearing and thread-free IUDs, and vanishingly low or zero rates of important infections anyway among thread-bearing device users in low-risk populations.

Pending more data, any adverse influence of the threads must be very small in practice, and more than outweighed by their usefulness during IUD follow-up and to simplify device removal.

9.65 How would you summarize practical implications, especially of the WHO studies (*Qs 9.54–9.59*)?

1 Monogamous parous women with monogamous partners as in China in the 1980s can use IUDs with absolutely no fear of PID.
2 Monogamous young nulliparae can definitely consider the option, but always as a second choice (WHO 2, or sometimes WHO 3, depending on

the discussion about sexual lifestyles of self or partner) because they do not have that cushion, of one or more babies already in the cot.

3 All potential and current users need to be informed/reminded where the infection really comes from because, as the 1992 WHO authors put it, 'exposure to sexually transmitted disease rather than type of IUD is the major determinant of PID'. Especially at times of partner change, users need to insist on condom use as well as their IUD.

4 Around the crucial time of insertion, the measures described in *Qs 9.54–9.58* need to be implemented.

5 There should be very vigorous treatment and contact-tracing of PID when it happens.

6 Providers should minimize the number of (potentially dangerous) reinsertions by choosing devices with the longest possible long-term efficacy (*see Q 9.134*).

9.66 How should significant IUD-associated pelvic infection be managed?

Laparoscopy is indicated in severe cases to establish the diagnosis. Ideally, full bacteriological screening at a GUM clinic should be performed. If such detailed bacteriology is impossible, often because treatment is urgent, at least endocervical swabs should be taken first into the appropriate transport media. The usual first choice of antibiotic would be a tetracycline (preferably for at least 2 weeks, to treat the most common and possibly most harmful pathogens, namely *Chlamydia* and *Neisseria gonorrhoeae*), with 5 days of metronidazole to deal with the frequently associated anaerobes.

9.67 Should the IUD be removed?

Data available do not support a better outcome to treatment if the IUD is removed (see the Grimes reference in *Q 9.51*) although, if there is not a good response within 48 h to appropriate antibiotics, I would have a low threshold to remove it, especially in young nulliparae. If it is removed, there should be urgent consideration of postcoital contraception according to the menstrual and coital histories (*see Qs 9.13 and 9.14*) – not omitting also, as gynaecologists so often do, to arrange with the woman a new long-term method of birth control.

9.68 Should there be any other action, after IUD-associated PID?

Regrettably, healthcare providers in most cultures still pussyfoot around this matter, but the sexual contacts of all such women should be traced and appropriately treated. There are a minimum of three individuals to be treated, the index case, her partner and his other partner.

Moreover, a very clear warning should be given about the disastrous effects of recurrent PID (reaching, after three hospitalized attacks, a tubal occlusion rate of one in two); along with advice about condom use to avoid another attack, leave alone that other risk she may also be running, of HIV infection. All this is not being judgemental, just good preventive medicine.

9.69 Is pelvic infection always a contraindication to an IUD?

If currently acutely or chronically present, this is an absolute contraindication (WHO 4). Moreover, all women reporting deep dyspareunia or with tenderness of the pelvic organs, whether on palpation or caused by cervical excitation, should not receive an IUD until infection has been excluded.

9.70 What about a history of past pelvic infection?

If this was not severe, more than 6 months ago and there has been no recurrence, and currently the woman is free of any symptoms or signs, then (after full discussion and counselling) IUD insertion is only relatively contraindicated (WHO 3). It would still be preferable that such a woman should have at least one living child.

Rescreening for STIs, especially *Chlamydia*, should be done and there should be serious consideration of tetracycline 'cover' for the insertion.

The woman might need to be advised to use condoms as well, subsequently. She should also be warned to return exceptionally promptly at the first sign of another PID attack.

Past severe or recurrent infection contraindicates the IUD (WHO 4) in a case at risk of endocarditis (*see* Q 9.90).

9.71 What does it mean when a cervical smear report says '*Actinomyces*-like organisms (ALOs) are present'. Is it necessarily *Actinomyces israeli*?

This bacterium is normally a harmless commensal in the mouth and gastrointestinal tract but has the potential to do harm (*see* Q 9.73). In the lower female genital tract it is almost never detected by cytology (or culture) except when a foreign body is present, the most common being an IUD or IUS. But not all reports of ALOs are necessary this particular organism.

There is also an association with bacterial vaginosis (BV) – which itself has been found more common in IUD users than controls (*see* Q 9.177).

9.72 How often are *Actinomyces*-like organisms (ALOs) found in the cervical smears of IUD users?

In some studies, the frequency with which ALOs have been reported in routine smears appears to relate in a linear fashion to the duration of use of the device: whether inert, copper or LNG-containing. After 1 year's use in one review 1–2% of smears were positive, rising to 8–10% after 3 years.

It was initially thought that copper prevented the carriage of these organisms. It is now believed that the main explanation for lower incidence is the shorter average duration of use of copper than inert devices (plus, in the past, more frequent changes, *see* Q 9.75).

9.73 What is the most serious potential significance of the finding of ALOs in the cervical smear?

Frank actinomycosis is an extremely serious and debilitating condition, featuring granulomatous pelvic abscesses. A fatal outcome has been reported in one IUD user and other women have been known to require pelvic clearance as a lifesaving measure. However, the incidence of this complication is extremely low, even allowing for underdiagnosis among women with severe IUD-related infections. In the context of millions of woman-years of IUD use there have been only a few hundred cases reported in the whole world literature.

In short, it seems clear that actinomycosis represents a very small part of the spectrum of pelvic infection associated with IUDs.

9.74 What action should be taken when a cervical smear from an established IUD or IUS user is reported as showing ALOs?

The protocol that follows is only partially evidence based but, substantially, it is that of the Faculty of Family Planning as first issued in January 1998 and subsequently reissued. Pending more data:

- The patient should be recalled without delay and questioned carefully about the occurrence of pain, deep dyspareunia, intermenstrual bleeding or excessive discharge, and dysuria.
- *She should always be examined*: if there is even mild adnexal or uterine tenderness on examination, or cervical excitation tenderness, or any mass is felt, in my view the knowledge that ALOs are present should markedly lower the threshold for IUD removal, whatever other action is taken.
- An ultrasound scan should be the norm in this assessment. If it shows adnexal mass(es) immediate gynaecological referral is indicated.
- If, as is the norm, she is completely asymptomatic and examination is normal, proceed directly to Q 9.75.
- Arrange appropriate referral for women with symptoms or signs. If actinomycosis rather than a 'normal' form of PID is suspected this should be generally to a gynaecologist rather than a department of GUM – again, especially if there is an adnexal mass.
- Investigations might include (preferably after personal discussion with the microbiologist): endocervical swabs and the removed IUD (threads

excised) for culture, and endometrial biopsies for culture and histology. If the laboratory recommends antibiotic therapy, penicillin or erythromycin are usual choices but in high dose often for several weeks. If other anaerobes such as BV are diagnosed, the usual course of metronidazole 400 mg bd for 5 days can also be advised.

■ The patient should be followed up to check for cure, and another method of birth control arranged.

9.75 What action should be taken if ALOs are reported and there are absolutely no symptoms or signs at all (pelvic infection not suspected)?

If so many long-term IUD users carry ALOs, and so very few ever develop symptoms, more morbidity (through resulting pregnancies) could be caused by insisting on ceasing the method than by simply monitoring the situation.

All asymptomatic women should first be counselled about the potential (small) risk and taught the symptoms of pelvic actinomycosis. At the Margaret Pyke Centre, we have a helpful leaflet describing the two management options:

OPTION A: REMOVAL OR CHANGE OF THE IUD OR IUS

This is a popular course of action, particularly for copper IUDs because it usually leads to a more reassuring situation for the woman. In 1984 a small study at the Margaret Pyke Centre, and a later study of 100 women in Newcastle upon Tyne, showed that device removal – *without* any antibiotic treatment – was followed by disappearance of the ALOs from the subsequent cervical smears. At the Margaret Pyke Centre this clearance occurred with or without immediate reinsertion.

Although later experience shows that such clearance is not invariable, we find that most women after counselling now elect to try device removal, with replacement or switching to another long-term method. The removed device does not need to be sent for culture.

After one case at the Margaret Pyke Centre developed full-blown actinomycosis – subsequent to being asymptomatic at IUD removal without reinsertion, and being discharged because she did not need contraception postmenopausally – I now recommend follow-up at 3 rather than 6 months in every case. The woman should also be counselled to return at any time should she have any of the symptoms in Q 9.74.

If at the follow-up visit a bimanual examination and repeat smear show no abnormality, she can simply return to having regular cervical smears on her local screening programme (e.g. every 3 years)

OPTION B: LEAVE THE IUD OR IUS IN SITU, WITH MONITORING BY REGULAR FOLLOW-UP EXAMINATION ARRANGED EVERY 6 MONTHS

The follow-up is for a *bimanual examination* and enquiry (and reminder) about relevant symptoms, i.e. pain, deep dyspareunia, intermenstrual bleeding or excessive discharge, and dysuria.

The woman is additionally advised, with backup written instructions, that if these should ever occur she must – without fail – return before her next routine visit. She should agree to be contacted at home or through her general practitioner if she defaults from follow-up.

Cervical smears are likely to remain showing the ALOs and are hence only repeated at the frequency of local screening guidelines.

In both cases, if BV is diagnosed (characteristic odour and history with pH more than 4.5) it should be treated with metronidazole 400 mg bd for 5 days.

COMMENT

Option A as compared with Option B has the potential to reduce both a woman's ongoing anxiety about harbouring a potential pathogen 'down below' and our burden of responsibility for long-term follow-up. But each case should be individualized and other factors, such as the cost of a new LNG-IUS when her existing one is suiting well, might also come into the equation.

PAIN AND BLEEDING

9.76 What is the most frequent complaint of copper IUD users?

 In practice, the most frequent problem is increased bleeding, frequently accompanied by cramp-like menstrual pain and the two are often considered together. However, it is a good working slogan that:

Pain plus bleeding in an IUD user has a serious cause until proved otherwise.

Thus, to label these as a 'side-effect' should only be after exclusion of the more important possible causes: pregnancy-related (miscarriage, ectopic) or otherwise (partially expelled, malpositioned or perforated device; or PID) (*see Qs 9.21 and 9.22*).

9.77 What types of bleeding pattern are observed by IUD users?

The loss at the menses might be heavier and/or longer: the latter typically because of light premenstrual bleeding, or spotting, before and after the flow proper. There might also be intermenstrual bleeding or spotting, too light to cause anaemia but often very troublesome to the woman.

9.78 How often do IUD users discontinue the method because of pain or bleeding?

About 5–20% of inert or copper IUD users have the device removed because of bleeding and pain within the first 12 months. Of the remainder, approximately half will admit to annoying bleeding symptoms that they have learnt to live with and some will subsequently discontinue the method for the same reason. (Measurement of the loss has shown that inert devices roughly double the measured volume of flow, whereas the smaller copper ones increase the amount only by about 50%, that is about 20–30 mL on average.) Nevertheless, removal rates were not dramatically improved when copper devices arrived. This is doubtless because none have eliminated the annoyance for some women of prolongation of duration of flow and intermenstrual spotting.

These last two bleeding problems are still features of at least the early months of use of progestogen-releasing devices like the LNG-IUS, even though they positively reduce the measured volume of loss and often eliminate pain. Perseverance is usually rewarded by frank amenorrhoea or infrequent light bleeds (*see* Q 9.147).

9.79 Is copper a haemostatic agent?

Menstrual blood loss measurement studies of my own in the 1970s, comparing Lippes loops with and without copper bands (but otherwise identical) showed clearly that the measured mean volumes were similar. Indeed, the duration of loss in the copper-using group was slightly but significantly increased. Hence it is possible to be definite that the reduced amount of bleeding with copper devices is a function merely of their smaller size and surface area (*see* Q 9.9).

9.80 What is the cause of the increased bleeding as an IUD symptom, with or without pain?

1   Various types of malposition can cause both symptoms.
2   The fact that the cavity of the uterus is distorted congenitally or by fibroids might be missed, causing pain as the uterus attempts to expel the device. Coincidental polyps are also possible.
3   Especially in nulliparae, whose cavities tend to be smaller, the fitting of a device that is too long or too wide (*see* Q 9.93) can similarly cause cramping pain. The stem of a device that is too long projects into the sensitive isthmic part of the uterus and pain might also result from penetration of the myometrium by the side arms.
4   Perforation of the cervix by the stem of the device can result from partial expulsion and also cause pain (see *Fig. 9.11* (p. 427) and Q 9.125).

In all these cases following bouts of cramping, some at least of the observed intermenstrual bleeding (IMB) can be caused by mechanical trauma to the endometrium. According to some X-ray studies, small-framed devices that float too loosely in a large cavity can also cause some IMB, but without pain.

The LNG-IUS (*see Q 9.145ff*) has the same mechanical limitations as the Nova T 380™, whose shape it shares, yet when properly located improves uterine pain in most women (as well as dramatically reducing quantity of bleeding).

GyneFIX™ (*see Q 9.141*) was expected to eliminate or minimize the problems listed above through its unique implantable technology. Surprisingly, however, a systematic review (O'Brien et al 2002 Cochrane Library, Issue 1. Oxford, Update Software) did not demonstrate improvement in bleeding/pain removal rates as compared with standard framed copper IUDs.

9.81 What is the uterine mechanism for IUD related bleeding and pain?

Insertion of IUDs leads to a high concentration of plasminogen activators, which increase fibrinolytic activity and hence lead to more blood flow. Linked in some way with these changes are alterations in the prostaglandin responses of the endometrium during menstruation. Prostacyclin activity is increased and this causes vasodilatation and inhibition of platelet function. An increase in other prostaglandins probably explains the increased menstrual cramps, but not why some users are affected so much less than others.

9.82 Are there any drugs that can reduce the menstrual flow and pain in IUD users?

There is no very effective therapy for the problem of prolonged spotting. However, for the heaviness of flow at the menses antifibrinolytic agents are certainly effective. Tranexamic acid is available but it is not certain whether the benefits of treatment outweigh its risks, particularly as it is not an analgesic. The pain-relieving PGSIs are therefore normally preferable for initial trial, particularly mefenamic acid (1500 mg), ibuprofen (1200 mg) and naproxen (1500 mg). (Amounts in parentheses are totals for each day, to be taken in divided doses.) These drugs need only be taken from the onset of menstruation for so long as the patient feels the benefit from treatment. Response is very variable (*Fig. 9.6*) but some women report that the flow diminishes rapidly within an hour of taking a tablet.

9.83 Do many women persevere for long with an IUD if they have to take drugs regularly to cope with bleeding and/or pain?

Not as a rule. Few women would be happy to continue for years taking powerful drugs with each menstruation and doctors too would be worried

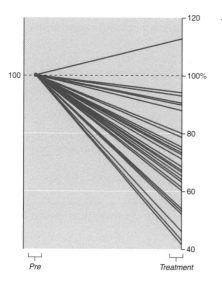

Fig. 9.6 Percentage change in menstrual blood loss with mefenamic acid. Q 9.83. The figure shows the percentage reduction in menstrual blood loss with mefenamic acid 1500 g daily for a maximum of 7 days. The mean of two treatment periods is compared for each individual woman with the mean of two previous control periods expressed as 100% (from Guillebaud et al 1978 Reduction by mefenamic acid of increased menstrual blood loss associated with intrauterine contraception. *British Journal of Obstetrics and Gynaecology* 85:53–62, Figure 1).

by possible long-term risks. Antiprostaglandin drugs are certainly very useful to reduce the cramps at IUD insertion, and both pain and bleeding over the first few cycles. In practice, however, few women continue to take them (except intermittently for dysmenorrhoea) and the majority either live with their symptoms or eventually give up the IUD method. A better alternative might be to exchange the IUD for an IUS (*see Q 9.145ff*).

SELECTION OF USERS AND OF DEVICES

Contraindications

If you are not fully acquainted with the WHO classification of contraindications, please see *Q 5.119*.

9.84 How are the absolute contraindications (WHO 4) to IUD or IUS use best classified?

These mostly relate to the adverse side-effects that we have already considered. They can be classified into *temporary* absolute contraindications, which imply some variable delay before possible later insertion, and *permanent* WHO 4 contraindications. In general, absolute contraindications apply to both IUDs and IUSs, but relative contraindications do not always apply to the IUS (see below).

9.85 What are the (possibly) temporary absolute contraindications to IUDs and IUSs?

1 Undiagnosed *irregular genital tract bleeding.* This is for fear of wrongly attributing postinsertion bleeding to the IUD when in fact it is due to important uterine pathology, such as carcinoma of the endometrium.

2 Suspicion of *pregnancy.*

3 *Postseptic abortion*, current *pelvic infection* or undiagnosed pelvic tenderness/deep dyspareunia or *purulent cervicitis* (*see Q 9.89*).

4 Therapy causing *significant immunosuppression*, i.e. more profound than use of low dose corticosteroids (*see Q 9.89*).

5 *Malignant trophoblastic disease*, with uterine wall involvement.

9.86 What are the permanent absolute contraindications to IUDs and IUSs?

1 *Markedly distorted uterine cavity*, or cavity sounding to less than 5.5 cm depth (see *Fig. 9.10* (p. 420) and *Q 9.92*). However, this finding signifies only category WHO 2 (broadly usable) for the GyneFIX™ frameless device (*see Q 9.141*).

2 Known *true allergy to a constituent* (*see Q 9.88*).

3 *Wilson's disease* (copper devices only).

4 Past attack of *bacterial endocarditis* in a woman with an anatomical lesion of the heart; or after any *prosthetic valve replacement* (*see Q 9.90*). This last can be weakened to WHO 3 in users of the LNG-IUS in the belief that the progestogen-altered cervical and uterine fluids reduce the risk of infection/bacteraemia (*see Q 9.90*).

9.87 What are the relative contraindications to copper IUD use?

These often do not apply to the LNG-IUS (see the note, below). They vary in their importance: the WHO classification is useful (*see Q 5.119*). WHO 3 means use very cautiously, other options usually being preferable, and WHO 2 signifies broadly usable, benefits outweigh risks. Unless otherwise stated, the factors listed here are WHO 2, meaning in the individual case that the IUD could even be her best choice, in comparison with alternatives. Some are considered in more detail at subsequent questions.

1 *Between 48 h and 4 weeks postpartum:* excess risk of perforation is WHO 3.

2 *Known HIV infection:* if controlled by drug therapy this is only WHO 2 (*see Q 9.89*). Eventual interference with the immune system by the virus in AIDS can be expected to increase the risk of severe infection (WHO 3). But the LNG-IUS is an excellent choice in either state

because of its added advantages of reducing pain and blood loss (WHO 1) – plus added condom use as routinely advised.

3 Recent *exposure to a high risk of a sexually transmitted disease* (e.g. after rape): ideally, the insertion should be delayed until after full investigation but in emergency situations, such as for postcoital contraception, a copper IUD is permissible (WHO 3) with full antibiotic cover (after swabs for bacteriology have been taken, *see Qs 10.24 and 10.28*).

4 *Structural heart disease* with risk (but not as Q 9.86(4) above); no past history of bacterial endocarditis. (Becomes WHO 2 once insertion with antibiotic cover is successful) (*see Q 9.90*): WHO 3.

5 *Past history of tubal ectopic pregnancy* (*see Q 9.32*) in *nulliparae*: WHO 3 if most effective banded copper IUDs or the LNG-IUS are used but it would be better still to use an anovulant method. Also, past history of tubal surgery, or other very high ectopic risk, in those still wanting a child would be WHO 3. Even among parous women the risk of recurrence of this dangerous condition implies some caution (WHO 2) and certainly the use of the banded-type most effective intrauterine methods. (WHO is less cautious, and calls past ectopic always WHO 1.)

6 With any prosthesis that can be prejudiced by blood-borne infection (e.g. *hip replacement*), IUDs are certainly usable, appearing in category WHO 2 solely to flag up that it might be a wise precaution to use antibiotic cover for the insertion.

7 *Benign trophoblastic disease*: WHO 3 but only when blood hCG is very high, with possible weakening of the uterine wall (*see Q 5.77*), otherwise WHO 2 (and WHO 1 when hCG undetectable). The same classification applies to LNG-IUS, pending more data.

8 *Past history of definite pelvic infection* (*see Q 9.70*).

9 *Lifestyle with frequent partner change*, risking STIs.

10 *Suspected subfertility already*: WHO 2 for any cause or WHO 3 if the questionable fertility relates to a tubal cause.

11 *Nulliparity and young age*, especially less than 20: the reason this is WHO 2 is both increased risk of infection and also the more serious implications thereof. But IUD or LNG-IUS, which do *not* cause PID, are very usable in selected cases (*see Q 9.20*). Summation with other factors in this list can make the caution stronger (WHO 3). Expulsion is also more common, although not with GyneFIX™.

12 *Diabetes*: WHO 2 allegedly for infection risk but the IUD is preferable to several of the hormonal methods for diabetics; and the LNG-IUS can be an excellent choice (*see Q 9.91*). (WHO says always WHO 1.)

13 *Fibroids or congenital abnormality without too marked distortion* of the uterine cavity (*see Q 9.92*): WHO 2 for framed IUDs or IUSs; WHO 1 for the GyneFIX™.

14 *Severely scarred uterus*, e.g. after myomectomy: WHO 3.

15 *Severe cervical stenosis*: Pretreatment with oestrogen can help (*see Q 9.34(3)*).

16 *Heavy periods*, with or without anaemia before insertion for any reason, including anticoagulation. This is an indication for the LNG-IUS: WHO 1.

17 *Primary dysmenorrhoea*: Offer GyneFIX™ (which at the least should not worsen this) or the LNG-IUS (which will probably benefit the dysmenorrhoea, (*see Q 9.146*), provided the uterus tolerates its frame) can be tried.

18 *Endometriosis*: there is no proven link but part of the mechanism of endometriosis might be retrograde menstruation. Hence prudence dictates it might be preferable not to increase this with a copper IUD. However, here again the progestogen-releasing LNG-IUS is a good option: WHO 1.

19 *Penicillamine treatment*, whether for Wilson's disease (WHO 4 for copper IUDs anyway) or rheumatoid arthritis: there are one or two anecdotes of in situ pregnancy occurring in penicillamine-treated copper IUD users – possibly due to interference with the contraceptive action of the copper. This is unproven; inert or progestogen-releasing IUDs would not be affected.

20 *After endometrial ablation/resection* (*see Qs 11.60 and 11.61* for more about this). LNG-IUS can be used in selected cases. Finally:

21 *Past perforation of the uterus* is only WHO 2 (*see Q 9.43*).

> The LNG-IUS (*see Q 9.145ff*) is actually indicated for (2), (16), (17) and (18) above, and poses no problem at all (WHO 1) for (19). The GyneFIX™ (*see Q 9.142ff*) normally poses no added problem for (13) or (17) and is indeed indicated whenever the expulsion risk is high – provided an expert 'GyneFIXer' is available!

9.88 Can copper IUDs cause local or systemic allergic reactions?

Definite cases have been reported, although they are rare. For instance, one case reported in 1976 presented with urticaria, joint pains and angioneurotic oedema, and positive scratch tests showed a true copper allergy. I had one clear case of marked reversible uterine pain and tenderness plus vaginal discharge, with no evidence of infection, resolving immediately after removal of the device. Referral to a dermatologist for specific allergy tests might be indicated, although most contact allergies to metal bangles or rings are not due to copper.

9.89 Is there evidence that antibiotics, antiprostaglandin or immunosuppressive drugs might impair the efficacy of IUDs?

As there is no evidence that the inflammatory reaction in the uterus and tubes of IUD users is normally caused by any infective process, the few reports of pregnancy occurring during antibiotic use can be dismissed as coincidences. One study comparing pregnancy rates in IUD users with and without rheumatoid arthritis has shown no evidence that interference with endometrial prostaglandin metabolism by PGSIs can impair IUD efficacy, although this had been suggested in a study from France.

There are reports that immunosuppressed transplant patients are more likely to become pregnant if they use IUDs. Probably more important is the risk of severe and silent infection. Hence other methods of birth control should be advised if such drugs must be used (not including corticosteroids, except for high-dose regimens).

9.90 What are the implications for IUD users of significant anatomical lesions of the heart?

This is WHO 3. It would often be preferable for such women to use another method because of the increased risk of bacterial endocarditis. The main time of risk for this being at insertion, the WHO gives heart lesions WHO 2 status.

The fitting of an IUD should be avoided (WHO 4) if there is a past history of endocarditis or in the presence of prosthetic valve(s) (although the LNG-IUS is seen as in the WHO 3 category for the latter). Intravenous drug abusers are also at higher risk of endocarditis if they have a relevant heart lesion.

Otherwise, if the method is selected the fitting should be done by an expert, under optimum sterile conditions, with antibiotic cover. Simple insertions with minor heart lesions can be given the minimal regimen of an oral sachet of amoxycillin 3 g, 1 h before the procedure. Otherwise, the more elaborate recommendations of the *British National Formulary* for 'special risk' cases should be followed, using intravenous ampicillin plus gentamicin.

Theoretically, the LNG-IUS would be preferable to reduce subsequent infection risk (*see* Q 9.146) though using a T-Safe Cu 380A™ or GyneFIX™ would helpfully reduce the need for reinsertions. The patient would need to be warned even more carefully than other IUD users to seek prompt medical advice should she develop pelvic pain, deep dyspareunia or excessive discharge. Any of these might herald a focus of pelvic infection and risk of bacteraemia.

Antibiotic cover for removal would only be indicated if it was difficult, and especially if intrauterine instrumentation were to be required.

9.91 What are the implications of diabetes for a potential IUD user?

It was suggested in a study from Edinburgh that diabetes rendered both inert and copper IUDs less effective. However, other workers, notably in Scandinavian countries, have completely failed to show this association.

More relevant is the fear that diabetes might make any pelvic infection more severe than it otherwise would be. However, the IUD, or perhaps even better the LNG-IUS, remains a valid option, particularly for diabetics at low risk of STIs. WHO is probably right to call this WHO 1.

9.92 Can an IUD or the LNG-IUS be used by a woman with uterine fibroids?

The answer is 'yes', provided the cavity of the uterus is not distorted by any submucous fibroid and (as will normally follow) she does not suffer from menorrhagia. After careful bimanual examination, and the usual discussion about future fertility, etc., provisional arrangements can be made for the device to be inserted. The woman should be warned that plans might have to be changed if, early in the insertion procedure, the uterine sound detects an obvious submucous fibroid (as in *Fig. 9.10*, p. 420).

Where the facilities exist, a preinsertion ultrasound scan is crucial, requesting specifically that the uterine cavity be checked for distortion by submucous fibroids. If there is distortion, a GyneFIX™ can still be tried or, in the absence of *marked* cavity intrusion, the LNG-IUS to control heavy periods – with warning about increased risk of expulsion and of malposition (this is where an implantable version of the latter would be so useful).

CHOICE OF DEVICE

9.93 How can one select the best IUD for each woman?

Feet come in different sizes and shapes, and shoes therefore come in many different fittings. Even without recognized distortions of the uterine cavity (see *Fig. 9.10*, p. 420), the sizes and shapes of uteruses similarly vary. There is no fixed relationship between total uterine length as measured with a standard uterine sound and uterine cavity length, which can comprise as little as one-third of the total (*Fig. 9.7*). Maximum fundal width also varies between individuals, and is less in vivo than when measured on hysterectomy specimens. The living uterus is a muscular organ, which contracts and relaxes and whose tonus also varies with the menstrual cycle (*Fig. 9.8*). Yet traditional framed IUDs come in constant shapes and in sizes that are sometimes too large for the cavity in which they are to be placed.

▲

Fig. 9.7 Measured endometrial and cervical lengths. Q 9.93. Eleven different combinations were noted in a series of 55 patients, all with the same total uterine axial dimension of 7 cm (from Hasson 1982 Uterine geometry and IUCD design. *British Journal of Obstetrics and Gynaecology* Supplement 4:3, Figure 3).

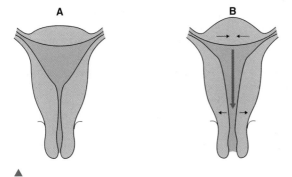

▲

Fig. 9.8 Functional changes in uterine shape. Q 9.93. A, postovulation; B, at menstruation (from Hasson 1982 Uterine geometry and IUCD design. *British Journal of Obstetrics and Gynaecology* Supplement 4:3, Figure 2).

In earlier editions I asked the manufacturers to produce a wider range of sizes for each design but this approach for smaller or distorted cavities has, I think, now been superseded by the implantable (frameless) technology of GyneFIX™ (*see* Q 9.141). This is more logical and will be applied increasingly to hormone-releasing as well as to copper devices.

9.94 Given the range of IUDs available in the UK, what is your normal first choice for a parous woman?

The main framed devices available are shown in *Fig. 9.9* (see also *Fig. 9.12*).

The UK version of the T-Safe Cu 380A™ – a successful series of banded devices – is now the 'gold standard' for copper IUDs, with one of the lowest cumulative pregnancy rates so far reported (*see Q 1.10*) and a UK-approved intrauterine lifespan of 8 years (and evidence-based for at least 12 years; Dennis et al 2002 *Journal of Family Planning and Reproductive Healthcare* 28:61–68) – meaning a bargain price of about £1 per year. None of the other framed IUDs available perform better, nor can they be left in situ for so long, which is a major advantage, given the risks at every insertion/reinsertion.

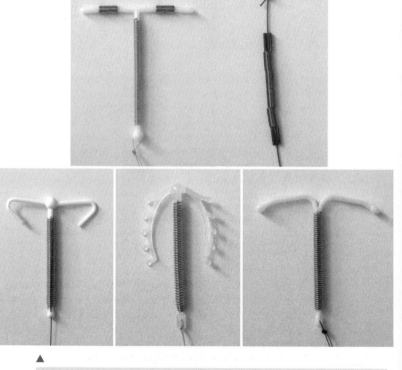

▲

Fig. 9.9 The main framed copper IUDs available in the UK (2003). Q 9.94. Clockwise from top left: T-Safe Cu 380A™ , GyneFIX™ , Nova T 380™ , Multiload 375™ and Flexi-T 300™ .

9.95 Is the new Nova-T 380™ with 380 mm² of copper wire improved as compared with the old Nova-T 200™?

Yes. The Nova-T 380™ is certainly more acceptable for use (at least to 5 years) than its predecessor. In the UK Family Planning Network study of 574 users its cumulative failure rate to 5 years was good, 2 per 100 women. But in the only RTC so far reported (Skjeldestad et al 2001 Abstract 38 at the British Congress of Obstetrics and Gynaecology, Birmingham, UK) among 470 volunteers its cumulative failure rate per 100 women at 3 years was 3.6, compared with 1.7 among 487 users of a clone of the banded T-Safe Cu 380A™.

Aside from its probable lower effectiveness, it suffers from not being evidence-based for use beyond 5 years. Its name is also somewhat confusing! But its small inserting diameter of 3.7 mm when loaded makes it easy to insert in nulliparae. This makes it a reasonable choice (like the Flexi-T 300™, below) for EC when required by a nulliparous woman, especially when the plan is for it to be removed in the next cycle when the woman is established on another method.

9.96 What do we know about the Flexi-T 300™ IUD?

In an RCT referenced in the Dennis article (*see* Q 9.94), among 300 users there was a failure rate of 2.5 per 100 to 3 years, which was higher (but not statistically so) than experienced by 300 users of the banded Cu T 380 A™ comparator. It also had a significantly higher expulsion rate.

Like the Nova-T 380™ it has a very narrow inserter tube and is exceptionally easy to insert, making it another, and cheaper, option for emergency use. But for all likely long-term users I still rate the T-Safe Cu 380A™ as first choice, if it can be fitted successfully.

9.97 When would you recommend use of Multiload IUDs?

We no longer stock these products. Multiloads tend to cause greater cervical discomfort (at removal as well as insertion) and are not well enclosed in a sterile tube while traversing the endocervical canal. Only the more effective 375 version should now be used: it is still licensed, only to 5 years though its effectiveness has been demonstrated to 8 years. However, its efficacy is lower than the banded Cu T 380 A™ comparator in most studies and even its expulsion rate does not (as used to be taught) show any comparative advantage.

9.98 Which IUD do you select for the nulliparous woman?

If the method is used, after discussion of all the young woman's options, the preferred choice for long-term use among marketed IUDs remains the T-Safe Cu 380A™, if it can be fitted – using local anaesthesia and dilatation as required (*see* Q 9.111).

The GyneFIX™ (*see Q 9.141*), with its small physical size (*see Q 9.62*), narrower inserter and low expulsion rate is also an excellent choice, above all for the tiny or distorted uterus. The special insertion skills it requires and its higher price are the main obstacles. So some services use it mainly for nulliparae who need a copper IUD for EC and then subsequently plan long-term use (alternatives being the Nova-T 380™, or the cheaper Flexi-T 300™ for that-cycle-only use). *See Q 1.44* for other indications.

The LNG-IUS (*see Q 9.150*) is even more expensive and, for the present (*see Q 9.147*), still has the problems of being on a frame rather than implanted. However, some data do suggest it would reduce (not eliminate) the risk of PID and hence could be a good choice, especially if the nullipara has heavy or painful periods.

The above devices all share the advantage of great efficacy, even in the highly fertile, against both intra- and extrauterine pregnancies.

By contrast the Multiload Cu-250 Short™ now has very little to commend it for nulliparae aside from price, and is superseded by the GyneFIX™, for its special indication for very short (< 5.5 cm) uterine cavities on sounding. It has a small copper load and therefore relatively reduced efficacy compared with banded devices, and is only licensed for 3 years' use.

9.99 Which device do you choose for women who have expelled a previous IUD?

The GyneFIX™ has the lowest expulsion rate but only if it is inserted by a healthcare provided with the required skill and experience (*see Q 9.141*). But the same kind of device as just expelled can be used if it is otherwise the best choice (e.g. LNG-IUS) and there are reasons for believing there was less than ideal placement of the first IUD.

INSERTION PROCEDURE

9.100 What is the importance of correct insertion?

This cannot be overstressed. A good 'revision test' is to check for yourself in *Qs 9.21 and 9.22* how it can be true that poor insertion technique is capable of producing every one of the eight IUD problems listed.

9.101 When should one perform so-called interval insertions?

COPPER IUDS, WHETHER FRAMED OR FRAMELESS

See Qs 9.15–9.17 for discussion of the optimum time in menstruating women, which is any time from around the end of the main menstrual flow through to day 12 of a 28-day cycle, normally. But this can be extended for copper IUDs to day 19 (adjusted for cycle length) even if contraception has been effectively non-existent up to that day, using it as a postcoital (anti-implantation) method. Thereafter, insertion could be even later if you are confident that there cannot already be an implanted pregnancy from intercourse earlier in the cycle, or up to 5 days after a single act of unprotected intercourse late in the cycle (*see Qs 10.15, 10.34*).

THE LNG-IUS

See Q 9.145. In brief, the speed with which this extremely effective method operates is not great enough within the first cycle for it to act as a postcoital method. Conception in the cycle of insertion would be of special concern because of the extremely high endometrial concentration of LNG hormone. Therefore, in cycling women it is recommended that insertion is performed within the first 7 days. If any later, there must be 'believable and really effective' contraception up to the day of insertion and condom use thereafter at least for the next 7 days.

Helpful tip

Ensure that, *as a routine*, all who plan to have an LNG-IUS are started on a more effective method than condoms (e.g. the combined pill or perhaps Cerazette™), so the insertion can be performed without that anxiety and on any mutually convenient date.

9.102 When should IUDs be inserted following a full-term delivery?

POSTPARTUM

Normal policy in the UK is for IUD insertion to be delayed until the postnatal visit, i.e. at about 6 weeks. This is fine for lactating women but, if she is not breastfeeding, the woman will need to use another method of birth control from the fourth week (*see Q 5.49*). Hence insertion during that fourth week by an experienced clinician may sometimes be contraceptively preferable, depending on the amount of lochia and satisfactory uterine involution (*see Q 11.22*).

POST DELIVERY

Immediate postdelivery insertion with careful fundal placement, manually or using a spongeholder or ring forceps, and directly after delivery of the placenta, has been shown in several studies to have high (but in some circumstances acceptable) subsequent expulsion rates. The GyneFIX™ is under development for this indication, with a biodegradeable enhancement to its implanted knot.

9.103 What is the optimum insertion time after lower segment caesarean section?

A T-Safe Cu 380A™ or other IUD or IUS can be sutured to the fundus with chromic catgut, by way of the lower segment incision. However, normal practice is to defer insertion at least to 6 weeks (some would say 8 weeks) to be sure of complete healing of the lower segment scar. As, after involution, this potential weakness finishes up very low – at the level of the internal os – there would in fact be no objection to the insertion by an experienced, careful clinician at the same time as for other women (i.e. at about 6 weeks).

Puerperal infection (with or without operative delivery) would indicate postponement – if indeed an IUD insertion were ever to be appropriate.

9.104 When should IUDs be inserted following any kind of abortion?

Careful studies have shown that immediate insertion at the time of evacuation of the uterus – whether for legal induced abortion or following an incomplete miscarriage – can be good practice in selected cases. Surprisingly to many, no statistical differences with respect to subsequent infection were found in RCTs comparing two groups of women, one receiving and the other not receiving a framed copper IUD at the time of uterine evacuation in the same service confirmed in a 2002 systematic review.

The expulsion rate in the above studies was higher than for interval insertions. So the current version of GyneFIX™ has been devised with a slightly larger polypropylene knot, to substantially reduce that risk.

The above studies were performed by experts; there is the fear that in less experienced hands a fragment of products of conception might be retained and the insertion of a foreign body might then both facilitate infection and render such infection more severe. But insertion of IUDs or IUSs at the time of the evacuation could be good practice almost routinely in parous women, and fairly often in nulliparae, if only there were:

■ preliminary full counselling
■ an ultrasound scan machine in the theatre to ensure no retained products
■ preliminary microbiological screening (for *Chlamydia* anyway)
■ antibiotic chemoprophylaxis (*see* Q 9.59).

9.105 Do you have any practical tips for IUD/IUS insertion in an older perimenopausal woman whose cervix might be tight despite previous parity – due to hypo-oestrogenism?

This is a very real problem that we faced at the Margaret Pyke Centre during our (highly successful) studies of the LNG-IUS as the progestogen component of HRT. The solution, which can dramatically improve (soften) the cervix, is to give a good dose of standard HRT oestrogen for one month before the planned insertion, systemically or to the vagina – followed by local anaesthesia and dilatation on the day.

9.106 What are the minimum practical requisites?

1 A firm couch at a convenient height.
2 A good adjustable light.

3   Sterile equipment, ideally from a central sterile supply department:
    (a) bivalve speculum
    (b) Stiles or Allis holding forceps, preferably not a toothed tenaculum, to reduce cervical pain (*and see Q 9.108(2)*)
    (c) sponge forceps
    (d) uterine sound
    (e) galley pot plus swabs for sterilizing solution
    (f) scissors
    (g) sterile gloves (if they are not sterile and a no-touch technique is planned, great care must be taken to maintain a 'sterile field' over one side of the trolley, ensuring the handle ends of all instruments that have been touched are systematically placed to the opposite side)
    (h) Spencer-Wells forceps.
4   In reserve:
    (a) local anaesthetic, needles and syringes
    (b) small cervical dilators up to 6 mm diameter
    (c) an emergency tray (*see Q 9.120*), and an oxygen cylinder and mask.
5   *An assistant in the room*: someone to aid sterile technique, for added reassurance – and to help in a rare crisis (*see Q 9.116ff*).

9.107 What are the characteristics and qualities of a good IUD doctor/nurse, whatever the devices, wherever inserted?

1   First and foremost, the clinician should be really well trained, which means excellent bimanual and speculum technique for a start, followed in the UK by the theoretical and practical training now organized by the Faculty of FP&RHC. This is in two stages: the basic Diploma is followed by a special advanced course leading to the Letter of Competence in intrauterine contraception techniques (including cervical local anaesthesia and the management of 'lost threads'). A separate additional training has been organized for GyneFIX™ because its insertion technique is so different – although not difficult when properly taught. This brief apprenticeship training with a good instructing doctor beats any amount of book learning.

2   Before attempting insertion in any patient, some initial practice with the same devices using a small plastic model and working through the manufacturer's instruction sheet is, in my view, essential. Such a 'dry run' should also never be omitted whenever a new device (e.g. GyneFIX™) or new inserter (e.g. recently for the T-Safe Cu 380A™ and LNG-IUS™) arrives on the contraceptive scene.

3   Initial competence with any device should be maintained by continuing experience, and this cannot be by inserting only one device every 3 months (12 IUDs or IUSs per year is the Faculty's accepted minimum).

4   During both examination and insertion, gentleness as well as competence should be the rule in all manoeuvres, especially when the sound or loaded inserter enter the uterine cavity (such gentleness is not the same as hesitancy or being excessively slow).

5   Last but not least, the clinician should be a good communicator, able to use plenty of that 'aural valium' whose route of administration is the ears – also known as 'vocal local'!

9.108 How does the insertion process begin?

Preferably by a good relationship developed during earlier counselling (*see* Q 9.121) and in an initial chat on the day. The woman should already have been offered/received a premed (*see* Q 9.111) and the result of screening for STIs, or at least *Chlamydia*, should be available. (If not, there need to be good grounds from discussion with that individual (*see* Q 9.58) for not giving chemoprophylaxis with, for example, doxycycline or azithromycin, *see* Q 9.59).

1   First, make yourself known to the woman. Even a brief initial conversation helps, followed by a matter-of-fact and informative commentary throughout the insertion procedure.

2   Offer to every case (in my practice) the use of local anaesthesia, at least at the 12 o'clock position on the cervix. This deals pre-emptively with that so unpredictable pain that a sizeable proportion of women get, when the holding forceps (of whatever design) are applied. A smaller group, where dilatation is likely to be required, often nulliparous or perimenopausal, might need a full paracervical block (*see* Q 9.111).

3   Make it explicit that *she is in control and that you are there for her, under her authority*. During the procedure give warning of any actions that might cause discomfort, e.g. the needle for paracervical block or the application of the Allis or Stiles forceps.

9.109 How important is the initial bimanual examination (BME)?

This is essential. It has two main purposes:

1   First, to ensure that there is no uterine or adnexal tenderness, especially on moving the cervix. (Check verbally that there is also no dyspareunia.) Positive findings mean that the insertion should be postponed.

2   The second essential purpose is to identify the size, shape, mobility and direction and position of the fundus.

9.110 Which is the best position for the patient to adopt during the insertion?

Most insertions in the UK are performed with the patient in the dorsal position but lithotomy or its near-equivalent working from the *end* of the couch is preferable for GyneFIX™ insertions. Sometimes access is radically improved by using the left lateral position, which after all is equivalent to lithotomy rotated through 90°. This is of particular value if the cervical canal is very flexed and the cervix points directly either anterior or posterior. The left lateral does lead to loss of eye contact with the woman, which must be replaced by better-than-average verbal communication.

9.111 What are the indications for preinsertion analgesia or local anaesthesia (LA)?

Most parous women questioned after an uncomplicated IUD insertion without LA reckon that the needle would have caused more discomfort than it would have removed. However, this is not always the case!

At the Margaret Pyke Centre, it is the norm that all women are offered premedication with a PGSI, normally mefenamic acid 500 mg, 30–45 min before the procedure (checking first for contraindications). If they are unusually anxious a short-acting benzodiazepine can be added. Personally, I always also offer local anaesthesia, at least at the 12 o'clock position on the cervix.

A sizeable proportion, often nulliparous or perimenopausal, especially where dilatation or intrauterine manipulation ('lost threads') are likely, will also need a good paracervical block: (about 10 mL in all 1% lidocaine injected first at 12 o'clock intracervically, and then through the cervical canal into the cervix, close to the internal cervical os at about 3 o'clock and 9 o'clock).

After training, this is not a difficult nor time-consuming addition to the procedure.

> Note that there are two distinct pains: the PGSI treats the (delayed) fundal cramps whereas LA (by gel or injection) is for the earlier somatic, cervical component.

9.112 Do you find 'Instillagel™' into the cervix is a helpful alternative to full paracervical block?

Frankly, in my experience, the answer is 'no' – I no longer use or recommend it. A pity, as it would be so good to have a 'non-needle' option. The technique uses 2% lidocaine antiseptic gel and just sufficient of this 'Instillagel™' is injected via a special Instillaquill™ to fill the cervical canal up to the internal os. If more than 1.5-2 mL is used it causes uterine pain.

There must then be a minimum wait for it to act. A significant ($p < 0.05$) benefit was shown in a small trial of this in 1996 in Leeds after waiting only 1 min before passing the sound. To me it is counterintuitive that it could ever work so fast, after all, EMLA local anaesthetic cream for skin is recommended for application a minimum of 1 h ahead. I wonder if the study was an example of a type 1 error (positive result by chance). Could any apparent benefit be through it being a bit of lubricant?

9.113 Should tissue forceps be applied to the cervix, and should the uterus be sounded?

Normally yes: Stiles or Allis forceps cause variable discomfort, reduced to nil if a little LA is injected as I recommend (*see Qs 9.108 and 9.111*) into the anterior lip of the cervix. X-ray studies have proved that gentle traction straightens the canal and very much assists in passing the sound. The latter is also essential to:

1 confirm the direction and patency of the cervical canal
2 estimate the length of the uterine cavity (*see Q 9.93*)
3 exclude obvious intrusion of any submucous fibroid or uterine septum (*Fig. 9.10*). *I teach that this should be done in all insertions by gently rotating the handle of the sound through a small arc.*

The sound should be passed with minimal force, rested between the finger and thumb like a loosely held pencil. Note that the anatomy of the cervical canal is variable. Be prepared to repeat the BME or to withdraw and reinsert

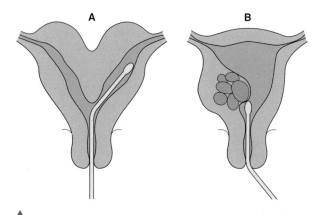

▲

Fig. 9.10 Uterine cavity distorted – congenitally or by fibroids. Q 9.113. *Note*: in A it is easy to obtain a normal sounding depth despite a septate uterus. Careful sounding will detect the abnormality, however, and will also identify a submucous fibroid, as in B. Such findings need to be confirmed by ultrasound. See also Qs 9.86, 9.87.

the sound if it does not pass readily *or* move on to using dilators (Hegar 3–6 should be available).

9.114 What about antisepsis?

This is much less important during the insertion than prescreening for specific pathogens and, as appropriate, antibiotic cover (*see Qs 9.58 and 9.59*). Remember that the flora of the endocervical canal is almost identical to that of the vagina.

All the same, even in the presence of a negative *Chlamydia* test and with no pelvic tenderness on examination, the cervix should still be inspected carefully at the time of the insertion. A purulent discharge could signify the need to postpone the insertion and arrange GUM referral to search for other pathogens.

Otherwise, the cervix should be cleansed thoroughly with a gauze swab usually dipped in aqueous antiseptic, concentrating on mechanical removal of any mucus at the external os.

9.115 What other practical points should be considered?

1   Only at the last minute, and after satisfactory sounding, should the device be loaded into its inserter, for fear that it should lose its 'memory'.

2   Some devices (e.g. Multiloads) are primarily 'pushed' into the uterus; most are inserted by a 'pull' technique in which the plunger is kept stationary and the inserter tube pulled back over it.

3   We all have a sensible paranoia about perforation but this leads to a tendency for the T-Safe Cu 380A™ or the LNG-IUS (or Nova T 380™) to be inserted rather low, risking expulsion and even implantation above the device. I teach that after the side arms of the above-mentioned devices have been released, you have an object that is most unlikely to perforate. Therefore, at that point in the insertion sequence for any of these devices, after the arms have just been released from the top of the inserter tube, the latter should be gently advanced towards the fundus. This might mean allowing the cervical stop to be pushed (caudally) by the external os, until the very top of the cavity is reached – always looking at the woman's face so as to be sufficiently gentle throughout. It has surprised me how often I have found that my initial estimate of the fundal depth was a centimetre or more less than the measurement from tip of tube to stop after this has been done.

4   Take care that the device finishes in the right plane, by observing the marker wings on the inserter, as well as in the correct high fundal position. If in doubt the device should be removed and a new one inserted.

GyneFIX™ has a very specific technique (changed since the new inserter was marketed in 2001) that must be learned with the help of the manufacturer's video, polystyrene models and then supervised insertions (*see also* Q 9.110 *re* the best position for the woman).

9.116 What about the prevention of the rare IUD insertion 'crises'?

1   First, so far as possible, they should be prevented by the presence of an assistant, a calm and relaxed atmosphere, combined with obvious competence and teamwork.
2   During the insertion, gentleness and accuracy while passing both sound and loaded inserter along the cervical canal reduce the incidence of vasovagal reactions.
3   Above all, starting at an earlier stage, good counselling and selection of cases, combined with a low threshold for premedication with an analgesic and perhaps a sedative, with or without paracervical block during the insertion; these are the essential prophylactic measures.

9.117 What if a vasovagal attack follows despite every precaution?

The patient becomes white, might sweat with a slow pulse and could faint. Occasionally there is no warning – be alert!

1   The first thing to do is to abandon the procedure, stop any cervical stimulation and remove a partially inserted device (but, unless symptoms persist, not one that is considered to be well located).
2   The woman's head should be lowered or her feet elevated, and she should be moved into the recovery position.
3   Oxygen (which should be available) can be administered by mask. An airway should be used if the subject loses consciousness. All this takes a bit of time and occupies anxious bystanders, which is excellent because the majority of attacks are self-limiting.
4   At this point, 500 mg of mefenamic acid should be given, if not used as a premed. If it was, a non-PGSI analgesic such as dihydrocodeine can be added.

9.118 What should be done if the woman continues to suffer severe dysmenorrhoeic pains?

I have no experience of the use of glyceryl trinitrate either sublingually or as a vaginal spray for severe uterine cramps, but it is said it might help (and it has also been used as a premed).

If the woman continues in severe pain with pallor for 30 min after the insertion, in my view even a fully inserted device should be removed. The chances of long-term successful use of the IUD/IUS in this situation are too low. If ultrasound scanning were routinely done most such cases would be explained by malposition or because of an unexpectedly small or even distorted uterine cavity. In an occasional case one might also be avoiding the later problems of a perforation.

A subsequent attempt with local anaesthesia, an expert practitioner and probably now using the GyneFIX™, is often successful.

9.119 What unusual complications of IUD insertion can occur?

PERSISTENT BRADYCARDIA

If the pulse is persistently less than 40 beats/min, the slow intravenous injection of atropine 0.3 mg repeated if necessary to a total of 0.6 mg might help, along with oxygen. If the pulse is absent and the patient completely unresponsive, any competent doctor or nurse ought also to be prepared to diagnose cardiac arrest, insert an airway and initiate cardiopulmonary resuscitation (fortunately, this is more than most clinicians will be called upon to do in a lifetime of inserting IUDs). Beware of vomiting and the risk of inhalation of fluid when consciousness returns – hence use the recovery position.

ASTHMATIC ATTACK, LARYNGEAL OEDEMA OR OTHER SEVERE ALLERGIC REACTION

Treat urgently with 0.5 mg (contained in 0.5 mL) adrenaline 1:1000, intramuscularly and repeatable, according to the response, to a total of 1 mg.

GRAND MAL ATTACK

This can occur even in the absence of any history of epilepsy or the subsequent development thereof. It is usually self-limiting. Diazepam emulsion 10 mg should be available, ready for intravenous use or as rectal tubes (e.g. Stesolid™, a good presentation for this situation). One 10-mg dose is administered, repeatable once if there is no response after 5 min. Epilepsy needs to be distinguished from:

ALKALOSIS DUE TO OVERBREATHING

This causes paraesthesia and carpopedal spasms. Treatment is by reassurance and instruction in (supervised) breathing in and out of a plastic bag.

9.120 In summary, what should be available in the emergency tray?

1   A well-fitting facemask and separate airways. Nearby, oxygen cylinder.
2   Diazepam emulsion 10 mg either for rectal (Stesolid™ tubes) or intravenous injection.
3   Atropine 0.6 mg for intravenous injection.
4   Adrenaline 1 mL of 1:1000 for intramuscular injection.
5   Mefenamic acid oral tablets – dose 500 mg.
6   Dihydrocodeine tablets – dose 30 mg.
7   Short-acting benzodiazepine tablets (temazepam 20 mg) for premedication.
8   Syringes, needles, etc. as appropriate.

This is all that is required, and most will never be used.

PATIENT INFORMATION AND FOLLOW-UP ARRANGEMENTS

9.121 What main points should be made in advance when counselling any prospective IUD user?

As usual, a balance has to be struck between creating unnecessary fears that might impair the woman's acceptance and satisfaction with the method, and the need to help her reach an informed and valid decision based on the likely benefits and risks for herself. During counselling, often rightly delegated to the family planning-trained nurse:

1   Mention first the many advantages of the method (*see* Q 9.19). Let her see and ideally handle the device she is to receive.
2   The possibility of failure including after unrecognized expulsion should be mentioned. Although expulsion ought to be particularly rare with GyneFIX™, the item itself is so small that it might well not be seen: learning to feel the threads is therefore even more important with this IUD than others.
3   Attention should be drawn to pelvic infection and ectopic pregnancy. Explain how both are linked with sexual transmission of infections. Take a full sexual history (*see* Qs 1.13 *and* 1.14), including a careful history of past PID or any treatments at a GUM clinic. Embarrassment should not stop good plain medicine, which is to go on to say something like: 'You know better than I can possibly know what your likely risk of (sexually transmitted) infection might be. This depends both on you and also your partner: have you ever wondered if he has other partner(s)?'. Stress also the importance of using condoms in all situations of risk especially at partner change – and of returning promptly to the clinic should relevant symptoms occur (*see* Qs 9.22 *and* 9.124).
4   Arrange at least a *Chlamydia* screen if at all possible, and usually antibiotic cover when no result is available (e.g. if the insertion is for EC, see the earlier discussion in Qs 9.58 *and* 9.59).
5   In my view, it should also be pointed out that some discomfort is common during insertion, helped by the use of premedication – with added local anaesthetic as she prefers (*see* Q 9.111), given that it is only fully effective by needle!
6   Problems like perforation are rare but should be mentioned with the aid of the leaflet (see (7)). Honest and accurate answers should be given to all questions (*see* Q 5.105).

7   Finally, counselling should be backed up by a user-friendly leaflet, such as the IUD or IUS ones from the Family Planning Association: 'To be read now before the insertion, but also for you to keep for future reference'.

9.122 What instructions should be given to the woman after IUD insertion?

1   She can be reminded that the method is effective immediately.
2   She should also be reminded that if she is ever in future in a very new or not mutually faithful relationship, she should use a condom as well (*see Q 9.18*), thereby reducing both the risk of failure and of infection.
3   She should be carefully taught palpation of her cervical threads and advised that this check should be done by self or partner postmenstruation, in each cycle, before the device is relied on. (LNG-IUS users with oligo- or amenorrhoea (*see Q 9.145ff*), should do this regularly, perhaps on the first day of each month). Q 9.174 offer some practical points about cervical palpation. If she becomes unable to feel the threads, or palpates the hard end of the device, she should be told to take additional contraceptive precautions and arrange an early examination.
4   As sperm can be bio-vectors of STI pathogens and the process of IUD/IUS insertion interferes with protective mechanisms at the cervix (*see Qs 9.55 and 9.56*) it is my personal policy to *recommend* abstinence for the next 3 days only.
5   Tampon use is also discouraged for 3 days, hopefully allowing enough time for the cervical barrier to be reconstituted.
6   *Important*: before leaving after the insertion she should be given instructions, preferably backed by a handout, concerning the new symptoms (arising after those from the insertion have subsided) that should lead her to telephone the clinic/surgery immediately, during the critical next 2–3 weeks (*see Q 9.60*).
7   If she has neither been prescreened for at least *Chlamydia* nor is being given antibiotic prophylaxis then it is best to arrange a follow-up visit at about 1 week (*see Qs 9.53 and 9.123*).

9.123 When and for what purpose should the first follow-up visit take place?

About 6 weeks after the insertion is usual, on a date planned to be after the first expected menses, so as to exclude (partial) expulsion.

However, the important data discussed in Qs 9.55–9.60 suggest that making the first visit routinely at about 1 week would be ideal, certainly if steps have not been taken to ensure a pathogen-free cervical canal! However, even if they were, the woman should be advised (*see Q 9.122*) to attend as an emergency for examination if she has pain or other symptoms that might be PID-related. Infections are so much more (six times) common in the first 20 days postinsertion that this protocol should permit more prompt, possibly tube-saving, antibiotic treatment.

At the routine 6-week visit the woman should be asked about all relevant symptoms (*see* Q 9.60). She should be asked whether she can feel her threads, and retaught as indicated.

On speculum examination the threads should be seen. As a general rule, in my view, but especially if the threads have apparently lengthened, the lower cervical canal should be sounded. This can be done with a sterile sound, or very simply using the omnipresent throat swab or even a Cytobrush™ (not advanced higher than the internal os). In this way partial expulsion of a framed IUD (so not a relevant check at GyneFIX™ follow-up) can be detected and the device replaced before an avoidable intrauterine pregnancy occurs. A BME should also be done to detect tenderness and adnexal or uterine enlargement.

9.124 How frequently should subsequent visits take place?

If the first visit is at 1 week, another at about 6–8 weeks is still logical, because expulsions are most common in the early months of use. Thereafter, in women without symptoms an annual routine visit is quite sufficient.

1   More important than any routine pelvic examination is an 'open house' policy and an IUD programme that makes it really easy for a user to obtain medical advice and help at once should a new problem occur, notably an attack of pelvic infection or an ectopic pregnancy or 'lost threads'. She should therefore be fully taught, with a leaflet, about all the symptoms that require prompt action and know where to obtain telephone advice.
2   Iron deficiency anaemia is very easy to miss in long-term users with heavy bleeding. This should be excluded or treated if present.

9.125 Are IUDs always easy to remove by simple traction on the thread(s)?

Not if the threads are absent in the first place (*see* Q 9.37) or 'lost' (*see* Q 9.35). But even without this problem the device might be malpositioned or embedded, or there might be a type of partial cervical perforation (*Fig. 9.11*). In such cases it is sometimes possible, under local anaesthesia, to grasp the device and push it in a cranial direction to disimpact it first. Excessive traction at removal must always be avoided, especially under general anaesthesia, for the reason noted in Q 9.48.

GyneFIX™ is removed by simple firm traction and is more comfortable done positively, not tentatively. A study at the Margaret Pyke Centre in

A   **B**

▲

Fig. 9.11 Two varieties of partial cervical perforation. Q 9.125. Both of these could cause difficulty in removal. Each is best treated (under appropriate anaesthesia) by grasping the end of the device and pushing in a cranial direction before traction.

2003 found the GyneFIX™ to require an unusually strong pull of 6 Newtons, compared with a mean of 2.2 Newtons for the comparator banded device (almost identical to the T-Safe Cu 380A™). There was no significant difference in the pain reported on visual analogue scales and with both devices the women anticipated more pain than they actually experienced. This result is worth using, to reassure women prospectively.

9.126 Do you have any tips for removal of IUDs that are a bit stuck after the menopause? Must they always be removed at all?

This is mainly a problem when removing inert IUDs or Multiloads 1 year after the last period. A solution is to prescribe natural oestrogen, e.g. one cycle of Premarin™ 1.25 mg daily beforehand; this will soften the cervical canal. Mefenamic acid 500 mg as a premed also helps (*see* Q 9.35(3)).

It is actually a matter of debate whether devices that are very 'stuck' (with or without avulsion of the threads) do have to be removed after the menopause – or an LNG-IUS that is found to be embedded, having been inserted at endometrial ablation. The postulated risk of a pyometrium is small and can be dealt with in the individual case. I would, personally, not now feel the risks of a general anaesthetic were justified for any difficult removal of IUDs postmenopausally, and would simply warn the woman to seek advice at any time later if she were to develop an offensive discharge.

An exception would be the presence of ALOs on a cervical smear in a perimenopausal woman (see the case reported in Q 9.75), where the device certainly must be removed and at least one follow-up visit at 3 months arranged.

9.127 Are IUDs a genuine cause of male dyspareunia?

Certainly, above all if a framed device is partially expelled so that its end just protrudes from the external cervical os! More commonly, some men notice the threads of the device.

If this problem is not resolved by slightly altering positions of intercourse, the threads should be trimmed – but not to within a few millimetres of the os, as this can actually worsen the situation. Rather, if necessary, they should be shortened to lie wholly within the cervical canal. Ensure that this is noted in the records and that the woman will report the fact to any future doctor. Long-handled Spencer-Wells forceps should easily retrieve the threads when removal is required.

9.128 Is short-wave diathermy treatment contraindicated in IUD users?

This treatment is now rarely given to patients with chronic pelvic pain, in whom removal of the device would normally first be tried. However, if there is an IUD present there is certainly a theoretical possibility that the copper wire might heat up. Experiments with devices in recently excised hysterectomy specimens have shown no obvious damage or charring to the endometrium, and the devices have merely become pleasantly warm. So this treatment is relatively contraindicated (WHO 2).

9.129 Are modern methods of imaging dangerous for the IUD-wearer, specifically nuclear magnetic resonance (NMR)?

Ultrasound is harmless, X-rays have no added risk, and provided the device is non-ferrous NMR would cause no problems. However, with steel devices (e.g. the M-device and Chinese rings) there would truly be a potential hazard of internal trauma, caused by movement of the ferrous metal caused by the magnetic field.

9.130 Are IUDs containing copper affected by any vaginal preparations?

There is no clear evidence that material from the vagina reaches the copper or affects the biochemical processes that cause the contraceptive effect (see Q 9.5).

DURATION OF USE

9.131 Do the white deposits on copper IUDs removed after varying durations within the uterus cause an increased risk of failure or have any other clinical significance?

These deposits have been studied intensively. They contain organic material along with calcium, sulfur and phosphorus and other inorganic elements.

They are not now thought to be linked with IUD failure. Many women's devices never develop this deposit. When present, if the IUD is copper bearing it seems that sufficient copper can pass through the deposit to continue the contraceptive effect. It is not an important factor in the rate of copper elution (*see Q 9.133*).

The explanation for failure of modern IUDs that are so effective when correctly located is, nearly always, less than ideal placement within the uterine cavity (*see Qs 9.11 and 9.12*).

9.132 How often should inert IUDs be replaced?

In the few women who still retain these, and with the exception of Dalkon Shields™, they should never be routinely replaced without a special reason. One possible reason would be ALOs on a cervical smear (*see Qs 9.71–9.75*).

9.133 How often should copper IUDs be replaced?

All the marketed devices have an officially approved duration, normally 3, 5 or 8 years. The reason for any limit is anxiety that the amount of copper available for release from the device might decline to a level at which the pregnancy rate would increase. Yet the recommended banded copper IUDs have shown no increase, and indeed a *decline*, in the annual conception risk for as long as they have been studied. So could they not be used for longer?

Aside from the Multiload 375™, for which there is evidence of efficacy to 8 years (licensed for 5), there is not good evidence to support any copper wire IUDs being left in situ for longer than their licensed duration. Unless fitted above age 40 (*see Q 9.138*), replacement of the old Nova T200™ at 5 years is of special importance because the ongoing failure rate thereafter is unacceptable (*see Fig. 9.2 and Q 9.137*).

9.134 What are the benefits of long-term use of IUDs?

Long-term studies (especially by WHO and the Population Council) have repeatedly shown a steady reduction with increasing duration of use in:

1 pregnancy rates (not with the Nova T200™, however)
2 expulsion rates
3 infection rates (overall)
4 bleeding/pain removal rates.

Exceptions that show a positive link with duration of use are carriage of ALOs (*see Qs 9.71–9.75*) and ectopic pregnancy – but the latter association is probably confounded by increasing age (*see Q 9.22*).

9.135 What are the explanations for the apparent improvement with duration of use of IUDs in the risks of pregnancy, expulsion, infection and removal for bleeding or pain?

It is too simple to interpret this as a genuine improvement due to the device 'bedding down'. The main point is that the long-term population of IUD users is highly selected and in all studies is a reduced proportion of those who originally had devices inserted. They are the 'survivors', so to speak. Their success in long-term use has less to do with the passage of time, as such, than with selection for features of the individual women themselves as compared with others earlier in the study:

1 They are likely to have been well fitted with an IUD, which was well matched to the particular shape and size of their uterus.

2 They are obviously well distanced in time from insertion-related expulsion, infection and bleeding/pain.

3 Much the most important factor: women with any side-effects or complications severe enough to have their device removed are by definition no longer in the study. For example, the most fertile become pregnant within the first year and have their devices removed, hence the reported pregnancy rates in later years are based on observation of a subgroup of the relatively infertile. Similarly, those whose partners are less likely to transmit a sexually transmitted infection to them are over-represented among long-term users.

4 They are also a little older, which helps most problems (*see Qs 9.22 and 9.53*).

9.136 What therefore is the view of the UK-FPA and the National Association of Family Planning Doctors (NAFPD; now the Faculty of FP&RHC) regarding long-term use of copper IUDs?

A statement published in *The Lancet* on 2 June 1990 remains substantially in force, except that the banded T-Safe Cu 380A™ has to be usable for twice the 5 years mentioned because its almost identical immediate predecessor in this country (Gyne T 380S™) was actually licensed for 10 years:

For routine management the modern copper-bearing IUDs … should be assumed to have an active lifespan of 5 years. … Beyond that interval, an experienced doctor or nurse should discuss with the client the option of changing the IUD or leaving it in *[it is wise to record this discussion in the notes]*

Basically, 'if it ain't broke, don't fix it'. But there is one thing specifically to record, that no promise was made that the device could not possible fail; only that the failure rate is believed to be no higher than during the preceding years of successful use.

9.137 Do you still follow the 1990 NAFPD statement for the older, < 250 mm copper wire IUDs, about usability in situ beyond 5 years? And what about the LNG-IUS (Mirena™)?

In general, 'no'. Studies in Manchester showed that standard (200 mm) copper wire devices like the Nova-T 200™ begin to lose copper at an accelerated (and linear) rate from an average of 27 months onwards. The rate of copper release was greater than average if the women complained of heavy uterine bleeding. After 4 years' use 28% of removed IUDs show fragmentation of the wire. Silver in the core of the Nova-T™ wire prevents that occurrence but would not otherwise reduce the rate of copper release. Indeed, it might even eventually increase it when silver becomes exposed, by a 'battery effect'. But none of this applies to the copper-banded devices, whose upper duration limit is not known but exceeds 10 years.

In the light of the above, most authorities would rarely apply the NAFPD *Lancet* advice in the case of young women under age 40, to use beyond 5 years any copper wire IUDs bearing less than 250 mm copper. This is because exchange to a more effective banded IUD (T-Safe Cu 380A™ or, as appropriate, the GyneFIX™) would be preferable, and both are evidence-based usable for at least 10 years.

The wire devices with > 250 mm copper, if fitted below the age of 40 might be usable on a 'named patient' basis (see *Appendix A*), especially the Multiload 375™, for which there is good evidence of efficacy to 8 years (licensed for 5). But there is no good evidence to support the other copper wire IUDs, including the Nova-T 380™, being left in situ for longer than their licensed duration. For duration of use of the LNG-IUS, *see Q 9.152*.

9.138 What about copper devices that were fitted above age 40?

This is a different matter! In a supplementary letter by the Chairman of NAFPD, it was also stated in the *Lancet* 1990 that:

… 'any copper device' (even one of the non-banded ones) 'which was fitted above age 40 may remain in situ until the menopause' …

(or until 1 year after for contraceptive safety, *see Q 11.34*). This has been widely accepted as UK policy ever since, because with diminishing fertility IUDs so very rarely fail above 40. Even when the copper wire has all gone the plastic frame seems to be sufficiently effective as an inert IUD in these late reproductive years.

That *Lancet* statement, like the later reports by WHO and others, points out that less frequent replacement would have enormous health advantages, in reducing all the insertion-related risks:

- ■ PID (the main time it happens!)
- ■ perforation (the only time it ever happens)
- ■ expulsion and
- ■ malposition, not to mention
- ■ inconvenience, pain, upset and costs for the woman!

However, for many IUDs and the IUS (and for all of them above age 40) this policy of long-term use well beyond 5 years is still unlicensed, so the criteria for 'named patient' usage must be observed (*Appendix A*).

9.139 How reversible is intrauterine contraception? Do IUDs cause infertility?

The conclusion of the section on this subject in the systematic review of 22 studies by Grimes in 2000 (*Lancet* 356:1013–1019), including large case–control studies, cohort studies and one RCT, states that 'fair evidence indicates no important effect of IUD use on infertility'.

Subsequent to that review, Doll et al 2001 (*British Journal of Obstetrics and Gynaecology* 108:304–314) concluded from the Oxford/FPA cohort study that 'long term intrauterine device use in *nulliparous women* appears to be associated with an increased risk of fertility impairment'. Later correspondence by Grimes and Guillebaud in 2001 (*Lancet* 358) highlighted several non-causal explanations for the association. In particular, long-term use over the period of the study necessitated frequent IUD replacements, but there was no prescreening of the cervix (*see Qs 9.53–9.59*): so that every reinsertion in the presence of undiagnosed cervical pathogens would equate in the study to an added risk that some long-term users would get tubal factor infertility.

Clearly, the women whose fertility might be impaired by IUD use are more likely to be those who drop out because of medical complications, which could include pelvic infection. However, in two cohort studies (from New Zealand and Norway), there were similar and good conception rates among those who had their IUD removed because of problems and those who discontinued the method in order to conceive. Two large American case–control studies reported in 1985 (references in Grimes 2000, see above) that past IUD use was significantly more common in primary tubal infertility cases than in controls. But most importantly, in one of them – the Cramer study – women who reported only one partner had no significant increase in tubal infertility, regardless of their choice of contraceptive.

For the vast majority of acceptors the IUD is a fully reversible method of contraception. Among those few who do suffer tubal infertility due to PID or ectopic pregnancy, the prime responsibility cannot lie at the door of the IUD itself (*see Q 9.51*). The frequency of this unwanted outcome can be minimized by careful selection of appropriate users by verbal screening (*see Qs 9.84–9.87*), careful IUD insertion (*see Qs 9.100–9.115*) with microbiological screening and consideration of antibiotic cover, and the best possible follow-up (*see Q 9.121ff*), with optimal management of any complications, of fully informed users.

9.140 Are there any special considerations if a woman wants to conceive after using a copper IUD?

It is usually advised that she uses condoms from the removal until the very next spontaneous period, to clear the endometrium of copper or levonorgestrel. This seems 'common sense' to some, although there are no data to support or refute that policy. *See Q 9.24* for the implications of in situ failure of copper IUDs, and *Q 9.147* for the LNG-IUS. Given the increased likelihood that IUD users might have BV, and the data that this might possibly increase the risk of amnionitis and premature rupture of the membranes, it might be worth at least considering excluding that diagnosis (and treating as appropriate) before IUDs are removed electively to conceive.

GyneFIX™

9.141 What is GyneFIX™ (*Fig. 9.12*), and how is it inserted?

This unique frameless device is the result of some good lateral thinking by Dirk Wildemeersch of Belgium. It is simply a single monofilament polypropylene thread, which dangles in the uterine fundus, bearing six copper bands similar to those on the Copper T-380™ (*Fig. 9.12*). A small anchoring loop and knot at the fundal end are inserted a measured distance of 9–10 mm into the myometrium by a special stylet, passed through the inserter tube, which is first pressed firmly against the fundus.

Fig. 9.12 The GyneFIX™ IUD in situ. Q 9.141.

Special training is vital for safe insertion of this IUD and is available through the Faculty of FP&RHC (*see Q 9.116*).

GyneFIX™ is licensed for 5 years, although this duration can now be extended to 10 years on a named patient basis (*Appendix A*) as a result of new data. There was just one failure among 274 users in two ongoing long-term studies (one in China and one run by WHO) between the fifth and ninth years. Copper release rates support much longer use even than 10 years for this banded copper IUD and an application for a 10-year licence is in the pipeline (Wildemeersch, personal communication, 2003).

9.142 How does GyneFIX™ compare with the gold standard, the T-Safe Cu 380A™?

Initial results were very promising. In short, it seemed to be about as good as the gold standard in most respects, and better in some:

■ After a learning curve for the practitioners there was a very low expulsion rate (only 0.4% in the first year when inserted by experts, the initial research team). The UK experience has not confirmed such a low rate; it is hoped the new inserter system (available since end of 2001) will lead to better results.

■ Although insertion was more painful during our own RCT of postcoital insertions at the Margaret Pyke Centre (in 2003), this was followed by significantly *less dysmenorrhoea pain* than with the T-Safe Cu 380A™ thereafter.

The above could be because GyneFIX™ cannot cause uterine pain of mechanical origin from a frame because it has no frame. So far there is not RCT proof of this advantage, however:

■ once correctly inserted, *partial expulsion* is almost impossible
■ movement of the device in the uterus to produce malpositioning (which is also one cause of lost threads) is not possible, unlike with a framed IUD.

With regard to efficacy when in situ, I expect it to be similar when the ongoing studies are concluded. The overall efficacy in a population will depend on how many unrecognized expulsions occur as there is evidence that they are more easily overlooked when they happen, leaving the woman exposed.

No difference in the rate of bleeding problems or pelvic infection has yet been established in a large enough RCT; we await better data. In the initial European study, infections were very rare and there were no ectopics. But this information is difficult to interpret because it might depend on recruitment of an unusually low-risk population plus unusually high expertise in the research doctors.

9.143 What are the possible or known problems with GyneFIX™?

Perforation is always possible with IUDs and this one has a sharp stylet within a quite narrow firm tube. The rate with the new (2001) inserter mechanism is unknown but unlikely to be lower than the 1:1000 rate usually quoted for framed IUDs – and it could be much higher in the hands of inadequately trained or inexperienced personnel.

If perforation occurs, the small size of the device can make it very difficult to retrieve laparoscopically. If that is unsuccessful it might be judged safer to leave it (being frameless) in the abdominal cavity indefinitely, rather than proceeding to laparotomy.

There was no evidence in one preliminary study of either implantation endometriosis or of more than an extremely localized inflammatory reaction at the site of the anchoring knot.

9.144 So what are the criteria/indications for use of GyneFIX™?

GyneFIX™ costs more than twice that of the gold standard T-Safe Cu 380A™, which is also currently licensed for longer, and so far no head-to-head comparison has confirmed the claimed better performance. For the time being, I therefore recommend it for second-line use as follows:

- Small uterine cavities sounding to less than 6 cm (framed devices being classified WHO 4 at 5.5 cm or less).
- Distorted uterine cavity on ultrasound scan (assuming an IUD is deemed an appropriate method at all). This includes distortion by fibroids or congenitally – in a bicornuate uterus there would be the option of inserting one GyneFIX™ thread into each uterine horn.
- Previous expulsion of any framed device, or other high expulsion risk (but with the implantation done by an 'expert').
- History of needing to remove another device within hours or days of insertion due to excessive cramping pain, where that is attributed to the frame.
- Significant spasmodic dysmenorrhoea in normal cycles, if the first choice intrauterine method in the presence of that symptom (the LNG-IUS) is unacceptable. At least the pain cannot be aggravated by the presence of a frame.
- Immediate insertion after therapeutic abortion (*see Q 9. 104*).
- Selected other nulliparae with light or normal periods upon request, particularly postcoitally.

THE LEVONORGESTREL-RELEASING INTRAUTERINE SYSTEM (LNG-IUS)

9.145 What is the levonorgestrel IUS/LNG-IUS/Mirena™ – also known as LevoNova™?

This Nova-T-shaped device is shown in *Fig. 9.13*. It releases 20 mg/24 h of levonorgestrel (LNG) from its polydimethylsiloxane reservoir through a rate-limiting membrane, over at least 5 years.

Its main contraceptive effects are local, by endometrial suppression and changes to the cervical mucus and uterotubal fluid, which impair sperm migration. The blood levels of LNG are about one-quarter of the peak levels in users of the POP, and so ovarian function is altered less. Most women continue to ovulate and in the remainder sufficient oestrogen is produced from the ovary even if they become amenorrhoeic as many do: this is primarily a local end-organ effect.

9.146 What are the advantages of and indications for the LNG-IUS?

1   It has unsurpassed efficacy: Pearl failure rate only about 0.2 per 100 woman-years, and in the RCT study by Sivin et al 1994 (*Fertility and Sterility* 61:70–77) a cumulative rate of only 1.1 per 100 women at 7 years. This was not different statistically from the 7-year rate of 1.4 for the T-Safe Cu 380A™, making them both entirely comparable to female sterilization: whose overall failure rate with a mix of methods in the American CREST study (*see Q 11.56*) was 1.8 per 100 women at 10 years!

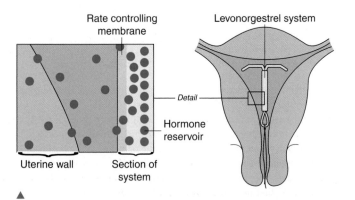

Fig. 9.13 The levonorgestrel intrauterine system (LNG-IUS). Q 9.145.

2 Return of fertility is rapid and appears to be complete.
3 It is highly convenient and has few adverse side-effects.
4 It is, in short, a contraceptive in which the 'default state' is one of contraception, unlike pills and condoms where the default state is the reverse – conception!

The above advantages are, of course, shared with the T-Safe Cu 380A™, which is the best current copper IUD. However, that is where the similarity ends. It fundamentally rewrites the textbooks about IUDs so that it really deserves a different category of its own (hence 'IUS' for intrauterine system, not IUD).

The user of this device can expect a dramatic reduction in amount (more than 90% in numerous studies now) and, after the first few months (discussed below), in duration of blood loss.

Dysmenorrhoea is also generally improved. The LNG-IUS is now the contraceptive method of choice for most women with heavy and/or painful menses. It is been licensed for the first-line treatment of menorrhagia even when there is no need for contraception.

It can also provide progestogenic protection of the uterus during oestrogen replacement therapy by any chosen route. For this use the 'named patient' criteria do need to be fulfilled (see *Appendix A*).

Although not yet proven in an RCT, the LNG-IUS might reduce the frequency of clinical PID, particularly in the youngest age groups who are most at risk (Andersson et al 1994 *Contraception* 49:56–72). This makes it possible to offer the device to some young women requesting a default state contraceptive who would not be good candidates for conventional copper IUDs (ALOs might still be reported, *see Qs 9.74 and 9.75* for management).

The data on file and published for this device show a definite reduction in the risk of extra- as well as intrauterine pregnancy, which can be attributed to its greater efficacy by mechanisms that reduce the risk of pregnancy in any site.

It is a good choice for epileptics and others on enzyme-inducing drugs (*see Q 9.149*), including nulliparae, for whom finding effective reversible contraception is essential and yet fraught with problems.

9.147 What are the disadvantages of the LNG-IUS?

It has the same risk of expulsion and of perforation and malpositioning as the Nova T 200™ or Nova T 380™, because it uses the same design. It has, in short, all the disadvantages of a frame, which are minimized with GyneFIX™ (and at last the form of hybrid LNG-releasing IUS that I have been campaigning for – using the same anchoring technique as GyneFIX™ – is being trialled, provisionally called FibroPlant-LNG).

A more important problem is the high incidence in the first postinsertion months of uterine bleeding, which although small in quantity can be very frequent or continuous and can cause considerable inconvenience. This usually settles to a very acceptable light monthly loss, but it can take 3–6 months to do so.

Later in the use of the method amenorrhoea is very commonly reported.

For both of these last effects, particularly the first, 'forewarned is forearmed': implying good counselling in advance of the fitting of the LNG-IUS. In my experience, women can accept the early weeks of frequent light bleeding as a worthwhile price to pay for all the other advantages of the method, if they are well informed in advance and coached and encouraged as appropriate while it is occurring. The amenorrhoea can even be explained and interpreted to a woman as a positive advantage of the method, rather than an adverse side-effect.

Women should also be advised that although this method is mainly local in its action it is not exclusively so: it is a hormonal method. Therefore there is a small incidence of steroidal side-effects, such as bloatedness, acne and depression. Blood levels are higher in the first 3 months than later and women can be informed that like the annoying bleeding, such symptoms usually resolve over that time.

Weight gain did occur, a mean 2.4 kg at the end of 5 years in the multicentre RCT by Andersson (referenced above). However, the increase was virtually identical (2.5 kg) in 937 copper Nova-T 200™ users to that in the 1821 LNG-IUS users. As no-one alleges that copper causes weight gain, it seems unlikely that the small dose of systemic LNG was to blame either.

Functional ovarian cysts are also more common but are usually asymptomatic and, if not, should be monitored because most resolve.

In the extremely rare event of in situ failure of the LNG-IUS, if the system were not removed well before organogenesis there is real uncertainty that the fetus might be harmed by the high local concentration of levonorgestrel. Because so few in situ failures have gone to term, there are no outcome data on this. Women must be so informed – so as to have full ownership of any decision about continuing with this unintended pregnancy (in which case the LNG-IUS should be removed at the earliest opportunity). *See also* Q 9.150 below for the implications for the insertion cycle.

9.148 What are the contraindications to the LNG-IUS?

There are very few absolute contraindications (WHO 4):

1 *Severe allergy* to a constituent.
2 Suspected *pregnancy*.
3 *Unexplained uterine bleeding*.
4 *Current breast cancer* (WHO 3 when in remission, defined by WHO as after 5 years, but could be sooner, in consultation with the oncologist and the patient).

5 Current active pelvic infection or pelvic tenderness, or purulent cervical discharge.

6 Recent proven STI, unless fully investigated and treated (can then be WHO 3).

7 Severely distorted uterine cavity, although it might be usefully inserted after preliminary hysteroscopic removal of a submucous fibroid, and occasionally after uterine ablation (*see Qs 11.60–11.61*).

8 Current liver tumour or hepatocellular disease (possibly WHO 3).

9 Current active arterial disease (this is arguable, probably WHO 2 in most cases).

10 Past attack of bacterial endocarditis.

11 Very severe immunodeficiency.

12 Current active trophoblastic disease with raised hCG.

13 In addition: *the LNG-IUS should not be used as a postcoital intrauterine contraceptive* (at least one failure has been reported – effective though it is in long-term use it appears not to act as quickly as intrauterine copper does).

9.149 What about relative contraindications to the LNG-IUS?

If you look through those listed in Q *9.87* for copper IUDs, most are irrelevant, or in the very usable category WHO 2, and some are indications!

Note in particular that the LNG-IUS is an option if there is a history of ectopic pregnancy (WHO 3). If there is structural heart disease and this IUS is chosen there should of course be full antibiotic cover for the insertion as in Q *9.90*. It would be preferable to a copper IUD if a prosthetic valve is present (WHO 3).

Although enzyme-inducing drugs have the potential to weaken the contraceptive effect of a hormonal method, the very high local concentration of levonorgestrel should not be lowered by any effect at the liver. And the Margaret Pyke Centre has now published a small collected series of over 50 such users with only one apparent failure, suggesting that the LNG-IUS does, at the least, retain very useful efficacy for these women (*see Q 9.146*).

It can be used during breastfeeding (like the POP, *see Qs 7.54–7.58*).

9.150 Are there any special points about insertion of the LNG-IUS?

There are indeed! It should be inserted no later than day 7 of the normal cycle, because it does not operate as an effective anovulant or postcoital contraceptive *and* because additionally it is potentially disastrous to conceive in the first cycle (*see Q 9.14*). Later insertion is advisable only if there has been believable abstinence or excellent contraception up to that time (best to not include condoms in that category!) with continued contraception (condoms OK) thereafter, for a minimum of 7 days.

Helpful tip

Ensure that, *as a routine*, all who plan to have this LNG-IUS are started on a more effective method than condoms (e.g. combined pill or perhaps Cerazette™), so that the insertion can be performed without the above anxiety and on any mutually convenient date.

The technique itself has changed with the arrival, in 2000, of the new inserter, although it is still based on that for inserting the Nova-T (200 or 380). However, the insertion tube is wider (4.8 mm rather than 3.7 mm), meaning that effective local anaesthesia and dilatation to at least Hegar 5 are not infrequently required (although rarely in multiparae, who remain, as for copper IUDs, the primary target population).

Two helpful tips (although, as always, no book can substitute for proper practical training):

1   Not only when loading the inserter but *also* later, when easing the loaded inserter through the internal cervical os, ensure with a finger that the green slider stays in the extreme forward position, nearest the woman. (Otherwise the external tube can slide back through friction so that the side arms of the IUS are prematurely released in the cervical canal …)
2   I see as a crucial step that, once the side arms are out, within the uterus, the healthcare professional doing the insertion gently eases the IUS device to the very top of the fundus (*see Q 9.115(3)*).

9.151 Which women might particularly consider a LNG-IUS?

If it were not for (frequently overestimated) price considerations, its duration of use only for 5 years and the initial postinsertion bleeding and hormone problems, this method could be reasonably selected not only by almost any IUD-acceptor but also by most women considering sterilization, not to mention hysterectomy or uterine ablation for dysfunctional bleeding. That it is not so selected tells us more about doctors and other healthcare professionals not sharing all the options – as a human right for women, I would say – and about irrelevant 'baggage' from the past about IUDs and infection (linked with the infamous Dalkon Shield™), than it does about any defects of the method.

Women are not going to know about the LNG-IUS unless we tell them: the media doesn't, paradoxically because adverse side-effects are so few and in general in the category 'nuisance' rather than hazardous. Thus there has been no 'Mirena™ IUS – scare' in the media to make people aware of it. Truly, much as we hate 'pill scares' it is also true that there is no such thing as bad publicity!

The LNG-IUS fulfils many of the standard criteria for an 'ideal' contraceptive (*Table 9.3*):

TABLE 9.3 A short list of features of the 'ideal' contraceptive
1   100% reversible
2   100% effective (with the 'default state' as contraception, fully 'forgettable')
3   100% convenient (and non-coitally-related)
4   100% free of adverse side-effects (neither risk nor nuisance)
5   100% protective against sexually transmitted infections
6   Possessed of other non-contraceptive benefits
7   Maintenance-free (needing no ongoing medical intervention)

1   It approaches to 100% reversibility, effectiveness and even, after some delay, convenience. This is because, after the initial months of frequent uterine bleedings and spotting, the usual outcomes of either intermittent light menses or amenorrhoea are very acceptable to most women who are properly counselled. Indeed, in Backman et al's 2000 post-marketing study (*British Journal of Obstetrics and Gynaecology* 107:335–339) of 17 360 users in Finland, the continuation rates to 3 and 5 years were amazingly high (81% and 65%, respectively) and 'the risk of premature removal was markedly lower among women who had occasional or total absence of menstruation'. Thereby demolishing the myth that women necessarily want to be regularly seeing periods!

2   Adverse side-effects are amazingly few and rarely dangerous.

3   Evidence continues to accumulate instead of its 'added value' through non-contraceptive benefits, including a useful reduction in symptoms of the premenstrual syndrome in about half of those receiving it.

4   Although it might be chosen by some young women with heavy menses or unable to accept alternatives, it is particularly suitable for women with heavy or just painful periods, or with contraindications to other options.

5   The LNG-IUS can often provide an excellent solution for the contraceptive dilemmas of many women suffering from a range of interacting medical disorders or risk factors, e.g. severe diabetes, SLE (*see Qs 5.134–5.137*) and epilepsy (*see Q 9.149*).

There is then the possible option, in the older reproductive years, of providing the progestogen component of a most useful form of 'contraceptive and no-period HRT' – to follow, if they are later prescribed oestrogen by any chosen route. Although so licensed in more than 30 countries, at the time of writing this remains an unlicensed use in the UK (see *Appendix A*) and for this indication it must be replaced every 5 years (*see Q 9.152*).

9.152 Can the LNG-IUS (Mirena™) be left in situ at the user's request beyond its licensed 5 years?

A qualified 'yes' to this question: Sivin's study (referenced in *Q 9.146*) in whom 174 users continued to the end of the seventh year, and another study from Brazil, do provide data that it is effective as a contraceptive for at least 7 years.

Copper IUDs fitted after age 40 work well indefinitely (i.e. up to final ovarian failure, *see Q 9.138*). After about 7 years the IUS-user will have, effectively, an 'inert' IUD. This is possibly acceptable on the woman's say-so for contraception, after her age then of over 47 (WHO 3).

Use beyond 5 years is not acceptable as part of HRT (*see Q 9.151*) because it is not evidence-based to protect the uterus beyond that time and use as part of HRT is at present unlicensed anyway.

To summarize, then, in three situations where prolonged use may be requested:

1 *For contraception*: use is evidence-based but unlicensed up to 7 years. Thereafter the older woman fitted above 40 *might* so proceed at her fully empowered request – but always on a named patient basis (*Appendix A*).
2 *As part of HRT*: current practice would be always to change at 5 years.
3 But if the LNG-IUS is not being, and will not be, used for either (1) or (2), it could be left in situ for as long as it 'works' in the control of heavy and/or painful uterine bleeding – and then removed after ovarian failure can be finally assured (say at age 58).

CONCLUSIONS

9.153 What are your ten commandments about IUD or IUS insertion?

See Qs 9.105–9.120 for more details:

1 Thou shalt never insert any IUD without training and without first having practised each step of the insertion procedure on a plastic pelvic model – and keeping in practice.
2 All manipulations of the cervix and uterus shall be performed gently – but not tentatively.
3 Thou shalt always consider and discuss the option of local anaesthesia – and always offer a PGSI, and always use 'aural valium and 'vocal local'.
4 Thou shalt ensure the best position of the patient for insertion (consider left lateral), always have an assistant and always use good equipment with a good light.
5 A preliminary BME will never be omitted.
6 The insertion will be postponed, pending diagnosis and treatment, whenever there is the slightest pelvic tenderness or other evidence suggesting infection.

7 The cervix will be thoroughly cleansed by repeated swabbing, and aseptic technique followed for all objects passed through the endocervical canal into the sterile uterine cavity.

8 Careful sounding of the uterus will not be omitted – to check the direction and patency of the canal and to assess the uterine cavity. Hegar dilators (3–6) will be available.

9 The device if it has a frame will be loaded into its inserter at the last possible moment – to preserve its asepsis and 'memory'.

10 The correct technique will be used to deliver the IUD in the right plane to the correct high fundal position.

9.154 What are your ten resolutions for the conscientious clinician providing intrauterine methods?

1 Remembering that one of the main times of action of IUDs is the last 9 days of the cycle I will follow the 7-day rule for elective IUD removal (*see Q 9.14*), to avoid 'iatrogenic pregnancies'. I will also be prepared to proceed with IUD insertion up to 'day 19' – adjusted for shortest cycle length – in selected cases (*see Qs 9.15 and 10.15*).

2 As the main IUD concerns and contraindications relate to threats to fertility, I will always make this the main point when counselling the nulliparous – but explain that the IUD itself is innocent!

3 As the rates of in situ pregnancy, expulsion and pelvic infection are inversely related to age, I will always make these potential advantages the main element when counselling the more mature.

4 As incorrect insertion/malposition can cause every category of IUD problem, I will ensure that my own insertions are competent, careful and gentle, and use the 'longest lived', appropriate IUD (*see Qs 9.134 and 9.138*). I will endeavour to fit well the right device in the right woman using the right technique.

5 I will maintain an 'open house' policy for them to discuss any symptoms with a healthcare professional by telephone or in person. Specifically, I will tell users that pain and bleeding are serious symptoms until proved otherwise, especially if sustained and intermenstrual.

6 More specifically, I will remember that any woman with menstrual irregularity and pelvic discomfort has an ectopic pregnancy until proved otherwise.

7 I will teach users that 'lost threads' means she is pregnant or at risk of pregnancy until proved otherwise.

8 In any continuing pregnancy I will ensure that the IUD is gently removed in the first trimester if feasible, and will teach users how to reduce the risks of abortion and preterm delivery. Moreover, I will follow the two equally important but opposite slogans in (9) and (10).

9 'Leave well alone' (often, after counselling, in asymptomatic long-term users).

10 'When in doubt take it out' when the woman does have troublesome symptoms; and also for her own reasons upon her request, so the method is never one over which (wrongly) only the clinician has control. But then I must not forget to ask about any intercourse in the preceding 7 days, and her plans for future contraception.

9.155 What problems of IUD use in the UK should be reported to the Medical Devices Agency?

The functions of this body have recently been taken over by the Medicines and Healthcare products Regulatory Agency (MHRA). The following should be reported:

1 Extrauterine pregnancy
2 All perforations/translocations
3 Severe pelvic infections – most especially actinomycosis (*see* Q *9.73*) or bacterial endocarditis (*see* Q *9.90*)
4 Apparent true allergy to any constituent of IUDs (*see* Q *9.88*)
5 Apparent interaction with a drug, or imaging technique (*see* Qs *9.128–9.130*)
6 Severe insertion reactions (*see* Q *9.119*)
7 Any unusual *possibly* related event.

 PATIENT QUESTIONS

QUESTIONS ASKED BY PROSPECTIVE OR CURRENT IUD USERS

9.156   How does the IUD or the IUS work? Is it often causing an abortion?

The answer depends on your own definition of when pregnancy begins (*see* Qs *9.7, 10.3, 10.4*). If your beliefs make you feel that contraception must never operate after fertilization then this method is not for you.

9.157   Can the copper be absorbed from copper devices into the body?

A tiny amount is absorbed, but very little so it is only just detectable in the blood. By far the majority of the small amount of copper that is lost over the years goes out in the vaginal fluid.

9.158   Why does the IUD or IUS have a tail? Can I pull it out myself?

Mainly to check that the device is present, but also to remove it when required. Deliberate self-removal is not recommended, but could be done. Removal by mistake has happened rarely, when chasing a 'lost' tampon perhaps.

9.159 Which is safer, the IUD or the ordinary pill? Could a woman die from using an IUD or IUS?

Overall, the risk of death or life-endangering disease is very low with both methods, but even lower with an IUD/IUS. Deaths have been caused but they are extremely rare. The problems are focused in the pelvic area and not all over the body, and they can all be minimized (*see Qs 9.153 and 9.154*). The main problems have to do with future fertility (*see Qs 9.22, 9.85, 9.87*).

9.160 Does the IUD or IUS cause any kind of cancer?

There is no evidence for this, whether for copper or hormone-releasing varieties (*see Q 9.21*). Indeed, there is a hint of protection against cancer of the endometrium (lining of the womb), especially by using the LNG-IUS (*see Q 9.19*).

9.161 If I get pregnant, will the baby be harmed?

There is no evidence of this with copper IUDs, even if the pregnancy occurs with the IUD still in position. There is more uncertainty with the LNG-IUS (*see Qs 9.101 and 9.147*). Either type of device should normally be removed in early pregnancy (*see Qs 9.24 and 9.147*).

9.162 What has using the IUD or IUS got to do with the number of sexual partners I have?

A great deal, because the main problem with IUDs is pelvic infection, and nearly all IUD-linked infections are actually caught sexually. Also relevant is the number of sexual partners of your own partner, even if you are entirely faithful to him (see also the question in $Q\ 9.121(3)$).

9.163 Do I need my partner's/husband's agreement to have an IUD or IUS?

No, the device can be inserted without his agreement. The threads can even be cut off if you so request, so he cannot know it is there unless you tell him. However, it is always ever so much better that any couple are both agreed, whatever method of family planning is chosen.

9.164 Should I ask to see which IUD or IUS I have before it is fitted?

Yes, most certainly, so you can't imagine something big and nasty ... Ideally, you should also write down its name and the date of fitting, in case you move to the care of a different doctor or clinic.

9.165 I think I'm allergic to copper; what should I do?

First, report the matter to your doctor. It might be possible to do special patch allergy tests. As most people who think they are allergic to copper turn out actually to be allergic to another metal, it might be all right to insert the device and see how you get on over the next few days. If you get marked discharge and pain within a very few days of insertion, you should return most promptly for advice (*see Q 9.88*).

9.166 I am told I have a cervical erosion (ectopy)/a tilted womb/a very tiny womb – can I have an IUD fitted?

If these are the only problems (i.e. there is no infection and the womb is not distorted congenitally or by fibroids) a device can normally be fitted (*see Qs 9.86, 9.98, 9.144*).

9.167 I have heard you can get very bad cramp-like pains when an IUD or IUS is fitted? What causes this and what can be done about it?

The pain people feel at insertion varies a great deal, from nothing to severe, and it is not easily predictable. Part of this is caused by the release of substances called prostaglandins, and you can ask your doctor for a specific painkiller that opposes their action. You should also discuss with him/her the possibility of having a local anaesthetic.

9.168 Does an IUD or IUS always have to be fitted during or just after a period?

No – not only can it be inserted later, provided contraception earlier in the insertion cycle has been brilliant, there might even be certain advantages to not inserting during heavy bleeding (*see Qs 9.15–9.17*).

9.169 Does being an epileptic increase the chance of my having a fit during the insertion?

Yes it does, and your doctor should arrange to have available the treatment to prevent/stop an attack (*see also Qs 9.119–9.120*).

9.170 How soon can I have sex after having the IUD or IUS fitted?

The protection from pregnancy by a copper IUD, or from the LNG-IUS if fitted before day 8 of your cycle is immediate, but although there's no proof it is important, it is my recommendation that you wait for about 3 days, to reduce even more any infection risk (*see Q 9.122*). If it was the LNG-IUS that was fitted on/after day 8, you will be advised to use condoms to ensure effectiveness in the first month (*see Q 9.150*).

9.171 Can I use tampons internally after being fitted with an IUD or IUS?

My usual advice is to use only a sanitary towel at first, for the bleeding that follows immediately after IUD insertion, until 3 days have elapsed. Subsequently sanitary protection can be entirely at your choice.

Prolonged use of the same tampon (more than 12 h) is always a bad idea, for fear of toxic shock syndrome (TSS).

9.172   Can an IUD or IUS fall out without my knowing?

Yes, this is certainly possible (*see Q 9.39*). The most likely time is during a heavy period, when it could be hidden within a large clot or on a tampon that is then flushed down the toilet. This is why it is best to check your threads after each period. Learning to feel for the strings is extra important with GyneFIX™.

9.173   How often should I feel for the threads?

Once a month is sufficient – best right at the end of a period. If you have an LNG-IUS and are not seeing regular bleeds, then do this on the first day of each new month. This is so that you do not begin to rely on the method each new month, until you have checked that it is still in position.

9.174   How do I feel the threads of the IUD or IUS? What should I do if I now can't feel them any longer?

Either squat down or put one foot on a bathroom stool. Insert both your index and middle fingers into the vagina and feel more in a backwards than an upwards direction until you come across the cervix. This feels rather like a nose with only one nostril, and you should then be able to find emerging from the opening one or two little threads feeling like ends of nylon fishing line. If that is all you feel, well and good. If, however, you feel something hard, like the end of a matchstick, this could mean that the device is on its way out. In that case, or if you can no longer feel the threads at all, you must assume that you are no longer protected and start using another method (e.g. condoms). Contact your family doctor or clinic urgently in case emergency contraception is required – most likely by urgent reinsertion (*see Q 10.23*).

By the way, some women don't learn to do all this, instead their partner does it for them each month – which is fine!

9.175   Can my IUD or IUS get lost in my body (perforation)?

Extremely rarely. It is 999:1 against this happening in your case. It is a rare cause of the problem of lost threads (*see Q 9.43*). Should it happen, the most that is normally required is a minor operation called a laparoscopy to retrieve it.

While your lost threads problem is still being sorted out, and you are perhaps waiting for a hospital appointment, make sure that you use another method of family planning (because the womb itself might be empty) and also take immediate medical advice if you get any pain in the abdomen.

9.176   Can I go back to using an IUD or IUS after a perforation?

This depends on the cause; but an IUD can often be reinserted with success, since the tiny hole in the womb heals up so completely.

QUESTIONS ASKED BY CURRENT USERS

9.177 Do women have more vaginal discharge with an IUD?

Yes. Sometimes the discharge has a specific and treatable cause, so it should always be reported to your doctor. If testing shows nothing specific and treatable, like BV or thrush, then it is probably caused by an increase in the usual vaginal fluid (which includes mucus, the fluid of sexual arousal and even semen). That needs no treatment.

9.178 Someone has told me the IUD can break into pieces inside you, is this so?

Years ago there was one dud batch of Lippes loop devices, which were distributed worldwide and were liable to fracture. No modern device will break up, except very rarely if removal is difficult. In that case a minor hysteroscopy operation might rarely be necessary to retrieve the missing portion.

9.179 My last period was very late and heavy; does this mean I might be miscarrying an early pregnancy?

Most probably not – heavy periods are not uncommon in regular use of an IUD, and the period could have been late just because your egg was released late in that cycle. However, you should visit the clinic for an examination and advice, partly in case your device was dislodged by the heavy flow. You might also ask about the LNG-IUS (Mirena™).

9.180 Can my partner really feel the IUD or IUS during lovemaking as he says, and what can be done about it?

Some men notice the threads, depending on which way the cervix points and perhaps on the position of intercourse. Many couples just adapt their sex lives accordingly, but otherwise it is possible to have the threads cut right off (*see* Q 9.127).

9.181 Can I use a sunbed with an IUD in place, or have vibromassage?

Neither of these can affect your IUD in any way.

9.182 If my IUD contains metal, will it make an embarrassing 'bleep' when I pass through security devices at airports or large department stores?

Despite rumours, this does not appear to be a problem either with copper-bearing or steel devices (or with any of the clips used to sterilize people) – presumably because the amount of metal is too small.

Another rumour that can be discounted is the one that was started by the woman who accused the magician Yuri Geller of causing the failure of her copper IUD. She claimed that the pregnancy was conceived when she made love on the hearthrug during a television demonstration by the above-mentioned showman of his metal-bending skills!

9.183 Can I cause my IUD or IUS to be expelled by vigorous aerobic exercises or intercourse in any unusual positions?

There is no evidence for this and plenty of ordinary and sexual athletes use the method with success.

9.184 Are there any drugs that might interfere with the action of my IUD or IUS?

Tell your doctor about the IUD if you are to receive any treatment. Should this be a corticosteroid in high dose or other drug(s) that could interfere with immune responses, it might be better for you to transfer to another method of birth control. However, there is no current concern about either antibiotics or painkillers (*see Qs 9.87(12) and 9.89*), or other treatments (*see Q 9.128*).

9.185 My girl-friend tells me I should have my device changed often, to prevent it getting infected or stuck inside me. My gynaecologist implies it would be better to have a new one before it officially runs out at 5 or 8 years, so as to keep it effective. Are these ideas true?

They are both 'urban myths', although still common, even what your gynaecologist is implying. Studies actually tend to show greater effectiveness the longer the same IUD or IUS is used, sometimes even beyond the end of the licensed time (*see Qs 9.131ff and 9.186*).

9.186 Do I really have to have my copper IUD changed at a set time, when it is suiting me well?

Nowadays this is becoming less and less necessary, and definitely not if your device was fitted above the age of 40 (*see Qs 9.131–9.138* for a full answer to this most important question).

9.187 How is an IUD or the IUS removed? Is it ever difficult?

Normally there is no problem; there is much less discomfort than having the device fitted in the first place. However, there are some situations in which it is more tricky and uncomfortable (*see Qs 9.35 and 9.125*).

9.188 If my IUD or IUS is removed so that I can try for a baby, should I wait, using another method for a set time?

It is recommended, but not vital, that you wait for one period to 'clear the womb' first. Even women who conceive immediately the device comes out (so it was still in place during the last period before the pregnancy) seem to be as likely as anyone else to have a normal baby.

Emergency (postcoital) contraception

10

BACKGROUND AND MECHANISMS

10.1 What is the definition of postcoital contraception, or emergency contraception (EC – the preferred term)?

In current usage this is any female method that is administered after intercourse but has its effects prior to the stage of implantation. The latter is believed to occur no earlier than 5 days after ovulation. Any method applied after intercourse that acts after implantation, even if this is before the next menses, should properly be called a postconceptional or contragestive agent.

The term 'morning-after pill' is not ideal because it could actually result in pregnancies by preventing women from presenting many hours later than the 'morning after' (*see Q 10.7*). Yet efficacy does appear to be greater the earlier hormone regimens are commenced (*see Q 10.6*).

10.2 Given all the new data and their implications, is there up-to-date guidance for clinicians about EC?

Yes, *Guidance, emergency contraception* was issued in April 2003 by the Clinical Effectiveness Unit of the Faculty of Family Planning and Reproductive Health Care (FFPRHC; *Journal of Family Planning and Reproductive Healthcare* 29:9–16). In the rest of this chapter this will be referred to as 'FFP Guidance'. As it includes all the most important references, these will not be referenced individually here, aside from the two seminal WHO studies:

1   Multicentre, double-blind RCT of 1998 women randomized to LNG 0.75 mg stat versus two tablets of a contraceptive containing 250 µg of LNG with 50 µg of EE, each repeated in 12 h. This will be referred to as 'WHO 1998 study' (*Lancet* 1998 352:428–433)

2   Multicentre, double-blind RCT of 4136 women randomized to 10 mg mifepristone as a single dose or two LNG regimens, which were for 1356 subjects standard progestogen-only emergency contraception (POEC) – two doses of 0.75 mg LNG 12 h apart – and for another 1356 the whole 1.5 mg was taken as a single LNG dose. This will be called 'WHO 2002 study' (*Lancet* 2002 360:1803–1810).

10.3 Is it ethical and legal to use EC contraception?

Yes. Legally in the UK a pregnancy is not recognized to exist until implantation is completed (Judicial Review of Emergency Contraception, Department of Health 2002; quoted in FFP Guidance). Although the methods usually work by preventing fertilization, it is undeniable that the mechanism might often be through blocking implantation.

The question is whether the prescriber and the woman concerned are happy to accept the view of most modern biologists and ethicists, that 'conception' is a process, which certainly begins with the fusion of sperm and ovum, but is not complete until implantation.

The situation is clarified by considering the status of the unimplanted blastocyst (*Fig. 10.1*). If it stays where it is in the cavity of the uterus it is in a 100% 'no-go' situation – unless and until it can stop itself being washed away in the next menstrual flow by secreting enough hCG into the woman's circulation to maintain the corpus luteum. The all-destroying menses cannot be prevented without successful implantation.

A second feature of the unimplanted situation is that the woman's physiology does not 'know' the blastocyst is present, yet. Only after implantation is there a two-way relationship, and for the first time 100% 'no-go' for the blastocyst becomes 'go'; now there is 'carriage'. As has been well said, at the earlier stage, when there is not yet 'carriage', how could application of any method of birth control be 'procuring a miscarriage'?

Finally, with at least 40% of blastocysts regularly failing to implant there seems little logic in putting a high value on something with which Nature itself is so prodigal.

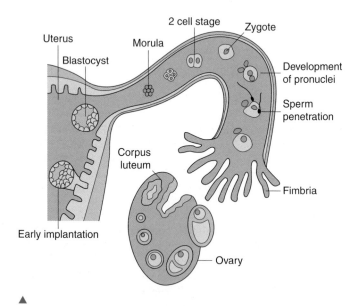

▲

Fig. 10.1 Ovulation, fertilization and early development to the stage of implantation. Q 10.3 considers the status of the unimplanted blastocyst, labelled above.

Prescribers must, of course, respect the views of their patients, and EC methods should not be used for any who are unhappy with the above interpretation. They should then, however, also understand the implications in relation to other methods (*see Qs 9.7 and 10.4*).

10.4 What are the implications of rejection of EC methods on ethical grounds?

In the main, this means that the woman concerned should also not use either IUDs or IUSs, or the old-type progestogen-only pill (*see Q 7.76*). All these methods although primarily working before fertilization, can operate – in a small minority of cycles – by blocking implantation.

10.5 What is the history of EC?

This is probably almost as old as the first recognition that semen is in some way responsible for pregnancy. Douching has been used since ancient times and remains in use today; 25% of women presenting for EC treatment in one UK study had first used a shower attachment, flannel or paper tissues, with or without a spermicide or household germicide. These methods are doomed to frequent failure; because sperm have been found in cervical mucus within 90 s of ejaculation.

The Persian physician Al-Razi suggested:

First immediately after ejaculation let the two come apart and let the woman arise roughly, sneeze and blow her nose several times and call out in a loud voice. She should jump violently backwards seven to nine times.

Jumping backwards supposedly dislodged the semen; jumping forwards would assure pregnancy.

A range of EC pessaries and douches have been described over the years, including wine and garlic with fennel, used in Egypt as early as 1500 BC; ground cabbage blossoms in the fourth century; and culminating in Coca-Cola™ in some developing countries even today. Diet Coke™ may actually have had some spermicidal action – but then they removed the quinine!

The history of more effective methods begins in 1963 with trials of diethylstilboestrol (DES) at Yale University. Because of the risks to any pregnancy should the method fail, DES should now never be used. After the mid-1970s the Yuzpe method (devised by a Canadian gynaecologist) became the first-choice method, using much less EE in combination with LNG.

Immediate insertion of a copper IUD is an alternative method first reported in 1972 and appropriate in some cases (*see Q 10.34*).

10.6 What are the currently accepted regimens of EC treatment?

See *Tables 10.1* and *10.2*.

TABLE 10.1 Choice of methods for postcoital contraception – a brief summary

Copper IUD	Levonorgestrel (LNG) method (Levonelle)	Combined hormone method
	Levonorgestrel 0.75 mg stat 0.75 mg 12 h later	(Yuzpe: NB used only when LNG method not available) Microgynon-30™ 4 pills stat, 4 pills 12 hours later
Normal timing Up to 5 days after earliest calculated day of ovulation or 5 days after earliest exposure in that cycle	Up to 72 h -- but usable to 120 h (see Q 10.9 and Appendix A) after earliest act of intercourse	Up to 72 h
Efficacy Almost 100% (timing as above)	98.5%* (within 72 h)	97% (within 72 h)
Side-effects Pain, bleeding, risk of infection through insertion	Nausea 23% (15%)* and vomiting 6% (14%)*	Nausea 51% and vomiting 19%
Contraindications (see Qs 10.28, 10.29) ■ Pregnancy and as for IUDs generally (Q 9.85– 9.87)	■ Pregnancy ■ Active acute porphyria ■ Severe liver disease ■ Severe allergy to a constituent	■ Pregnancy ■ Current focal migraine, jaundice, active acute porphyria, sickle-cell crisis, severe liver disease or serious past thrombosis ■ Severe allergy to a constituent

References: WHO (1998) *Lancet* 352: 428–33 and *WHO (2002) *Lancet* 360: 1803–10
Numbers rounded to one decimal place.

1 Immediate insertion of a copper-bearing IUD (*not* the LNG-IUS, *see Q 9.148*), not more than 5 days after the most probable calculated date of ovulation, even if there have been multiple acts of unprotected intercourse; or 5 days after any single (earliest) exposure.

2 The Yuzpe method: this is started within 72 h of the earliest act of unprotected intercourse, its efficacy being greatest in the first 24 h and declining thereafter (although not to nil after 72 h). Two tablets of a contraceptive containing 250 µg of LNG with 50 µg of EE (Schering PC 4 or Ovran) are given at once, followed by a further two tablets 12 h

TABLE 10.2 Efficacy of Yuzpe (combined oestrogen-progestogen) compared with POEC (progestogen-only emergency contraception) WHO findings (1998 and 2002)

Coitus-to-treatment interval	Pregnancy rate		Of those truly at risk % of conceptions prevented
72 h or less	*WHO 1998 Study*	*WHO 2002 Study*	
Combined oestrogen-progestogen	3.2%		
POEC	1.1%	1.5% (to 120 h if abstained after treatment, *Q 10.17*)	80%
24 h or less			
Combined oestrogen-progestogen	2.0%	–	95%
POEC	0.4%		
25–48 h			
Combined oestrogen-progestogen	4.1%	–	85%
POEC	1.2%		
49–72 h			
Combined oestrogen-progestogen	4.7%	–	58%
POEC	2.7%		
72–120 h			
LNG-only (both regimens, see *Qs 10.8, 10.9*)	–	2.5% (? as small nos in 2002 study)	

In the WHO trial, it is calculated that with just the single sexual exposure, only about 8% of all those treated would have conceived without treatment. Percentages in the last column use these as the denominator.

later. Although in the UK this has been supplanted by POEC and will be little discussed below, practitioners in some countries are forced – where there is no source of oral LNG (i.e. no appropriate POPs on the market) – to continue to recommend the Yuzpe method. This commonly entails using four tablets of Microgynon-30™ or local equivalent brand stat, repeated in 12 h.

3 Use of LNG alone: this is referred to here and in the FFP Guidance as POEC. If started within 72 h of the earliest exposure it again has its greatest efficacy in the first 24 h, declining thereafter but, not to nil, at

72 h (*Table 10.2*). It requires 750 µg LNG stat, normally repeated in 12 h. In the WHO 1998 study it proved to be more effective, with fewer side-effects (especially vomiting) and there are also fewer contraindications. In the UK this is now marketed to clinicians as Levonelle-2™ and to the public over the counter as Levonelle™. In the US a version of POEC EC has the excellent brand name Plan B™! Outside Europe and the US practitioners are usually forced to construct the dose from marketed POPs (e.g. by giving 25 tablets of the local equivalent of Norgeston™ stat, repeated in 12 h). If this can be done it is still preferable (with much reassurance of the woman that 50 tablets is not an overdose!) to constructing the less effective Yuzpe regimen in (2), above.

Other methods previously in use are now of historical interest only (*see also Q 10.50 and 10.51* for variants and methods being researched).

10.7 What is the mechanism of action of EC contraceptive methods?

The IUD operates by blocking implantation (*see Q 9.7*) when, as commonly it is, inserted after ovulation, although if applied earlier in the cycle it will use its primary action (as in more usual long-term use) to block fertilization. The mode of action of POEC is incompletely understood. If taken before the LH surge it will usually inhibit ovulation, and it is probable that the uterine fluid/genital tract mucus can also be rendered hostile to the sperm. After ovulation, other effects on LH levels and the length of the luteal phase might be important but there is little evidence to support a direct anti-implantation effect (FFP Guidance). Most authorities now believe that if POEC is not administered in time to block ovulation or fertilization, the method is much more likely to fail.

It is important to remember that fertile ovulation might simply be postponed in that cycle, hence the requirement to use a method such as the condom until the next period.

10.8 Does the second dose of POEC have to be given accurately 12 h after the first?

No. The SPC, based on the pharmacokinetics of LNG, already suggests that the doses can be given 12–16 h apart. WHO has now reported on its second (2002) double-blind RCT of EC, in which 4136 women at 15 different centres worldwide were randomized to 10 mg mifepristone as a single dose or two LNG regimens (FFP Guidance). They showed no difference in pregnancy rates (or side-effects, see below) between 1356 women randomized to standard POEC – 2 doses of 0.75 mg LNG 12 hours apart – and another 1356 randomized to take the whole 1.5 mg as a single LNG dose.

I understand that by 2004 the CSM will have advised a change to the licence to permit this single dose regimen. Until then, the FFP Guidance recommends that the two-dose regimen remains normal practice. However the new data make it no longer necessary for any woman to take her second dose in the middle of the night. She can avoid this by taking the second dose either up to 4 h late, or early, or both doses when she is first seen (but in the two latter cases, until the licence is changed, follow *Appendix A*). But she should never delay the first dose.

10.9 Will POEC work if given later than 72 h?

Yes, but less well. Although many prescribers have treated it as such, the 72-h time limit as licensed has never implied an absolute contraindication. From the data of the first WHO trial (1998), it appeared (although not well confirmed in the later 2002 trial) that POEC worked best if started in the first 24 h, and the failure rate increased with time thereafter.

In the second WHO (2002) trial (*see Q 10.8*), the two-dose POEC regimen had a 1.7% failure rate for treatment in the first 72 h, rising to 2.4% for treatment between 72 and 120 h. Given that so many would not have conceived anyway, calculations based on the best available data for conception risk by cycle day before or after ovulation showed that this corresponds to a fall from preventing 79% of actual conceptions to 60%. The results for the single dose were very similar at both time periods of the intervention, and if the two LNG regimens were pooled, treatment from 72 to 120 h had an overall failure rate of 8/314 cases or 2.5% (equating to prevention of about 60% of actual conceptions expected).

Most clients, if they have rejected the alternative of having a copper IUD inserted, will see those numbers as considerably better than doing nothing. Moreover, the WHO researchers concluded: 'Even if a declining trend in efficacy with time were verified, the regimens studied still prevent a high proportion of pregnancies even up to 5 days after coitus'.

Only 12% of the WHO subjects were treated on days 4 and 5, confidence intervals were wide including zero effect, so and the FFP Guidance is cautious saying only 'a recommendation for use beyond 72 hours cannot be given'.

10.10 Do you consider it is now adequately evidence-based (although unlicensed) to use POEC between 72 and 120 h after UPSI in selected cases?

Yes, I do! In the WHO 2002 study for the POEC and single-dose LNG groups combined, the conception rate was only 1.5% in all those who claimed abstinence after treatment when it was up to 5 days after the unprotected sexual intercourse (UPSI, although only about 12% were treated on days 4 or 5). However, it should be recorded that the woman understands that:

■ She needs to be completely transparent about any possible earlier exposure, so that you can then proceed in good faith, in the belief that you will not be disturbing an already implanted pregnancy

■ Insertion of a copper IUD would be more effective (indeed, I agree with the Faculty that that should always be said, even to women presenting within 72 h of exposure)

■ This late treatment ought certainly to be better than nothing, stopping at best 6 out of 10 actual pregnancies to be expected with no treatment (contrast about 8 out of 10 if she had been treated earlier) and:

■ The treatment must be on a 'named patient' basis (see Appendix A) until the SPC changes, as it will.

10.11 Can POEC be given more than once in a cycle?

Yes (*see also* Q 10.43). The FFP Guidance is in full agreement about this one!

10.12 Might other progestogens be effective?

Other progestogens such as desogestrel or gestodene, or even DMPA by injection, might well be effective but neither their efficacy nor the best doses have so far been evaluated in proper trials.

The antiprogestogen, mifepristone, in a single 10-mg dose was shown definitively, in the third arm of the WHO's 2002 trial, to work as well as either LNG regimen (*but see* Q 10.51).

EFFECTIVENESS

10.13 What is the overall efficacy of the two main EC methods?

1   For the IUD method the failure rate is very low indeed. We have reported one failure with the device still in situ at the Margaret Pyke Centre and another, with partial expulsion of the device, has been reported from elsewhere. This represents two failures in about 1300 insertions reported in the literature to that date, or about 0.3%. Considering that in this context the risk of pregnancy applies only for the cycle of insertion, this is a rate of 1–2 failures/1300 cycles; so entirely compatible with the usually quoted failure rate of the IUD at that time of about 1/100 woman-years (100 woman-years equals 1300 cycles).

2   *Table 10.2* summarizes the basic data on efficacy of POEC from the 1998 and 2002 WHO studies. Data from the second study has already been given in Q 10.8. The first was a randomized comparison after single exposure of the combined (Yuzpe) versus the LNG-only method. Note the greater efficacy of early presentation within the 72 h, for both methods. Indeed, WHO stated from that database (FFP Guidance) that each 12-h delay raised the pregnancy risk by almost 50%. But it was clear

that the Yuzpe method worked less well and it should now therefore only be used if POEC in some form is not available.

10.14 Should one be prepared to withhold EC treatment?

This can often be unwise. As the FFP Guidance says, 'there is no time in the menstrual cycle when there is no risk of pregnancy following unprotected sexual intercourse (UPSI)'. As discussed at some length in *Q 2.13ff*, there is a fertile window of about 8 days, beginning about 7 days before the date of ovulation, but no woman can know when in a given cycle she will ovulate. The probability of conception in the first 3 days of the cycle appears to be negligible, but after taking an accurate menstrual and complete coital history the decision to treat depends on many factors, not least the amount of anxiety present.

The treatment is very safe, if not entirely risk free, so in the words of the FFP Guidance 2003 'if a woman is very anxious and wishes to use EC ... where the risk of pregnancy is assessed as very low, this may be appropriate after counselling'.

In future it might be possible to discover, simply and accurately in the clinic, what stage of the menstrual cycle the woman has reached. At present, although treatment is not always indicated, it is not easy to be sure that ovulation will not occur on an atypical day in that particular cycle. Your patient could be having an amazingly short, or long, menstrual cycle out of the blue.

So when in doubt, in the normal cycle, treat. When pills have been missed in the pill cycle, on the other hand, this treatment is much less often indicated (*see Q 10.23*).

10.15 What are the time limits for successful treatment?

1 *The IUD method*: the time limit of 5 days relates either to 120 h after the first episode of UPSI at any time in the cycle *or* after the most likely expected day of ovulation, i.e. expected date of next menses, subtract 14 days and add 5. This is calculated in good faith from the menstrual data given by the woman and applies irrespective of the number of earlier acts of unprotected intercourse. Five days is well within the time limits from intercourse to implantation, according to the consensus of medical opinion. It will not be construed in law as possibly procuring an abortion. My view is that, depending on the woman's own views about the ethics of the situation, the calculation should be based on the shortest likely cycle. This is strengthened by a judgement that suggests some leeway: in the case of Regina *v.* Dhingra, 24 January 1991, Mr Justice Wright did not convict a GP accused of illegal abortion achieved by inserting an IUD 11 days after intercourse because it was day 18 and thus prior to implantation:

I further hold, in accordance with the uncontroverted evidence that I have heard, that a pregnancy cannot come into existence until the fertilized ovum has become implanted in the womb, and that stage is not reached until, at the earliest, the 20th day of a normal 28-day cycle, and, in all probability, until the next period is missed.

2   *Single act of intercourse*: if this was after calculated ovulation, the copper IUD method can be inserted (if indicated at all) up to 5 days after that act or earliest unprotected act. But exposure once only at, say, day $x - 4$, before ovulation occurring on day x, allows treatment at $x + 5$ days (follows from (1), above).

3   *The Yuzpe and POEC methods*: there is an increase in the failure rate if treatment is initiated more than 72 h after exposure. But given the new evidence from the WHO 2002 study, incomplete though it is, the method is usable up to 120 h in selected cases (*see Q 10.9*).

10.16 Is it always preferable to treat at the earliest possible moment?

1   *The IUD method*: this is so effective that delay (any time up to 5 days after ovulation) is unlikely to lead to failure. This can be helpful in practice, if the facilities are not present for IUD insertion where and when the woman first presents (e.g. in a pharmacy or some GP surgeries). Referral to an appropriate session a day or two later might be well within the time limit (*see Q 10.38*).

2   *The hormonal methods, specifically POEC*: given the WHO data (*see Q 10.6*), it is best practice to start treatment as soon as the woman presents. But there remains some flexibility of dosing, according to the circumstances of presentation and the woman's own views (*see Q 10.8*).

10.17 What reasons can account for 'failure' of POEC

1   Unasked-about or unadmitted other exposure earlier in the cycle. It is essential always to question each woman most closely about the possibility of inadequate contraception earlier than the index event.

2   Treatment initiated more than 72 h after first UPSI – or late in the cycle, when it has lost the chance to interfere with fertilization.

3   Vomiting within 2 h of tablet-taking (*see Q 10.25*). This is an obvious efficacy as well as comfort advantage of POEC in contrast to the old Yuzpe method. In practice it is a relatively rare cause of failure. Some authorities have argued that there is no need to replace the second two tablets if they are vomited back because the occurrence of vomiting implies a particularly strong pharmacological effect. There are no data to support or refute this view. Women should be instructed to contact the clinician for consideration of some action, particularly in a high pregnancy-risk case. Such action could be the provision of further tablets along with an antiemetic (*see Q 10.26*) or more rarely the insertion of an IUD.

4   Non-compliance leading to inadequate dosage. For this reason, given the data of the WHO 2002 Study, the FFP Guidance advises that clinicians can sometimes prefer to see the whole POEC dose swallowed in their presence.

5   Unprotected intercourse subsequent to the treatment, which might simply postpone ovulation (*see Q 10.17*). In the WHO 2002 study, after treatment within 5 days of a single UPSI, for the POEC and single-dose LNG groups combined, the conception rate was 6.6% among those who had unprotected sex between treatment and the expected menses but only 1.5% in those who claimed abstinence during that time.

6   In the real world, this raises the important question of 'quick start': should a planned long-term method, such as the COC or injectable, more often than currently, be rightly started immediately after the emergency method (*see Q 10.42*)?

Points (1) and (5) are probably more common explanations than true method failures.

10.18 What are the risks if the EC treatment fails? What about ectopic pregnancy?

This is a vitally important aspect of counselling, dealt with here and in *Qs 10.19 and 10.20*. Ectopic pregnancy should be mentioned. Whenever any of the methods operate at the uterine level, if the woman has pre-existing tubal damage (known or unknown), tubal implantation will clearly not be prevented. In other words, she will get her ectopic whether she has EC or not.

Additionally, there is the small possibility that the hormonal methods might interfere with tubal transport. This is disputed and, I would say, unlikely to be important, given only one ectopic in 2712 women treated with either of the two LNG regimens in WHO 2002.

Actually, all the methods reduce the chance of fertilization, so the overall number of ectopics should be reduced, even if the percentage among the pregnancies goes up (*see Q 9.30*).

In practice, any woman presenting for EC might have tubal damage and, because she will be at risk with or without treatment, it is certainly safest to warn her to seek prompt advice if any pelvic pain occurs.

10.19 If the pregnancy is in the uterus, will it be harmed in any way (hormonal methods)?

A small teratogenic risk cannot be ruled out because insufficient pregnancies have gone to term after hormonal EC treatment failure, especially with POEC. In a series collected in the early 1990s by the UK National Association of Family Planning Doctors/Faculty of FP&RHC, there were 178 full-term pregnancies whose outcome was known following the previous (Yuzpe) EC therapy, which did of course contain the same progestogen LNG (along with EE). Reassuringly, the rate of and distribution of abnormalities was no different from what would be expected in a normal population, delivering without the Yuzpe EC therapy (Cardy, personal communication). Similarly, spontaneous reports to drug regulatory authorities after POEC do not suggest any consistent teratogenic effect.

Moreover, even if there were a potential adverse effect, exposure will be negligible if the hormonal methods are correctly used, and very little if any of the artificial hormone(s) could reach the blastocyst via the uterine secretions, because it is not yet implanted. Also:

1 The blastocyst is very resistant to partial damage by noxious agents. Research in animals suggests that it is either destroyed or else, because its cells are 'totipotent', it can recover and develop entirely normally.

2 It is very much accepted clinical practice for women to continue to full term when they have taken the combined or progestogen-only pill for several weeks during organogenesis: a more critical time, and there would also be more exposure (see (1) above). Yet meta-analyses and registers of fetal abnormality have failed even in those circumstances to show any significant increase in major fetal abnormalities.

In practice, the woman can be told:

The risk of a pregnancy being harmed is believed to be extremely small, less than that when the ordinary pill is inadvertently taken in early pregnancy – but no one can ever be guaranteed or promised a normal baby (1 in 50 have an important birth defect). Research so far, looking at babies born after failure of the emergency pill, has not proved any harmful effects. The risk is so low that after failed EC an abortion should never be recommended solely on fetal grounds.

The circumstances of the failed postcoital conception mean that, in practice, most women request a therapeutic abortion. If a woman wishes to continue to full term, very detailed records should be kept, documenting that she has fully understood the italicized statement above.

10.20 What about failure of the copper IUD method?

In the ultra-rare event of continuing pregnancy following EC insertion of an IUD, management should normally include removal of the device after a preliminary ultrasound scan, as discussed in *Q 9.24* (*see also Qs 10.37 and 10.40*).

INDICATIONS AND ADVANTAGES OF POSTCOITAL CONTRACEPTION

10.21 What are the advantages of EC contraception?

1 It provides a way of escape from an unwanted pregnancy at a time of high motivation after (for whatever reason) unprotected intercourse has taken place.

2   By definition, it is non-intercourse-related.

3   All three methods are effective; the copper IUD most.

4   The methods can be applied well after exposure to the risk with a good chance of success: up to 5 days (now) after a single (earliest) UPSI if the hormone method is used and, in an extreme case, if an IUD is inserted up to 12 days (after exposure on, say, day 7 of a 28-day cycle).

5   The methods are very safe, although sharing the potential hazards of hormonal/intrauterine contraception respectively. No deaths have been reported.

6   Presentation for the EC treatment gives a welcome opportunity to discuss future contraception; in the case of the IUD, solving the woman's immediate problem can also provide for her long-term needs.

7   The method is under a woman's control (i.e. its use cannot be prevented by her partner, if she can find a sympathetic provider).

8   The method can be prescribed in advance in many cases, for example, a young woman about to travel abroad and anxious about rape or other circumstances of unprotected intercourse in foreign parts.

> However, the present hormonal methods are not yet advised for regular ongoing use, for several reasons (*see Q 10.47*).

10.22 What are the indications for the treatment?

On presentation, depending on time of the cycle that exposure took place (*see Q 10.14*), whenever the clinician feels that the small risks of the method are outweighed by the risks of pregnancy and other relevant factors such as the woman's level of anxiety.

10.23 How do women present for treatment?

In the WHO 2002 study, 52% presented reporting that no contraception had been used, and 44% that there had been a condom failure. Outside of a research environment these would still be by far the most common groups, but there are numerous smaller presentation categories to consider:

NO METHOD USED

1   'Moonlight and roses' summarizes the most common presentation in this category, where intercourse was consensual but unpremeditated. It is often with a new partner, especially first-time-ever intercourse or extramarital affairs (e.g. where the husband has had a vasectomy). Or there could have been an unexpected reconciliation with an ex-partner. Even today, and worldwide, far too few men consider that birth control is any of their business whatsoever.

2 Intercourse under the influence of alcohol or drugs.

3 Total misunderstanding of the 'safe period' approach, or disregard of the mucus signs (or red light of Persona™ (*see Qs 2.28–2.29 and 10.34(7)*): these likewise equate to no method used.

4 Special situations:

  (a) Rape and sexual assault: here, counselling and management must be even more sensitive than usual and continuing emotional support is likely to be required. Involvement of the nearest Rape Crisis Centre and the local police force may be necessary. Avoid destroying forensic evidence if an accusation is to be made, and arrange tests and prophylaxis (and follow-up) for STIs.

  (b) Incest.

  (c) Women with learning disorders (taken advantage of).

  (d) Recent use of teratogens: drugs, or live vaccine such as polio or yellow fever.

CONTRACEPTIVE FAILURE (OF THE METHOD OR OF ITS USE)

5 The most common category here is the split or slipped condom. In a study from the West Midlands no fewer than 48 out of 80 women reported a broken sheath. In more than one case a fragment of rubber was retrieved from the upper vagina, proving that not all such reports are fictions to appear respectable in the eyes of the provider.

In such cases, always discuss whether the (rubber) condom might have been exposed to any mineral or vegetable oil (*see Q 3.21*).

6 Complete or partial expulsion of an IUD or IUS, identified midcycle – or where midcycle removal of the device is deemed necessary (should be rare, *see Q 9.14*). Here, careful reinsertion of another IUD is preferable, especially if there has been repeated intercourse since the last menstrual period. But occasionally POEC might be preferred.

7 If there has been recent intercourse and deliberate removal of an IUD at midcycle is essential as part of therapy for infection (*see Q 9.14*).

8 Errors of cap use, e.g. the discovery after intercourse that it was in the anterior fornix; or its too-early removal.

9 *Gross prolongation of the pill-free week in a COC user*: normally through the pill cycle, when pills are missed, the woman should simply follow the advice of *Q 5.17 and Table 5.3*. However, if intercourse has occurred during the pill-free week and it has been extended to more than 8 days, or the equivalent, meaning two or more pills missed during the first 7 days of a new pack: the FFP Guidance recommends hormonal EC treatment, followed by return to pill taking within no more than 12 h;

and also the use of a condom for the next 7 days (*see Qs 5.15–5.25 esp. Q 5.24*). *What about midcycle or end-of-pill-cycle omissions?*

(a) Extra hormonal EC treatment is usually redundant for midcycle pill omissions, provided at least seven tablets were correctly taken; although the Faculty of FP&RHC suggests it be given empirically if four or more tablets were missed. (WHO would only consider this for five or more missed, *Q 5.18*).

(b) At the end of the pill cycle the standard advice to run on to the next pack will nearly always make the woman contraceptively even safer than usual: having only had 'her own' PFI. However, the history of missed pills (e.g. through a severe vomiting attack) might sometimes not emerge until *after the next PFI has already been taken on top*: and this does justify proceeding as above (*see also Q 5.24*).

(c) FFP Guidance is also that POEC would be indicated if pills were 'effectively' missed either side of, and thereby lengthening, the PFI, through inadequate additional contraception or UPSI during and for 28 days after use of liver-enzyme inducers (*see Q 5.40*).

10 In a POP-user:

(a) Sexual exposure: any time from the first missed tablet (by 3 h) through until the mucus effect is expected to be restored after retaking it for 48 h, justifies hormone EC treatment, followed by condom use until pills have been taken correctly for a minimum of 2 days; but not during full lactation (*see Q 7.23*).

(b) If there has been a contraceptive accident or UPSI during or in the 28 days following, use of liver enzyme inducers (*see Q 5.34ff*).

11 In a DMPA user: here, the FFP Guidance is to give this only when it is more than 14 weeks since the previous injection. I prefer the more conservative protocol that first uses this at 13 weeks (*see Qs 8.53–8.54*).

12 In a user of Implanon™: inadequate additional contraception or UPSI during and for 28 days after use of liver-enzyme inducers.

13 Other contraceptive accidents involving, for example, spermicides or unsuccessful withdrawal.

DISADVANTAGES OF POSTCOITAL CONTRACEPTION

10.24 What are the disadvantages?

THE HORMONAL METHODS (NOW JUST POEC)

1 Nausea, and vomiting (*see also Q 10.27*).

2 Failure rate, especially if the woman tries to use it frequently as her main long term method.

3 Contraindications: very few (*see Q 10.28*). There is no age limit.

4 Further unprotected intercourse following therapy must be avoided, in case of postponement of ovulation (*see Q 10.7*).
5 The next menses are sometimes be delayed beyond 7 days – in 5% of POEC users according to WHO 2002 (*see Q 10.44*).
6 Interacting drugs must be allowed for (*see Q 10.30*).

COPPER IUD

1 A 'surgical' procedure is involved, when what the woman is primarily requesting is a quick medical 'fix it'.

2 Pain might be caused to the woman at insertion or subsequently.
3 Risk of causing or exacerbating pelvic inflammatory disease (PID). Where the method must be used and the risk is judged high from a carefully taken sexual history, for whatever reason (including exposure through rape), then after the relevant tests – appreciating that the latter cannot identify *Chlamydia* for a minimum of 5 days after first exposure – antibiotic cover should be given (*see Qs 9.58, 9.59, 10.38*). And removal after the next menses might sometimes be best, after the woman is established on a more appropriate long-term method.
4 There is a risk of causing all the other known complications of IUDs, because these are so often insertion-related (*see Qs 9.21, 9.22, 9.100*).

10.25 What is the incidence of nausea and vomiting after the currently used hormonal methods?

In the WHO studies the incidence of these symptoms was as shown in Table 10.3. It is interesting that, for POEC, the WHO 2002 study results were different from those in 1998. But it is difficult to interpret this difference because there were very large variations between the study centres in 2002: for example, nausea within 7 days of treatment was reported by only 2% in New Delhi but by 28% in Manchester!

The 2002 rate of vomiting (call it under 2%) seems a more accurate estimate than 5%, based on our clinical experience at the Margaret Pyke Centre.

TABLE 10.3 The incidence of nausea and vomiting after hormonal EC methods (WHO trials)			
Study year	**1998**	**1998**	**2002**
Nausea	Yuzpe 50.5%	POEC 23.1%	POEC 15%
Vomiting	Yuzpe 18.8%	POEC 5.6%	POEC 1.4%

10.26 What can be done to minimize the nausea/vomiting problem? Should one give antiemetics?

1 In the first place, forewarned is forearmed.
2 Where the timing of intercourse and presentation permit, the second dose should be followed by sleep if possible.
3 With respect to possible use of an antiemetic, domperidone maleate 10 mg with each dose is now recommended because it does not readily cross the blood–brain barrier or cause extrapyramidal side-effects. But nausea and vomiting are so much rarer with POEC than the old Yuzpe method (*see* Q 10.25) that at the Margaret Pyke Centre, antiemetic treatment is given selectively, not routinely:
   (a) where there is a history of vomiting in the past following POEC, or
   (b) along with second dosing in the current cycle when vomiting occurred within 2 h.

10.27 What other symptoms are associated with EC treatment?

 'Fatigue' was reported by about 15% of all groups in the WHO studies. Fairly commonly reported is breast tenderness, plus a range of other symptoms including dizziness, headaches, eye symptoms, etc. The association with therapy is not necessarily causal.

A few women report a 'withdrawal bleed' following treatment even with POEC, and the woman should be instructed not to assume that this is her next period (unless she was treated very late in the cycle), but to take advice.

PATIENT SELECTION AND CHOICE OF METHOD

10.28 What are the absolute contraindications (WHO 4) to EC contraception?

WHO says there are none, and I (almost) agree:

ALL METHODS

1 *Pregnancy*: WHO states there is no known harm from EC to the fetus, but every effort should be made to avoid exposure by taking a careful history, and, where indicated, doing the most sensitive pregnancy test available.
2 *Severe allergy to a constituent*: i.e. LNG or EE or an excipient in the tablets, or to copper (*see* Q 9.88). A dubious history, or moderate allergy, is WHO 3.
3 *Patient's ethical objection to a method possibly operating after fertilization*: this should not always be presumed absent because she has presented. Note also that her concern might not apply if she presents at risk early in the cycle, when the method is so likely to work by a prefertilization mechanism.

HORMONAL METHODS: POEC

1 *Acute porphyria*, with past attack (WHO 4): predisposition alone is WHO 3 (*see Qs 6.42 and 6.43*); other porphyrias are WHO 3 or 2.
2 *Severe liver disease* with abnormal function tests (usually WHO 3).

There is no upper nor lower age limit (given sufficient risk of conception).

NON-HORMONAL METHOD: IUDS

In addition to the three applicable absolute (WHO 4) contraindications listed above, the majority of both the temporary and permanent absolute contraindications listed in *Qs 9.85–9.87* would also apply. However, it is acceptable practice in selected cases to insert a copper IUD with screening and full antibiotic cover (*see Q 10.24*) when PID has not been excluded; or in women at high risk (especially after rape).

If the IUD method is thought inappropriate for long-term use (e.g. in a nullipara who has had a previous ectopic pregnancy), it can always be removed after the next period when she is on a method such as DMPA.

10.29 What are not contraindications to the use of POEC?

1 Presentation *more than 72 h after unprotected intercourse*: this is an option, discussed above (*see Qs 10.9 and 10.10*).
2 *Previous ectopic pregnancy* (*see Q 10.18*).
3 *Postpartum*: if an ovulation risk exists, which might be negligible if the LAM criteria apply (*see Q 2.36*). POEC is also usable (WHO 2) if hCG is persistent following trophoblastic disease (*see Q 5.77*).
4 *Lactation*: the woman can also be reassured that POEC should not impair this. She might be concerned to avoid the vanishingly small but unquantified risk through the artificial hormones entering her breast milk. This can usually be done without prejudicing lactation by expressing the breast milk and bottlefeeding the infant for 24 h.
5 *Current breast cancer*: this is WHO 2, for such short term use.

10.30 What if a woman taking an enzyme-inducing drug (which could be by her own supply of St John's wort) should require hormonal emergency contraception?

See Qs 5.34–5.36 for a full discussion of this important question in relation to regular use of the COC. The solution here, in the Faculty Guidance of 2003, is simply to increase the dose of either method by 50%: two tablets (1.5 g) of Levonelle™ stat followed by one 12 h later, or three tablets at once. The woman should also be advised of the alternative choice of an IUD.

10.31 What if she is on a non-enzyme-inducing antibiotic?

There is not even a theoretical problem (*see Qs 5.34 and 5.35*) with POEC, like all progestogen-only methods.

10.32 Can other drugs interact with POEC?

Concern has been raised in respect to warfarin (FFP Guidance): the anticoagulant effect might be altered, more probably increased so the woman should be warned and advised to have her INR test carefully checked, initially 3 days after the treatment.

10.33 What are the relative contraindications to EC IUD insertion?

1 All the relative contraindications listed in *Q 9.87* might apply if it is intended that the method will be used long term, but some (e.g. history of dysmenorrhoea or menorrhagia) are irrelevant to the very short-term option, just until the time of the next period with initiation of a different long-term method thereafter (*see also Q 10.28*).

2 Past ectopic pregnancy: even in nulliparae this is only a weak relative contraindication (WHO 2) to very short-term use in selected cases (*see Q 10.18*) – and only WHO 2 for long-term use of banded copper IUDs (*see Q 9.32*).

10.34 As the majority of women presenting for EC prefer and expect oral treatment, when should the intrauterine method be offered instead?

As the question implies, POEC is the normal first choice except where there are special reasons for a copper IUD. These are:

1 Where she desires the most effective available option, which this is (*see Q 10.13*). The FFP Guidance rightly makes a special point of this offer being made to all women attending for EC, even if they present within 72 h of UPSI, and especially when the assessed risk of conception is high (e.g. 20–30% periovulation).

2 The woman's desire to use the IUD as her long-term method: this could be a very good indication in a parous woman, for instance, and also some who are nulliparous (*see Q 9.19ff*). However, it is always permissible (and sometimes to be recommended) that the device is used purely to solve the immediate problem, and is removed at the next menses (this also means screening and often antibiotic cover, *see Q 10.38*).

3 Where there is an absolute contraindication to the progestogen (i.e. severe allergy, acute porphyria, very severe liver disease).

4 Where there has been multiple exposure, and the clinician inserts the device in good faith no more than 5 days after the most probable calculated ovulation date (*see Q 10.15* and below).

5 Where presentation is more than 72 h since a single episode of unprotected intercourse: the upper time limit any time in the cycle being 5 days – but it could be considerably longer so long as the calculation for the day of implantation (length of shortest likely cycle, subtract 14 and

add 5 days) does not mean giving the treatment might be given to an implanted pregnancy.

6 Rarely, after vomiting of the tablets when either the Yuzpe or POEC regimen was initially selected. IUD insertion is only indicated if the woman is a high pregnancy-risk case and if the vomiting occurs within 2 h of ingesting a dose, especially the first dose. Otherwise it is more usual to give additional tablets, perhaps along with an antiemetic (*see Q 10.26*).

7 Rarely, in a woman who has taken a risk but wants to go back to using Persona™ and does not wish to wait the added 2 months-plus after taking hormones before she can return to use of that method (*see Q 2.30*).

See also Q 10.38.

COUNSELLING AND MANAGEMENT AT THE FIRST VISIT

10.35 How important is counselling for EC?

1 The treatment is simple and very safe: POEC has almost no absolute contraindications. Obviously, if there has been a simple condom rupture or dislodgement occurring in a stable relationship, the woman will just want her EC in a non-judgemental way with minimum delay and hassle. The amount of emotional support she needs will be far less than in cases of rape or incest, although the availability of such support should always be clear. In every case without exception:

2 *Confidentiality must be real and must feel real, to every attender – most especially to young teenagers* (*see Qs 11.5, 11.11*).

3 Every woman needs information and clear instructions sympathetically given. In practice, much of the information can be conveyed by a good leaflet and the counselling – including on the crucial subject of future contraception – most appropriately delegated to a family planning-trained nurse, and often now commercially by a pharmacist.

With Patient Group Directions, nurses (including school nurses) and pharmacists have been empowered to take the whole emergency contraception workload, which with good training they often do better than doctors – and this can also assist access for young women who feel they cannot afford the charge for normal over-the-counter provision by pharmacists. The FFP Guidance rightly stresses the importance of managed clinical care pathways to ensure 'joined-up' working between different service providers.

10.36 In summary, what aspects should be covered in taking the medical history?

1 Date of the last menstrual period, and whether it was in any way abnormal.

2 Details of the patient's normal menstrual cycles: shortest, longest and most usual lengths.

3 The calculated date of ovulation.

4 The day(s) in the cycle of all unprotected intercourse.

5 The number of hours since the first episode of unprotected intercourse.

6 The current method of contraception: Persona™ and LAM are particularly relevant (*see Qs 10.29(3) and 10.34*). In pill-takers who have missed pills, the timing relative to the PFI is critical (*see Q 10.23(9)*).

7 Any contraindications (from the history), use of any enzyme inducers (including St John's wort, *see Q 10.30*), all risk factors for the COC (because it might be going to be used in future), and any past PID or ectopic pregnancy.

8 Take a sexual history in every case (*see Q 1.14*) and 'offer STI screening to *all* [my emphasis] those attending for EC' (FFP Guidance). Depending on the case this might mean referral to a GUM department, or perhaps a *Chlamydia* test on site.

It should be stressed to the woman that the whole 'contract' to give this kind of treatment depends on utmost mutual good faith and honesty, especially concerning the menstrual/coital history.

10.37 What are the ten main points to cover in counselling for emergency contraception?

1 Assess the menstrual and coital history and sexual history as in *Q 10.36*, and hence whether any treatment is necessary. Offer the recommended STI screen.

2 Discuss, backed by a good leaflet, the methods available and their mode of action, medical risks and side-effects.

3 The failure rate of each method, and the implications, i.e. the IUD being the most effective option, ectopic pregnancy risk (*see Qs 10.18 and 10.29*) and to return if she experiences any pain.

4 Explore her attitudes to possible failure of the regimen and continuance of the pregnancy: the small risk of fetal abnormality, which could happen although the method applied preimplantation is most unlikely to be causative (*see Q 10.19*).

5 Discuss the consequential importance of follow-up. Suggest that she brings an early morning urine sample if her next period is surprisingly light or absent.

6 *Above all*: let her make her own final decision – about whether to use EC treatment, and which method – when the above have been discussed.

7 If a hormonal method is selected, advise her to telephone the clinic or surgery for advice if she vomits within 2 h of either dose. Consider domperidone, based mainly on past history (*see Q 10.26*).

8 Discuss contraception for the rest of the current cycle (*see Q 10.7*): this is not a problem if the IUD is used.

9 Discuss long-term contraception. *See Q 10.41* for the advice to be given if the combined pill is selected.

10 Keep an accurate record, written at the time, dated and signed, especially (and see *Appendix A*) if the use will be unlicensed (e.g. use of POEC more than once per cycle).

10.38 What is different about insertion of a copper IUD as an emergency in this way rather than electively?

First, it is more like an elective insertion than some imagine, i.e. usually the 'emergency' pressure is off because there are several days until it would be 5 days after ovulation. So the actual procedure can and often should be done later in the day or the week, at a more convenient time and place – for the woman as well as the service.

Using the terminology of the Sexual Health Strategy (2001), if she presents at a Level 1 service in primary care there should be a well-organized local referral channel to the specialist Level 2 service practitioner or clinic. However, the Faculty Guidance makes two wise suggestions:

1 to give POEC as a 'holding manoeuvre' while waiting for the fitting. The FFP says: 'Should she fail to re-attend the woman has had the benefit of oral EC'. FFP recommends this only 'if within 72 hours of the UPSI', but I would be happy to extend that to 120 h, based on the WHO 2002 study (*see Q 10.9*).

2 According to FFP, 'Ideally an emergency IUD should be fitted at first presentation': implying she has presented at a Level 2 service. Although even then she could have a sandwich and cup of coffee, and return for her premed with a PGSI, possibly at the end of the surgery.

The medical eligibility criteria are similar to routine IUD insertions *except* that nulliparity, young age, risk status for STIs and previous ectopic pregnancy are all just reasons for caution in such short-term use, balanced by risks of a likely pregnancy without the treatment. There can often be a plan to remove the IUD altogether when the woman is established on what might be a more appropriate long-term method.

If a carefully taken sexual history reveals the woman to be in a high-risk group – as it very often will among those attending for EC (FFP Guidance says as much), it is recommended, after screening at least for *Chlamydia*, to give either azithromycin 1 g stat or doxycycline 200 mg twice daily for 7 days and recommend abstinence pending results (FFP Guidance).

However, if the woman is not in a high-risk group (monogamous, no recent partner change, condom accident) 'the use of prophylactic antibiotics *routinely* [my emphasis] at the time of emergency IUD insertion cannot be recommended' (FFP Guidance). This whole issue of whether to give antibiotic cover at IUD insertion is discussed in some depth in and before Q 9.59.

After the insertion, warn about any excessive pain or other manifestations of PID in the days ahead (*see* Q 9.60).

The Faculty recommends an IUD bearing at least 300 mm surface area of copper (FFP Guidance). If the woman is at all likely to become a long-term user I would favour more specifically the only banded IUDs available: the T-Safe Cu 380A™ where possible or GyneFIX™ if the uterus is small or distorted. Otherwise, a Flexi T-300™ is easy to fit, and cheap.

10.39 Should these women always be examined vaginally?

This is obviously mandatory to allow safe assessment for and insertion of a copper IUD. But otherwise in my view the answer is normally 'no'; the anxiety so caused, for example, to a young teenager presenting after her first-ever sexual experience rules it out. But there might be a clinical or screening indication:

1   To exclude a concealed (advanced) clinical pregnancy.
2   To screen opportunistically, especially for *Chlamydia*, or more comprehensively at a GUM department, according to need. EC attenders under 30 are a high-risk group (FFP Guidance). Pelvic tenderness or a purulent discharge suggestive of active infection might also be discovered.
3   Sometimes a baseline can be usefully established, e.g. if an irregular outline of the uterus is noted (suggesting small fibroids), this will assist a follow-up examination.

Examination at follow-up is similarly only rarely required, on clinical grounds (*see* Q 10.45).

10.40 Should the woman be asked to sign any type of consent form?

This is deemed unnecessary, even for emergency IUD insertion, provided accurate contemporaneous records are kept, the clinician asserting that the woman gave verbal informed consent. It is most helpful to supplement the counselling including about the chosen method for the future with an appropriate leaflet, such as that produced by the FPA (*see* Q 5.106).

FOLLOW-UP

10.41 If the woman selects an oral contraceptive subsequent to EC treatment, when should she take the first tablet?

It is usual for both the COC and the POP to be commenced on the first day of the next menses. However, there is rarely a light (and not relevant) withdrawal bleed just after the POEC hormones, and a light 'threatened abortion' loss might also occur very early in pregnancy. The FFP Guidance states the woman should be advised about menstrual irregularity (*see Q 10.44*).

It has been practice at the Margaret Pyke Centre, therefore, that both the COC and POP should be started when the woman is convinced that the flow is within her own normal range, commonly on the second day rather than the first. This slight delay still allows the woman not to be required to use extra contraceptive precautions (*see Qs 5.49, Table 5.4, Q 7.25 and Table 7.4*).

It is important, however, to ensure that, even if in doubt about her period, she does start the COC or POP before day 3 and then take advice – or if later uses condoms additionally for 7 days.

10.42 Might she be instructed to start the combined pill or injectable immediately after PC treatment?

This 'quick start' approach might indeed be acceptable in selected cases. There is a medicolegal concern: if the woman were to conceive, and the baby have an important fetal abnormality (as occurs in 2% of cases), a legal claim that the abnormality was caused by the extra packet of combined pills being given after implantation might be submitted. It would, of course, be highly unlikely that such an abnormality was truly caused by the COC (*see Q 6.46*) or injectable. However, it would be even more unlikely that teratogenesis would follow the POEC regimen alone, given, as it should only be, preimplantation (*see Q 10.19*).

There are certain circumstances in which this might be acceptable management, provided there has been a thorough and documented discussion of all the implications with the woman concerned – especially in a case where the risk of EC treatment failing is considered to be particularly low and the risk of conception through poor condom use before the next period is high.

A proper RCT is under way at the Margaret Pyke Centre, comparing immediate starting of the COC versus starting at the next menses! *See also Q 10.23(9) for a form of 'quick start' that is already normal practice: if the PFI has been lengthened an immediate (re-) start of the COC is advised.*

10.43 Can POEC be given more than once in a given cycle, if a woman has already received EC treatment and reports further exposure?

Yes. Because in clinical practice we cannot be sure when ovulation occurs, and it might have been postponed by the earlier treatment, it might well be right to represcribe, for a second or even a third time. The same dose of LNG as Postinor™ was used in Hungary and elsewhere for many years, with a recommendation to use it postcoitally up to four times per month. The failure rate was reported as 0.8% for each treatment cycle (FFP Guidance) along with irregular bleeding problems, and women should be so counselled.

The main problem when additional dosing is clinically indicated is attempting to exclude the possibility of early conception already present (implantation having already occurred through exposure earlier in the cycle). Irregular bleeding might also follow. And once again this is an unlicensed use (see *Appendix A*).

10.44 What is the usual time of onset of the next period after EC treatment?

In the WHO 2002 study, over half of the subjects had their next menses on the expected day plus or minus 2 days and all but 5% of the non-conceivers in the two LNG groups came on early or no later than 7 days late.

It is believed that late onset is more likely when treatment was early enough in the cycle to postpone ovulation. When it acts to block fertilization, the method tends to bring the next period on early, whether or not there is withdrawal bleeding immediately after the treatment (the latter being quite uncommon). It is useful to be able to tell the woman that her next period is likely to be on time or early, so she will not need to be in suspense for too long.

No obvious impact on cycle length has been reported following postcoital IUD insertion.

10.45 How important is it to follow-up EC women after treatment?

A defined follow-up visit is essential after IUD insertion, normally set for about 6 weeks. But it is not now insisted on after hormonal EC if the next period comes on normally. What matters is that the woman clearly understands that she can return without an appointment:

- If she has any worrying symptoms, particularly pain or irregular bleeding.
- If her menses are delayed by more than 7 days (*see Q 10.44*). A pregnancy test might then be necessary and, if there is any clinical doubt, especially concerning an ectopic, a pelvic examination and possible referral.
- As needed to continue her ongoing contraceptive care – in all cases if she has been fitted with a copper IUD. Beware of the occasional pressure with the latter to 'leave well alone' in circumstances in which the IUD is a poor choice for long-term use (*see Qs 9.84–9.87 and 10.28*). The original and better plan to transfer to another method (such as DMPA) might need to be encouraged.

10.46 What if the method does fail?

Good pregnancy counselling should follow. After POEC there should be no real difference in the content of this counselling from that when any other method of birth control has failed (see the full discussion in Q 10.19).

Unless the woman is having a termination, if she is pregnant with an IUD in position the device should normally be gently removed (see Qs 9.24 and 9.25).

10.47 Should the POEC method be provided in advance of need?

Yes, indeed this is WHO 1 in the WHO's eligibility criteria book (WHO 2000). As the FFP Guidance reports and references, RCTs have shown that, for selected women, advance supply is safe. It can reduce the rate of unintended pregnancies, is used correctly by the majority of women, does not reduce the use of other contraceptive methods and even (perhaps surprisingly) is not associated with an increase in unprotected sex.

If provided ahead of need, women need reminding that even with very early use of the POEC method after UPSI, a lunar-monthly failure rate of, say, 0.4% would mean an annual failure rate of over 5%. However, given that a sizeable group of women requesting advance prescribing might have intercourse once a month or less, on a rather unpredictable basis, increasing availability in this way should reduce the unacceptable continuing high rate of unplanned pregnancies.

10.48 So what is your view on EC being now available additionally over the counter?

I consider that the advantages of over-the-counter supply of EC definitely outweigh its risks. And given the answer to the last question, perhaps the time is right for the pharmacist simply to sell the product in advance of need and without all the detailed questioning required by Royal Pharmaceutical Society's Practice guidance (as referenced in Faculty Guidance). However, for best practice, pharmacists should offer:

1 Excellent user-friendly labelling/leaflet and a checklist of important information for the client.
2 Adequate privacy.
3 Easy local arrangements for transfer for the insertion of a copper IUD, as sometimes indicated.
4 Easy arrangements for long-term contraceptive follow-up (via clinic, or family doctor) and to investigate STIs as required.
5 Details of a parallel location for free NHS supply, for those who might not be able to afford the retail product (priced, in 2003, at a fairly steep £24).

6 Details of a 24-h telephone hot-line for clients' queries – NHS Direct now supplies this, and there is also the FPA's excellent service, accessed by telephone during working hours:

■ FPA UK: tel. 0845 310 1334, Monday to Friday 9 a.m. to 7 p.m.
■ FPA Scotland: tel. 0141 576 5088, Monday to Thursday 9 a.m. to 5 p.m., Friday 9 a.m. to 4.30 p.m.
■ FPA Northern Ireland: tel. 028 90 325 488 (Belfast) or 028 71 260 016 (Derry) Monday to Thursday 9 a.m. to 5 p.m., Friday 9 a.m. to 4.30 p.m.

10.49 What would be the features of an ideal future EC method?

These would be similar to those of any reversible birth control method (*see* Q 1.15), but the following aspects would require particular emphasis. The ideal EC treatment would:

1 be so effective each cycle that on a cumulative basis the annual rate of failures was less than 1/100 woman-years (*see* Q 10.47)
2 be effective for the remainder of each cycle as well as in relation to the particular act of intercourse
3 require only a single dose
4 have no contraindications (at all) – POEC gets very close
5 have a very low incidence of side-effects, whether dangerous or annoying (such as nausea)
6 cause no disturbance of the menstrual cycle
7 be free of teratogenic effects.

10.50 What are the prospects for the future of EC?

A really reliable postovulatory contraceptive agent with the features listed in Q 10.49, coupled with a simple and reliable method of determining whether the exposure had been before or after ovulation, would be a considerable advance. Indeed, in the distant future it might be possible for regular release of an EC agent (e.g. from an implant) to be actually triggered by a biological event such as the LH surge.

Another potential approach, although one fraught with ethical and legal difficulties, is the regular use of a postconceptional or contragestive agent to be administrated only when the woman is just overdue her period. Given average fertility, this approach would mean exposure to the potential systemic risks of the agent only on a few (four to six) occasions each year; but it would be out of order for many because it would be seen as a regular early abortion.

10.51 Specifically, what agents are being studied?

The greatest current interest is in progesterone receptor-blocking agents, such as mifepristone. In the third arm of the WHO 2002 trial, a single

10-mg dose was shown definitively to be as effective as either of the LNG regimens – indeed even more so when complete abstinence followed the treatment until the next menses. However, delayed ovulation with menses delay beyond 7 days in almost twice as many women as with POEC poses a real practical problem; so, given also its 'aura' as an abortifacient, I think mifepristone is unlikely to be marketed for EC.

Many would be particularly interested in a product, perhaps an implant, effective if applied up to the time of nidation, which went on to give ongoing long-term contraception thereafter (on the model of copper IUD insertion).

PATIENT QUESTIONS

QUESTIONS ASKED BY PROSPECTIVE USERS OF POSTCOITAL CONTRACEPTION

10.52   Is the 'emergency pill' the same as the 'morning after pill'?

Yes, it is. The reason for the new name is that the treatment (although most effective when started in the first 24 h) can be given much later than the morning after – at least 72 h, and sometimes after many days if the IUD method is chosen. So the old name was extremely misleading. It should be abandoned!

10.53   And isn't the emergency pill just the same as the contraceptive pill?

An out-of-date kind – still used abroad – did contain the same two hormones as in a combined pill; the current one Levonelle™ is the same single hormone as one of the POPs. But both are given in a different way, i.e. in two larger doses, 12 h apart, following intercourse.

10.54   If my sex life is erratic, why can I not be given pills in advance for use on a regular basis?

An answer to this common question is given in Q 10.47. There are some special reasons why it should not be used at all by some women, or why the alternative IUD method would be medically preferable (see Qs 10.28 and 10.34).

However, because the POEC pill method (Levonelle™) is so remarkably safe, and there is such an epidemic of unplanned pregnancies in many countries, I feel the benefits outweigh the risks of it being much more available, including through school nurses and over the counter, supervised by pharmacists (see Q 10.48).

10.55   I shall be travelling alone in the Far East and South America for the next 6 months. Could I take a supply of EC treatment for emergency use?

It could certainly be appropriate for you to be prescribed a supply in advance (*see Q 10.47*) but you might, alternatively, consider arranging a regular method like the pill or even an IUD, along with a good supply of condoms of course!

10.56   Can I wait a few hours for my own or the surgery's convenience or should I be treated just as soon as possible?

There should not be any undue delay; treatment in the first 24 h is best for the pill method (POEC). Certainly there is no need to disturb anyone within a few minutes or an hour of intercourse! See also *Q 10.8* regarding the timing of the second dose.

If the best method for you is going to be the IUD (*see Qs 10.61 and 10.34*), as *Q 10.38* points out, waiting at least for some hours is usually not a problem – it might even be recommended. If it will be on another day you would often be given POEC first as well.

10.57   Should I mention any earlier times when we made love (since my last period), when I attend for EC advice?

Yes, this is essential. The decisions as to whether to treat and how to treat successfully all depend on your being entirely forthcoming about every relevant fact. This also includes telling the pharmacist/nurse/doctor the correct date of your last period and how normal it was. The whole 'contract' between you and the healthcare professional depends on what is called 'utmost good faith'.

10.58   Will I need to be examined before EC treatment?

Usually not (*see Q 10.39*) unless – after discussion – you choose the IUD method.

10.59   Why might the practitioner or pharmacist tell me the EC treatment is not necessary?

The main reason might be that, after considering the time of the month and every other aspect, they judge that there is an almost-nil risk of you conceiving; and that this does not justify the (small) risks of the EC treatment. This is mainly only true when COC pills have been missed, especially in the middle or at the end of a packet – as explained in *Q 10.23*.

10.60   What should I do if I vomit within 2 h of either of my doses, especially if I actually bring back pills?

Take urgent advice. If there is a high risk of conception in your case, it might be right then to insert an IUD. But more usually it will be enough just to give you additional tablets with an antiemetic, or even no special treatment at all (*see Q 10.26*).

10.61   Why did the doctor/nurse recommend a copper IUD for me when I really wanted pills?

For one of the reasons in *Q 10.34*. Depending on you, this might be a good method to continue using long term, but remember that you can choose to have it removed after your next period if you then plan perhaps to transfer to another effective method such as the combined pill or an implant.

10.62   Why should I use another method of family planning between EC treatment and the start of my next period?

The reason is that sometimes the method might be working not by blocking the fertilized egg from establishing itself in your womb, but instead by blocking egg release. There is then a high risk of fertilizing that later egg if your partner does not use another method such as the condom.

10.63   Should I expect a period immediately after using EC pills?

A few women do get what is known as 'a withdrawal bleed' within a day or two of POEC treatment. This will not usually seem like a proper period and, unless you were due one so early, it is important to continue using the condom or any other effective method you were recommended to use, until you do have a definite period – or you might need to arrange follow-up at the surgery or clinic.

Fortunately, your proper period normally arrives either on time or a little early. It is still best that you keep your follow-up appointment(s), and this is even more vital if the next period is delayed or unexpectedly light.

10.64   For what reasons should I see the doctor sooner than arranged, following EC treatment?

The main reason would be because of any pain in your abdomen, because of the small risk of pregnancy outside the womb in your fallopian tube (*see Q 10.18*).

10.65   Does morning-after treatment cause an abortion?

No, not according to the modern view of when pregnancy starts (*see Q 10.3* and *Fig. 10.1*).

10.66   Must I have an abortion if EC treatment fails?

Not necessarily. It is thought that this treatment will not significantly increase the risk of an abnormal baby above the surprisingly high 2% risk that all women run. So the decision (always very difficult) about what to do about the unplanned pregnancy is really just the same as it would be if any other method of family planning were to fail (*see Q 10.19*).

The present and the future

CONTRACEPTION FOR THE OLDER WOMAN

THE FUTURE

This chapter includes much that is useful revision of the information elsewhere in the text. I am particularly indebted to Toni Belfield, Director of Information of the UK Family Planning Association (FPA). She has allowed me to use sections of her own text from an article in the *British Journal of Sexual Medicine*, but supplemented and much rearranged in this book's question-and-answer style. See also Belfield T 1999 in Kubba et al. *Contraception and Office Gynecology* London: Saunders.

11.1 What factors influence the observed great variability in the choices of contraceptive methods actually made by couples?

Please refer to *Fig. 11.1* and *Table 11.1*, along with *Tables 1.1* (p. 11) and *1.2* (p. 14).

The relative importance of the two main factors – maximum health safety as opposed to maximum effectiveness and independence from intercourse – and hence the appropriateness of different methods, varies greatly according to all the factors shown in Dr Christopher's 'factors wheel' (*Fig. 11.1* and see also *Appendix B*).

Choice, it seems, is seldom based on rational or objective information – the fact that a friend had a dreadful time with an IUD will weigh far more heavily than any amount of statistics that show this is not usually the case. It is also influenced by age and the particular stage of an individual couple's reproductive lifetime. Decisions are made at specific times:

- at the beginning of sexual experience
- after an accidental pregnancy or 'near miss'
- with life changes, e.g. a career change
- after a planned birth
- when there are problems with a particular method
- when the family is complete.

Initially, while the relationship is being established, a high degree of efficacy might be considered most important. However, if their sexual experience is infrequent or sporadic, male or female condoms may be ideal provided they are used correctly, especially as they have the bonus of some protection against sexually transmitted diseases (STIs).

For child spacing, less efficient methods with reduced health risk might well be preferred. Once the family is established but the couple are not sure whether it is yet complete, the IUD can have particular merit. These points are summarized in *Table 11.1*, which is derived from Table 15 of my book *The pill* and also looks forward to the near future.

This changing pattern of reproductive desire, in the couple's total life situation, places a big responsibility on the doctor or nurse to be themselves flexible and fully informed about the whole range of methods available. They

TABLE 11.1 The seven contraceptive ages of women

Age	Suggested method
0 Birth to puberty	No method required. Responsible sex and relationships education (SRE) is essential, *started by parents* and continuing through schooling
1 Puberty to marriage (or equivalent)	Either (a) a condom method, with emergency contraception back-up available; (b) the combined pill/near combined options (skin patch or ring)/Cerazette™/injectable/implant: always with a condom outside of mutual monogamy (or, one day an effective chemical virucide); or, if acceptable (c) abstinence until the final life-partner if found. The choice depends on factors like religious views, perceived risk of sexually transmitted diseases, the frequency of partner changes and of intercourse
2 Marriage (or equivalent) to first child	First choice probably a pill, but could be one of various patches/rings/injectables/implants followed by a fertility awareness method for some months before 'trying' for the first child
3 During breast-feeding	Either lactational amenorrhoea method (LAM) or any progestogen-only method or reversible male method with breastfeeding or a simple barrier method. Intrauterine device or system, male or female injectable or implant likely to be appropriate only if a long gap is expected between pregnancies
4 Family spacing after breastfeeding	Continue with any method started during 'age' 3, or shift to Cerazette™/the combined pill/injectable/implant from an old type progestogen-only pill for greater effectiveness. Later, a banded copper intrauterine device or system is progressively more appropriate, for a combination of the least long-term health hazards, efficacy and reversibility
5 After the (probable) last child	The first choice is an intrauterine device or system; other possibilities are any progestogen-only pill, or a combined method, if free of arterial or venous factors, or injectable/implant according to choice
6 Family complete, family growing up	First choice still as 5: banded copper IUD, or IUS if periods at all heavy or painful. Vasectomy would be generally preferable to female sterilization as more effective and easier to perform (Q 11.56ff)
7 Perimenopausal (no sterilization)	Contraceptive hormone replacement therapy will become more available (continuous combined methods being the norm, as trail-blazed by the intrauterine system plus oestrogen implant). It is important to recognize that, at this age, a weaker contraceptive (e.g. foam or sponge) may be fully effective when combined with very reduced fertility.

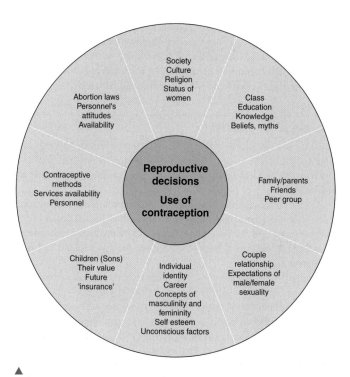

Fig. 11.1 Reproductive decisions – the factors wheel (courtesy Elphis Christopher).
Q 11.1, see also Appendix B.

must also be able and willing to spend time finding out what sort of person they are actually dealing with under the headings summarized in *Fig. 11.1*!

COMPLIANCE WITH CONTRACEPTIVE METHODS

11.2 Don't the words 'compliant' and 'non-compliant' sound rather 'bossy', and as though we prescribe and then everything else is the fault of those silly contraceptive-users?

Yes, but if we can ourselves agree not to mean anything of the sort, other words that are sometimes used – 'concordance' and 'adherence' – to me seem rather poor substitutes. What we are talking about is the user's responsibility to avoid user failure. More on the healthcare provider's responsibility follows later.

Regardless of whatever professional hat we wear, we are all also consumers when it comes to thinking about or using contraception, so our own experiences have the potential to make our counselling less objective than it should be. But how contraception is considered, discussed and, more importantly, delivered will determine just how well it is accepted and used.

11.3 How big is the problem?

This big: in a completely anonymous 1998 Sexual Health Matters survey, after a night on the town 1:5 young men admitted to sex that they now regretted, 1:7 had had unsafe sex and 1:10 were unable to remember if they had had sex!

Today, contraceptive choices and services are freely available, and research shows that people have the facts (in their heads) about contraception. Yet the behaviour that would be the logical outcome of that knowledge stubbornly refuses to follow! See the apocryphal story at the start of *Chapter 2*.

Young people deserve encouragement to make sexually responsible choices, which start with either having or not having sex – and their views should be sought on all matters that affect their sexual health. Abstinence is one of the valid choices but, in recent surveys, applies to less than half of all girls who were 16 at their last birthday (just 48% claimed to be virgins in study from the South-west of England in the 1990s, and only 12% by age 20). Given the potential emotional and psychosocial trauma of very early coitarche, quite apart from the risk of STIs and cervical neoplasia, this group (and the boys too) should receive our encouragement – as providers – to continue to resist peer-group pressure and to wait for 'Mr or Ms Right'. They should not be labelled a minority group because this has an implication of abnormality. Yet, if abstinence is fairly obviously the 'best', the best must not become the enemy of the good – which in the real world is to optimize the provision of sex and relationships education (SRE) and to provide totally confidential and appropriate reproductive and sexual health services.

Unintended pregnancy rates and requests for abortion remain persistently high. Although the under-16s achieve more publicity, older teenagers and women aged 20–25 are together responsible for far more unplanned pregnancies. A 1990s study of recent mothers by Anne Fleissig showed that, in the UK, as many as one in three of the last pregnancies was unplanned. In the same year, it was estimated in *Population Trends* that one in five clinical pregnancies ended in legal abortion. Cumulatively, about one woman in three in the UK now has at least one termination before the age of 30.

In another 1990s study of teenage mothers, 84% had no intention of becoming pregnant but were using no contraception when they conceived.

Although in some studies where there was good compliance, the COC has had failure rates of well below 1/100 woman-years (see *Table 1.2*, p. 14), in typical use failure rates of 3% are commonly reported, rising to up to 20% in inner city areas. Worldwide, it has been calculated that if – by improved pill taking – we could reduce the failure rate of this one method by 1%, at least 630 000 fewer women would have accidental pregnancies each year.

11.4 What is the most important single reason for unwanted conceptions?

Sex! But it has been well said that the biggest sex organ is the head! Other reasons then follow.

1 Sex is embarrassing: contraception is inextricably linked with emotional and sexual well-being and it is impossible to talk about contraception without addressing sexuality – the two are inseparable. Research shows that contraception continues to be a source of considerable embarrassment and anxiety for both men and women, and this has implications for its uptake and usage. It can have an inhibiting effect on people's willingness to seek information and advice from professionals.

2 Also, in Elphis Christopher's memorable phrase (see *Appendix B*), 'sex is hot, and contraception is cold'. And any method that is chosen is always 'the least worst method'! Snowden wrote in 1990 that whereas it can be argued that the prevention of pregnancy is beneficial, the use of contraception is not a pleasant experience for most people, which is a marked contrast to the sexual behaviour that prompts its need! Actual choice results from a negative process of 'seeking the least bad' among the options. The methods not chosen were even more disliked than the method chosen.

3 Sex is now – the possible problems resulting from sex seem unimportant. As we have seen, 'head' knowledge can be superb but still does not affect behaviour in the heat of the moment. The brain and the genitalia are not often used at the same time (see p. 21)!

Risk-taking and AIDS are not unlike risk-taking and pregnancy. Neither AIDS infection nor fertilization are certain, the gambler often survives, and the penalty is remote: 9 months in the case of pregnancy, maybe years in the case of AIDS.' (Malcolm Potts, 1988)

So, like safer sex the built-in problem of family planning is the 'planning bit'. This highlights the potential advantages of the postcoital methods. But their potential are not being realized. A 1992 study by Nigel Bruce of unplanned pregnancies in North London showed that more than half of those who could have sought such emergency help because they (a) knew about it and (b) knew there had been a contraceptive risk, did not do so! Asked why, the reason given amounted to that they 'had got away with it before'. So, strong in matters of sex is the gambling instinct! Plus inertia …

4   The early years of reproductive life are not that fertile, through anovulation. In the first year after the menarche 85% of cycles are anovular, but this falls to an average of 30% after 5 years. So young people's experience of 'getting away with it' in early years is likely to catch them out a little later, as their fertility peaks in the late teens and early 20s.

5   Finally, 'the fact that contraception has to do with sex seems to set up an environment where risks are exaggerated or misunderstood' (Malcolm Potts). So 'sex' even explains some of the risk-illiteracy of our clients about, say, the pill – ordinary, unprotected sex (and even the cigarette that follows) all seem so natural and safe by comparison!

11.5 In the many studies of compliance in developed countries, what background factors have been shown to correlate with non-use, poor use or early discontinuation of contraceptive methods?

Here is a list, longish but doubtless not complete, relating mainly to the COC:

■ Young, immature: after the very first years, youth also means optimum fertility, hence a greater likelihood of not getting away with any of the more frequent compliance errors. According to Jones and Forrest in 1989, failure rates of the pill in the first 12 months of use are more than five times higher in the under-20s than in the 35–44 age group.
■ Unmarried.
■ Nulliparous.
■ Early coitarche.
■ Multiple sexual partners.
■ Previous contraceptive failure/abortion.
■ Perception of low personal risk of conception (especially because of previous 'scares' that resolved).
■ Erratic daily timetable.
■ Cultural or religious opposition to birth control.
■ Poor social conditions.
■ Parents not married.
■ Lack of parental support.
■ Low evaluation of personal health.
■ Low educational attainment and goals.
■ Feelings of lack of personal self-worth and self-determination.
■ Feelings of fatalism (babies happen, rather like death, 'when your number comes up').

- Cigarette smoking (unplanned conception more likely, but in several studies of young teenagers also likely to start sexual activity younger).
- Alcohol: 'drink in – wits out!': 53% of 16–24-year-olds in a study in the South-west of England felt they were more likely to forget about the risk of pregnancy after drinking alcohol. The same applies to other drugs of addiction.
- Media 'scare stories' and misinformation/myths.
- Fear of side-effects.
- Experience of side-effects: above all, bleeding side-effects. Also other side-effects, perceived or real, especially weight gain, headaches, nausea, depression, breast tenderness, acne.
- Wrong or incomplete information (e.g. about missed or vomited pills).
- Poor service delivery/counselling/advice, particularly when combined with lack of assurance of confidentiality for the client. This is the (preventable) provider contribution to compliance problems (*see Qs 11.16 and 11.17*).

There is some considerable overlap between these risk factors, but more importantly and very relevantly in practice, there is synergism. Ensure more time for counselling when combinations of the above apply! See also Appendix B.

11.6 What situations/circumstances correlate with unprotected intercourse?

Here are a few, which are well documented:

- First ever intercourse (or first with a new partner).
- Around the start or the end of any relationship – another good argument for long-term relationships, because there will be fewer 'bust-ups' (when the pill packets are thrown away) and then rebound relationships which are unprotected. This also argues for long-term, 'forgettable', methods that, if there are no troublesome side-effects, are much more likely to be continued with across the gap between relationships.
- Times of major life stress, e.g. bereavement, unemployment.
- On holiday, or trips away from home: indeed any situation where the individual or couple feels anonymous, a bit mad and so liable to behave out of character.

11.7 What are the factors in non-compliance and discontinuation in the developing world?

Everything above, only more so – wrong information, for instance. A recent survey in Egypt found that the most common error of providers, leave alone users of the pill, was the belief (as often in the UK, *see Q 11.8*) that the next packet of pills should routinely be started on the fifth day of the withdrawal bleed! Fatalism and cultural and religious obstacles to good compliance are often very strong.

But the biggest single factor is the basic one of non-availability of the actual methods, or the drying up of supplies once a good method like DMPA has been initiated. Even when available, contraceptives are seen as an expense and inconvenient (as they are in many poor communities of the developed world, too).

11.8 What do surveys show about more specific aspects of COC compliance?

A 1986 general practice survey in a mainly low social class (inner city) area showed that only 28% of women were taking the pill in accordance with the makers' instructions. Much of the confusion related (most crucially, *see Q 5.15*) to when to start the next packet after the PFI:

- ■ 12% believed they should wait until the fifth day of the withdrawal bleed
- ■ 11% thought they should start the next packet only when the bleeding stopped, or after 1 week but only if the bleeding had stopped.

Starting late with the next packet was not perceived as anything to do with missing pills (*see Qs 5.15 and 5.24*)! Two-thirds of the pill-takers in a similar GP study thought the most contraceptively risky pills to miss were in the middle of a pack. There is little to suggest any improvement during the 1990s in such settings.

By contrast, in 1988 in a semirural setting of higher social class, 89% were found to take their pills correctly. But could this in part be because those women had much more personal attention from the providers, explaining specifically things like the crucial importance of the PFI? We must admit that medical error – and especially not providing enough time for counselling and questions – can be significant components of user failure (*see Qs 11.15 and 11.16*).

11.9 Do we expect a lot from pill-takers?

Yes!

Correct pill use means that a healthy woman has to take a pill daily for months or years at a time, whether her intention is to delay or prevent pregnancy, and whether she is consistently sexually active or not. She must know how long to wait between pill packets, how to make up missed pills, and when to use another method as a back-up. She then must have the back-up method available and actually use it. Finally, she must be confident about the pill's effectiveness and safety, despite frequent rumours and negative reports in the press. In short, the pill is a more complex method to deliver and use than we previously thought. (Linda Potter, Family Health International)

According to an NOP survey in the UK in 1991, 'on average women seem to forget a pill about eight times a year'! And young teenagers seem to be late with their pills up to three times per month.

11.10 Teenagers are mentioned a great deal in the context of compliance. What are the important medical and legal considerations when prescribing a medical method like the pill to girls before the age of consent (16 in the UK)?

MEDICAL

Although early cycles after the menarche are anovulatory, very early conceptions can still occur and are becoming ever more common. Aside from that, there is the risk of STIs, cervical neoplasia and much potential emotional trauma. But it must be made clear that the risks are those of precocious sexual activity and multiple partners, not of the pill or any other contraceptive.

A modern low-oestrogen combined pill is usually a suitable method, although its 'default state' (i.e. of conception if errors are made) is not ideal. As far as we know, once periods are established it poses no special problems in teenagers, as compared with women in their 20s (including with respect to breast cancer or cervical cancer, *see Qs 5.79 and 5.81*).

Injectables and implants (especially perhaps the new Implanon™, *see Q 8.64ff*) are somewhat preferable to IUDs or the LNG-IUS because of the pelvic infection anxieties about the latter, although these are exaggerated and these methods too are definite options. *Re* progestogen-only injections, *see Qs 8.24 and 8.25.*

Because this age group are now the most at risk of all sexually transmitted agents, including *Chlamydia* and HIV, it is essential to promote use of the condom in addition, often, to the selected main contraceptive ('Double Dutch' – so-called because the Dutch give the lead here, as they do in so much to do with teenage reproductive health). Unfortunately, reliance on the condom alone for pregnancy prevention by teenagers usually gives poor results. If it is selected, take every opportunity to promote the emergency pill.

LEGAL AND SOCIOETHICAL

Sexual intercourse before the age of consent represents a major category of technical law-breaking, not by the girl but by the male partner(s). Yet prosecutions are very rare if they are about the same age.

Any GP faced with an under-16-year-old needs first, as appropriate, opportunely and non-patronizingly, to raise the advantages – both psychological and physical – of delaying intercourse until later. Next, if this rings no bells, seek agreement by the young person that they will tell, or allow you to tell, at least one parent. This is vastly preferable.

11.11 But what if under-16s completely refuse the involvement of a parent/guardian?

In 1985 the House of Lords overturned an Appeal Court judgement in the celebrated case brought by Victoria Gillick. In the new ruling, Lord Fraser of Tullybelton produced the 'Fraser Guidelines', which are the basis for assessing what is sometimes termed a young person's 'Gillick competence'. They are also in the revised DHSS *Memorandum of Guidance* (DHSS HC(FP)86). In the summary that follows, note that the highlighted initial letters spell out the words:

UnProtected Sexual InterCourse

It is good practice to proceed to prescribe a medical contraceptive without parental knowledge and consent if:

1 the girl, although under 16 years of age, will **u**nderstand the doctor's advice
2 she cannot be persuaded to inform the **p**arents or allow the doctor to inform them
3 she is very likely to begin or to continue having **s**exual intercourse with or without contraceptive treatment
4 her physical or mental health or both are likely to **s**uffer unless she receives contraceptive advice or treatment
5 her best **i**nterests (therefore) require the doctor to proceed without parental consent
6 at all times the young woman's entitlement to 100% assurance of **c**onfidentiality is the same as for any adult. This must not only be real, as goes without saying, but it must also be explicit to her, e.g. even if she recognizes that the receptionist is a friend of her mother's!

11.12 How are compliance, side-effects and discontinuation connected?

In a complex way. To quote Linda Potter again, referring primarily to pill users in poor communities (i.e. in inner cities of rich countries as well as in the developing world):

Poor compliance can lead directly to pregnancy. However, incorrect use can also contribute to discontinuation. Studies indicate that as many as 60% of new OC users discontinue use before the end of the first year, most within the first 6 months, and most of these because of menstrual irregularities and other side-effects.

The side-effects may be either the cause or effect of incorrectly taken pills, and may lead to either discontinuation or failure, making the relationship a complex one. For example, nausea in the first few months may lead to intermittent use, which in turn may provoke breakthrough bleeding, which in turn may lead to discontinuation.

11.13 According to the UK FPA's National Information Service, what – to help them to use contraceptives well – do potential consumers themselves consider most important?

Above all, information. Some professionals feel consumers cannot deal with 'too much information' but the number of enquiries to the FPA (about 100 000 per year) suggest that consumers want more information, not less.

Sadly, in the FPA's experience, too many professionals do not provide full information about the range of options, fully explain the side-effects or discuss risks and benefits of contraceptive methods.

Many professionals make assumptions, often underestimating a person's degree of motivation, ability or needs and 'censor' or limit information, and many use a variety of ways to pressure a woman to use certain methods. In a word, paying lip-service to 'client choice'; they are much more into 'provider choice'. So women often express to the FPA feelings of anger, frustration and powerlessness because they feel they are not listened to, not spoken to on equal terms and given neither time nor 'permission' to voice fears or anxieties.

Family planning advisers need to be aware of how far they might go in determining choice rather than influencing it, i.e. there is a need to consider the differences between informed consent and informed choice.

There are fears, worries and doubts about potential, perceived and currently known side-effects. What consumers consider important when choosing a method are:

- effectiveness – will it work? (emphasis on failure rather than success)
- suitability
- risks and benefits
- how to use a particular method
- how the method works.

11.14 What mnemonic is a good guide to comprehensive, client-centred counselling?

In US Family Planning circles the recommended word is 'GATHER'. This stands for:

G: **greet** each young person warmly.

A: **ask** the young person about herself (himself) and why they have come.

T: **tell** the young person about each available family planning method. Then demonstrate the method(s) that most interest her.

H: **help** her to choose the method she feels will best suit her and her partner.

E: **explain** how to use the chosen method, using a user-friendly leaflet to be taken away and for reference.

R: **return** for follow-up. Agree on a time to meet again routinely *or* at short notice upon request.

The very first word – greet – conveys a client-centred approach beautifully. It is worth remembering the response from a member of a focus group (run by Brook, who provide user-friendly services for young people) to the question 'Who would you want to see?' – 'Someone with a SMILE would be your best bet' was the reply.

11.15 How should the information be conveyed?

Verbally and by the written word, supplemented these days by videos, computer games and websites. The onus is on providers to give information that is accurate. It should update, reassure and demythologize – all without embarrassment. Knowledge is power.

Providing written information, and currently the best brief source in the UK is the FPA leaflets, offers privacy, anonymity and time to absorb information at leisure. People can remember only 20% of what they hear and only 50% of what they hear and see.

The length of the text is not a barrier to communication for consumers, provided the material is well organized, well laid out and well signposted. Indeed, the more comprehensive FPA leaflets that are now available should be given with the words 'keep this in a safe place for reference'.

Contraceptive manufacturers and family planning organizations are at last actively working together to standardize and simplify the information given. Providers can already choose, selectively, to offer some of the better manufacturers' literature, which has been much improved in recent years. Possibly even more important is creative packaging, whereby user-friendly design assists compliance, and some companies' packets now convey valuable information like what to do in the event of missed or vomited pills. The increasing use of video and audio recordings is also to be welcomed because they can save time and be discussion openers, ensuring the ground is covered fully, especially the bits the provider might find 'boring' and so forget to mention at the crucial first visit.

11.16 As an overstretched but well-intentioned family practitioner, how might I improve my family planning service?

Generally, more people attend GPs for contraception than community-based family planning clinics. But you might lend support to the view that availability of the choice of service is paramount – including the clinic service, which is, moreover, an essential resource for the practical training of doctors and nurses in this field. Availability of complementary (not rival) and accessible services is important; at present, with repeated 're-disorganizations' of the NHS, potential users of contraception might have to run a bit of an obstacle race to find the service that meets their specific needs. One of the most useful improvements that many health authorities still need to make is to implement the recommendation of the 1991 RCOG Working Party on Unplanned Pregnancy, that there should be 'a senior specialist to oversee the provision of contraception and sterilization, both by community clinics and in general practice' – a coordinating community gynaecologist or Head of Reproductive Health Services, in fact.

Doctors and nurses tend to put birth control methods into five main categories: barrier, hormonal, intrauterine, sterilization and termination of pregnancy. But to our clients there are primarily just two categories: those methods you can get on with yourself and those where you have to involve (get 'permission' from) other people, possibly rather bossy people, and so lose privacy and control. Given this context, therefore, in our own services we must set aside any illness-oriented style and adopt an information-providing and counselling mode for these healthy couples.

There are a number of very practical questions you might consider:

FAMILY PLANNING, THE SCOPE
In our practice, do we provide:

- a full range of contraceptive methods, on site or easily arranged, including postcoital contraception and condoms (discuss with the local AIDS budget-holder)?
- pregnancy testing and support and counselling for unplanned pregnancy?
- counselling and referral for male and female sterilization?
- advice and help with regard to 'safer sex'?
- help or referral for sexual and relationship problems?
- advice, treatment or referral for STIs?
- advice, help or referral for infertility?
- comprehensive well-woman/well-man services?

SERVICE PROVISION
Do we:

- work as a joined-up team (I include here receptionist, health visitor, school nurse, practice nurse, partners)?
- provide flexible clinical services, with rapid access/walk-in facility for urgent first visits (postcoitally) and adequate support to those with follow-up problems (e.g. side-effects of IUDs or pills)?
- provide sufficient time for all family planning consultations, especially the first or the postcoital visit? Have we fully thought through the pros and cons of a dedicated session?
- provide an assurance – especially to the young – of confidentiality in

visits, communications and record keeping? In short, from reception onwards, can we consider ourselves to be fully teenage-friendly? (The RCGP and RCN provide an excellent green laminated card for practices, issued in 2002, including a brief questionnaire to assess this).

■ provide (where possible) a choice of male or female doctor?

TRAINING

Do we ensure that all staff (including reception/clerical staff, but most especially nursing staff) are appropriately trained?

INFORMATION

Do we:

■ always provide standardized, complete, up-to-date and objective information? That is, the information we ourselves would expect to receive?

■ use suitable language that both enables and informs? Thus, do not talk about coils, rhythm method or morning-after contraception, but do talk about IUDs, natural family planning and emergency (postcoital) contraception.

■ make it clear during counselling for pills and barrier methods that there is a profound difference between the failure rates for perfect use and typical use?

■ always discuss risks and benefits?

■ recognize that people are not always comfortable and might feel too shy to ask questions? (It can help to 'ventriloquize' some questions, and to ask certain others to check that the most important facts have been retained.)

■ always provide good written information that backs up and reinforces any verbal advice?

■ publicize our services so people know about them?

Ensuring compliance is, after all, not about professionals 'telling' consumers what to do – it is about enabling consumers to make informed choices through a partnership with health professionals. (Toni Belfield)

IATROGENIC CAUSES OF UNPLANNED PREGNANCIES

11.17 How wrong can we, the providers, sometimes be? Can a doctor or nurse be an accessory in causing 'iatrogenic' unplanned pregnancies?

Very much so. We have just been reviewing, in a contraceptive context, plenty of evidence for the saying: 'you can take the horse to the water but you cannot make it drink'. But is it not also clear already that we as providers can fail in the first place to 'take the horse to the water'?

Many 'sins of omission and of commission' by providers are obvious in Qs 11.13–11.16. The list that follows, of over 30 more specific errors, primarily medical or prescribing errors, is by no means complete. Indeed, I would be interested to receive other examples to use in my next edition!

Although probably more important than all of them is summarized in the response 'Someone with a SMILE would be your best bet' (see Q 11.15), the prescriber can be an accessory to an unwanted pregnancy in any of the following ways:

1 First and foremost, by not allowing enough quality time for the contraceptive consultation, backed by good literature. This leads to one of the most common – most basic – errors, which is when the practitioner simply says 'you must stop the pill' without any adequate discussion of the future method (see (7), below).

2 When changing methods, by not ensuring an appropriate overlap. For instance, when changing from progestogen-only pill (POP) or IUD to condom, failing to advise use of the condom for 7 days before the POP is discontinued or device removed. Or if a woman is transferring to a (for her) untried method like the diaphragm or Femidom™ (see Q 4.55), removing an IUD before she has found it to be satisfactory. And, prior to female sterilization, failing to advise abstinence or extra care with barrier methods for the cycle leading up to the surgery risks a clip-induced ectopic or an intrauterine conception (see also Qs 9.13 and 9.14).

3 Especially postpartum, if any amenorrhoeic sexually active woman wants to start using a hormonal or intrauterine contraceptive, by insisting on waiting (a) for a 6-week postnatal visit (see Q 11.22) or (b) for the next period (which then never comes because she conceives during the wait!) – when there other are ways of minimizing the risk of fetal exposure (see Qs 8.53, 8.54, 11.22).

Many studies have shown that confusion about irregular bleeding, and its nuisance-value as a side-effect, are among the most frequent causes of pill-taking errors, discontinuations and unwanted conceptions.

CHAPTERS 1–3

4 After a bad attack of PID, overstressing that the woman might be infertile – so she is inefficient with subsequent contraception.

5 Overstressing the ineffectiveness of coitus interruptus (see Q 3.6) so that it is not used when it would be a very great deal better than nothing in an 'emergency' situation.

6 Failure to warn about the 300+ million sperm in each man's ejaculate, and the unpredictability of sperm survival in the female genital tract. Hence failure to explain the consequences: that a tiny 'leak' of semen can cause pregnancy, and that the postmenstrual 'safe period' is of a completely different order of potential efficacy from the properly identified postovulatory phase (*see Qs 2.4–2.17*).

7 With Persona™, recommending the method to the 'wrong' kind of couple ('limiters', when they should be 'spacers'); failure to offer the option of relying only on the second infertile phase (as described in *Qs 2.31 and 2.32*) and failure to explain the preliminary need for two natural cycles of barrier method use after any hormones (including for emergency contraception).

8 Failure to advise about effective condom use, and especially about common chemicals/prescriptions that damage rubber (*see Q 3.21*).

9 Regarding caps, giving such a profusion of other instructions about spermicide, etc. (most of which have never been validated) that the woman fails to get the most important message: namely that she should make a secondary check that her cervix is covered following every insertion of her diaphragm or cap, however comfortable it feels.

CHAPTER 7 (CONSIDERED HERE BECAUSE REGULARLY INDICATED THROUGH FAILED USE OF ABOVE METHODS)

10 Failure to inform male and female users of barrier contraceptive about the existence of emergency contraception, and failure to offer it when appropriate (e.g. if an IUD has to be removed midcycle, *see Q 9.14*).

11 Use of the incorrect term 'morning after pill', and failing to stop its use by others (*see Q 10.1*).

12 Failure to inform women that the postcoital 'emergency pill' can be used up to 72 h after exposure.

13 Not being prepared to insert an IUD postcoitally up to 5 days after ovulation, as calculated in good faith (*see Q 10.15*). With exposure on day 7 this could mean, quite legally and ethically, insertion up to 12 days after unprotected intercourse! And with a solitary exposure, 5 days after intercourse is acceptable at any time in the cycle.

CHAPTERS 4 AND 5

14 Giving erroneous starting instructions for the combined pill (see p. 133 and *Q 5.49* for the correct ones, including the 'Quick start' option in selected cases (*Table 5.4 and Q 10.42*)).

15 Failure to explain the significance of the pill-free week in the initial pill consultation, in advance and alongside the FPA's COC leaflet (*see Qs 5.15–5.27*) as well as supplying the manufacturer's PIL.
Understanding at the outset the simple idea that the COC is bound to

work least well at the end of the regular time when it hasn't been taken at all (i.e. the contraceptive-free time), helps to stop the common notion that 'being a bit late starting' is not 'missing a pill'! Detailed examples:

(a) not stating clearly that starting the new packet on time is critically important and that the first pill is the most 'dangerous' if missed

(b) not explaining that, if pills are missed at the end of a packet, the next following PFI should be shortened or eliminated

(c) giving implicitly wrong instructions for subsequent packs, e.g. 'the doctor said [he/she probably didn't, but was the point clarified?] that I should wait until the fifth day of my next period – or until it is finished – before I restart each packet'

(d) instructing the woman to start a new brand of pill on day 1 of the WTB after the last one without advising her what to do if, by chance, she gets no WTB in that cycle. She might well then wait beyond 7 days unless otherwise instructed.

16 Failure to check at follow-up whether pill takers still have a copy of the FPA leaflet as well as the PIL, and replacing as necessary (this is routine at the Margaret Pyke Centre).

17 Simply represcribing the COC (perhaps with a 'pep-talk' about compliance) after true pill method failures, or even when only one or two tablets have been missed. Instead, the tricycle method should be offered (*see Qs 5.27 and 5.31*).

18 Inadequate explanations at pill discontinuation. Examples:

(a) Failure to inform a woman that the pill-free week is only a safe time for unprotected intercourse if she does in fact restart a new packet. If she is discontinuing the method, it is very common for a woman to assume that the condom is unnecessary for the first week. In reality she might well ovulate early in the second week (*see Qs 5.15 and 5.24*).

(b) Failure to explain that calendar calculations, of even the potentially safer second phase of the safe period, are completely invalidated during the first cycle following pill discontinuation, which can be very variably prolonged.

(c) Failure to dispel the myth: 'I heard that women often take a long time to get pregnant after stopping the pill, so I thought I would be safe'.

19 Failure to forewarn and explain that the occurrence of BTB should not be considered as a period (and the pill therefore stopped in midpacket) – and that it might subside over time. Choosing brands that produce good cycle control is obviously helpful too.

20 Failure to demolish the myth that you should not restart with a new pack until a 'period' has occurred. Not explaining, in fact, that absent

withdrawal bleeding is very rarely because a pregnancy has occurred. (Some women become pregnant through failure to restart the pill after the first episode of absent WTB and hence become unnecessarily pregnant solely because they thought they already were.) A useful check of good pill taking is to ask the user which day of the week she regularly starts each new pack: beware if she says 'it all depends!'

21 Ovulation induction in a woman who presents with oligoamenorrhoea but definitely does not (yet) want to be pregnant! (*see Q 5.64*). 'No-one ever asked me if I wanted my fertility problem treated!'

22 Unnecessarily avoiding the COC in cases of past secondary amenorrhoea from which there has been a complete recovery (*see Qs 5.63 and 5.67*).

23 Unnecessarily instructing the woman to discontinue/avoid the COC because of the medical myths in *Qs 6.56, 6.77, 6.78*, including for minor surgery like laparoscopy (*see Q 6.15*).

24 In the case of a healthy woman who really wants to continue pill taking, agreeing too readily to her 'taking a break' when idea comes only from a friend (*see Qs 6.72 and 6.73*).

25 Unnecessarily instructing a woman to stop the POP (or any EE-free method) before any surgery, however major (*see Qs 7.41 and 7.73*).

26 Telling the woman – correctly – to stop the COC before major surgery (*see Q 6.14*) or because of migraine with focal aura or other valid reasons, but failing to discuss and organize an alternative such as DMPA.

27 Failing to explain to a woman transferring to the POP that she should cease to take 7-day breaks.

28 Failing to discuss with a lactating old-type POP user that her chance of breakthrough conception will greatly increase whenever she begins weaning her baby. So if efficacy is very important to a woman, she should be offered Cerazette™ or advised to start the COC on the first day of the first of her returning periods (*see Q 11.29*).

29 Failure to advise appropriately (*see Qs 5.34, 7.28, 8.11*) when prescribing any of the hormone methods of *Chapters 5, 6, 7 and 8* in the event of use of interacting drugs, whether short term (e.g. rifampicin just for 2 days) or long term.

30 Bad handwriting (a real problem in practice). One of the most dangerous examples of this is when Femodene™ is intended but Femulen™ is read by the person issuing the pills. I am aware of at least one pregnancy caused this way because the woman continued to take routine pill-free breaks of a week's duration! Preventive recommendation, as practised at the Margaret Pyke Centre: Always write: Femodene-30; Femulen POP.
Also easily misread: Marvelon-30/Mercilon-20 and EVRA/Evorel.

CHAPTER 6

31 Failure to observe the 'do not rely on the IUD for 7-days pre-removal rule' recommended in Q 9.14. Avoidable intrauterine or 'iatrogenic' extrauterine pregnancies in IUD users following clip sterilization can also result. Barrier method-users should abstain during the same 7 preoperative days.

32 Failure to insert an IUD on presentation around midcycle, if necessary up to day 5 following the most probable day of ovulation. As explained in Q 9.15, a much more generous interpretation of the term 'postmenstrual' could lead to a worthwhile reduction in the number of conceptions caused by clinicians who wait for the woman's elusive next period. Leave alone always insisting on inserting IUDs during menses as, despite the very strong counter-arguments (Q 9.19) according to the FPA's helpline (2003) many doctors still do!

33 Failure to warn women that if they fail to feel the threads of an IUD, until proved otherwise, their uterine cavity is IUD free (*see* Q 9.34).

CONTRACEPTION/STERILIZATION AFTER PREGNANCY

11.18 When should counselling start?

It should not be an afterthought: it should be initiated antenatally. Counselling should be non-directive, with the doctor or midwife acting as an adviser and facilitator and never making the decisions. It is true that most women are more motivated towards family planning just after childbirth than at any other time, and in many parts of the world postnatal follow-up is weak or non-existent. However, although it might be correct to 'strike while the iron is hot', caution is necessary, especially regarding sterilization, and all kinds of pressure are to be avoided. For all women this is a time of emotional turmoil as well as one of rapidly changing hormonal status.

11.19 What is known about sexual activity in the puerperium?

See the brilliant section on this in the book by Esther Sapire (see Further reading). According to Masters and Johnson, writing in 1966, after delivery almost 50% of women have low levels of sexual interest for at least 3 months. In another study, the same percentage had resumed sexual activity as soon as 6 weeks, but possibly with little enthusiasm on the woman's part. However that may be, the onset of sexual dysfunction reported much later can often be traced back to this time. Sleepless nights, exhaustion and limited time together can affect both partners. The man might resent exclusion from the intense bond between mother and baby, compounded by the woman's fatigue and diminished libido. In the woman, there might be multiple anxieties about the baby and about adjustment to motherhood. All these can be worse if there is a true postpartum depression.

Physical problems include breast and nipple tenderness, or dyspareunia from the site of perineal suturing, monilial vaginitis and diminished vaginal lubrication.

11.20 When does fertility return after pregnancy? What is the earliest postpartum day on which ovulation can occur, without and with breastfeeding?

Despite much research it remains impossible to predict this accurately for any individual woman. This is due not only to normal biological variation, racial or genetic factors, but also to the effects of:

1 the nutritional status of the woman
2 the stage of gestation at which the pregnancy ended
3 whether indeed she is breastfeeding – and in that case the timing, frequency and duration of nipple stimulation, the amount of supplementary feeding and the time elapsed since delivery.

Although fertilization is the only proof that an ovulation is fertile, research suggests that in the absence of breastfeeding fertile ovulation could possibly and very rarely occur on day 28, and contraception of some kind should therefore be started by then (*see* Q 5.49).

It is even more difficult when attempting to answer the same question for lactating women, because the variability in intensity of baby-induced nipple stimulation is superimposed on woman-to-woman variation. But avoiding all freak ovulation events is perhaps asking too much: a better question is 'For how long can lactation be expected to provide the same kind of contraceptive protection as other acceptable birth control methods, such as the IUD?' (one answer is contained in LAM, *see* Q 2.36).

The essential caveat is that LAM still has a 2% failure rate even when well-applied: no promise of complete efficacy should be implied – as should be the case with all methods.

11.21 Isn't there a two-way interaction between lactation and contraception?

Yes. Lactation can affect contraceptives, primarily by greatly increasing the efficacy of the old-type POP and all non-hormonal methods like barriers and spermicides. Conversely, the COC for example can affect lactation adversely by altering the quantity and constituents of breast milk.

Breastfeeding should also be advocated and promoted by clinicians because it is so good for babies – and might give some protection against breast cancer.

11.22 In an amenorrhoeic woman seen postpartum, say at 6 weeks, if breastfeeding has stopped and contraception has been questionable, how can one safely start a medical method (e.g. avoid giving DMPA or fitting an IUD after a new conception)?

Some doctors are so paranoid about this that they insist on the arrival of a period. But they thereby risk in the long wait for this an 'iatrogenic' conception (*see Q 11.17(3)*).

One fairly obvious practical preventive of this problem is: Why do we perpetuate the tradition of postnatal checks at 6 weeks: they could be arranged instead routinely at or just before 4 weeks, when the risk of a fertile ovulation having occurred is negligible (*see Q 11.20*), even if the woman has not managed to breastfeed?

Availability of one of the ultrasensitive slide or dipstick pregnancy tests now marketed for use in the surgery is invaluable here (e.g. Clearview™). On an early morning urine this will diagnose pregnancy at or before the 14th day after ovulation; but not of course one very recently conceived, due to fertilization within that time. If that is a relevant possibility, one useful protocol is the following:

1   Request that the woman agrees to avoid all risk of conception (by abstinence, combinations of methods, whatever) for 12 or 14 days since the last intercourse (depending on whether the sensitivity of the available test is to 25 or to 50 IU/L of hCG).
2   She then returns with an early morning urine. If it gives a negative result this can be interpreted as 'no' conception – implanted or 'on the way':
    (a)   up to 12 (or 14) days previously (this by virtue of the sensitivity of the test), plus:
    (b)   since then also, on her responsibility, as she had agreed to be 'safe' during that time.
3   After discussion (recorded in the case notes) of the tiny risk that an early conception might still be present, the COC could be started, or one could proceed at once to a DMPA injection or Implanon™ or IUD insertion. If any hormones are to be used, or an IUS inserted, for extra security the couple should use the condom for a further 7 days. And there must be an early follow-up visit to finally exclude conception.

11.23 Can natural family planning be used successfully after childbirth (after LAM, *see Q 2.36*)?

The fundamental problem, throughout reproductive life, is how to recognize fertile ovulation far enough in advance to allow for the capriciousness of survival of the very best among the millions of sperm deposited at intercourse. The problem is compounded after pregnancy by the very variable effects of lactation, as discussed above.

With or without breastfeeding, postpartum the oestrogenic changes of increased quantity, clarity, fluidity, slipperiness, elasticity and good Spinnbarkeit occur well in advance of the first fertile ovulation. Hence, if cervical mucus is used there are numerous false alarms.

Users of natural family planning who begin mucus observations from the cessation of lochia and who do abstain or switch to another method from the very first appearance of oestrogenic mucus onwards will most probably avoid pregnancy. But they will also be avoiding unprotected intercourse for an unnecessarily long time. Changes in the cervix – dilatation, softening and elevation away from the introitus – might help (*see Q 2.35*).

To date, newer techniques using various biochemical changes are still disappointing for ovulation prediction far enough ahead.

11.24 Do you recommend an IUD for family spacing?

Yes, and it is an even better choice when the family might prove to be complete but the couple aren't sure yet. See *Chapter 9* for more details. Particularly relevant points at this postpartum time are:

1 *Infection*: this can be caused by lack of screening or poor technique during insertion (*see Q 9.56*) or exacerbated if uterine tenderness due to postpartum endometritis is overlooked. The individual's risk of sexually transmitted conditions still poses the main threat for the future, however.

2 *Perforation*: this has been a particular concern in relation to postpartum IUD insertion. However, no significant additional risk for T-shaped IUDs was shown by Chi (1993 *Contraception* 48:81–108) rate 1 in 1632 during lactation. Perforation postpartum seems to be primarily a problem of linear (e.g. Lippes loop) devices and can be almost eliminated by withdrawal insertion techniques – and by extra care by an experienced inserting doctor. Ideally, postpartum clinics should not be used routinely for training purposes because lack of expertise markedly increases this risk.

11.25 What is your advice on the timing of postpartum IUD insertions?

See Qs 9.102 and 9.103. Good results are reported whenever this is between 4 and 8 weeks after delivery. I favour 4 weeks to avoid all the 'hassle' discussed in *Q 11.22*, although the postcoital contraceptive action of the IUD method does provide some leeway.

After lower segment caesarean section (LSCS) the scar will have healed by 4 weeks and is situated at the level of the internal os. So there is no need to delay insertion beyond say 6 weeks. After elective LSCS the cervical canal might require gentle dilatation, often with local anaesthesia, as for nulliparae. These insertions are not for beginners.

IMMEDIATE POSTPLACENTAL INSERTION

See Q 9.103. A new GyneFIX™ IUS (*see Q 9.141*), bearing a biodegradeable enhancement of its retaining knot, is being studied for this indication. It shows greater promise with respect to expulsions than previous designs. Follow-up arrangements should be good, so that women can have their now elongated threads shortened or a new device inserted if expulsion is noted.

IMMEDIATE INSERTION AFTER CAESAREAN SECTION

Modern IUDs can similarly be inserted via the lower segment incision immediately the placenta has been delivered, with superb results reported from China. Some researchers suture the device to the fundus with chromic catgut but this appears to be unnecessary.

IMMEDIATE POSTABORTION INSERTION

This can be appropriate (*see Qs 9.104 and 9.144*).

11.26 Are COCs suitable immediately postpartum?

Despite their efficacy, convenience and many other advantages, COCs should not be used during lactation. Most studies report some adverse impact on breastfeeding performance and milk volume composition. And in any case the COC cannot improve upon the near 100% efficacy of the POP plus full lactation.

11.27 When should the COC be started in women who do not breastfeed?

If a COC is started too late, some women will become pregnant before their first period. If it is started too early, there is the risk that the oestrogen content will increase the already increased risk of thromboembolism in the puerperium. So, ideally, COC taking should not begin until the similar changes induced by pregnancy have returned to normality. This starts dramatically with delivery of the placenta but fibrinogen concentrations actually increase at first until a decline starts around day 5. Dahlman and others found that both blood coagulation and fibrinolysis were significantly increased during the first 2 weeks, but by 3 weeks both were in general normal. This literature might be interpreted as implying that oestrogen-containing pills should normally not be commenced earlier than day 21 of the puerperium, and this would be the optimum time for those perceived as being at high conception risk (*see Q 5.49*).

Selective delay beyond 4 weeks using an alternative contraceptive might be safest where known risks apply, particularly in combination. These factors are obesity, preceding severe pregnancy-related hypertension, the HELLP syndrome, operative delivery, especially caesarean section, restricted activity, age above 35 and grande multiparity. A good rule is to wait until full mobility and normality of any previously abnormal biochemical or other tests.

11.28 What if the woman had pregnancy-related hypertension?

It used to be thought that women with hypertension in a preceding pregnancy would be unusually prone to oral contraceptive-induced hypertension. This was disproved by Pritchard and Pritchard in 1977. However, it is definitely a relative contraindication (*see Q 5.136(1)*), requiring judicious use of the COC method with extra careful subsequent monitoring (WHO 3).

Why? Because the RCGP study showed that this past history is linked for unknown reasons with an increased risk of arterial thrombosis – and seriously so if they also smoke (risk ratio of over 40!). If no alternative to the COC as subsequent contraception is acceptable and the 'pre-eclampsia' was severe at the preceding delivery, starting the COC should be delayed for at least 8 weeks.

11.29 Where should the POP fit into any scheme for postpartum contraception?

Very prominently. This is discussed in detail at *Qs 7.54–7.58*. Unlike the combined pill, POPs, including Cerazette™, have not been found to impair the quantity or the quality of breast milk.

1 *Timing of postpartum use*: as there is no anxiety about enhancing the risk of thrombosis, it is medically safe to start the POP in the early puerperium. However, studies have shown an increased risk of puerperal breakthrough bleeding in POP users, despite the expectation that they should have amenorrhoea during lactation. It is therefore now suggested that women (whether or not breastfeeding) should begin to take the POP after about day 21 following delivery. Any amenorrhoeic woman in whom cyesis has definitely been excluded, if necessary by the routine described above (*see Q 11.22*), can start the POP at any time, with 7 days additional contraceptive precautions.

2 *Efficacy*: it is important to bear in mind that because there is the additional contraceptive effect of breastfeeding, less than perfectly compliant old-type POP-takers will 'get away with it': until, perhaps, weaning and hence fertile ovulation commences (*see Q 7.57*). Two successive women in one of my own clinics gave the history that their next baby came 'too soon' that way, because the suggestion that they might prefer to switch to the COC at weaning had not been made to

them! This point needs making in advance: if efficacy is very important to a woman, she should be prescribed Cerazette™ or the COC so she can start in good time.

11.30 What about injectable contraception postpartum? Does the same apply as with the POP?

Most studies of DMPA show either no change or an improvement in both quantity of milk and duration of lactation. Both DMPA and NET-EN and their metabolites cross from maternal plasma into breast milk, and to a greater extent than with the POP, so it is not a first or frequent choice in the UK. Yet it has been calculated that a child would have to breastfeed for 3 years to receive as much DMPA as the mother receives in 1 day. And, to date, no morbidity and no adverse effects on growth have been found.

1 *Timing of the first dose*: because, in some countries, contact with medical personnel is limited to delivery, the first dose of DMPA is often given within 48 h of delivery. Injectables do not increase the risk of puerperal thrombosis; but this is much earlier than necessary for contraception and it has been noted that such early administration increases the likelihood of heavy and prolonged bleeding. Hence, in the UK, the first dose is now preferably (but not always) delayed to 5–6 weeks postpartum. In a woman who is not breastfeeding I would be quite happy to give DMPA early, at any mutually convenient time before day 21 – so it could be sure to prevent the earliest likely ovulation – but with forewarning about the increased risk of bleeding.

2 *Efficacy*: here there is no concern that the method will become less effective as breastfeeding frequency diminishes. Instead, the woman must be warned to plan well ahead if she wants another baby because of the well-recognized delay in return of fertility – although this has often been exaggerated (*see* Q 8.39).

11.31 What is the policy about hormonal methods if there was trophoblastic disease in the last pregnancy?

This is fully discussed in Q 5.77.

11.32 What considerations apply to male or female sterilization in the early puerperium?

It often appears convenient for all concerned if the woman is sterilized at this time. But Professor Robert Winston showed that the decision is more commonly regretted at this time of emotional instability for many couples. So there is a welcome trend to offering laparoscopic sterilization as an interval procedure about 12 weeks postpartum. The inadvisability of routine postpartum procedures is well shown by the observation that a distinct minority, around 15%, change their minds during that 12 weeks, preferring to keep their contraceptive options open longer.

There then still remains the risk of early death of the latest child (e.g. by the sudden infant death syndrome). Many vasectomy services therefore prefer to defer the procedure until the youngest child is 6–12 months of age. It is not clear why such admirable caution is less commonly observed by obstetricians with regard to female sterilization, especially as there is a strong suspicion of an even higher failure rate at that time.

For more about all forms and timings of sterilization, *see Qs 11.56–11.59* and the excellent RCOG evidence-based Guideline No 4 *Male and female sterilisation*: this can be readily viewed or obtained via the RCOG website (www.rcog.org.uk).

CONTRACEPTION FOR THE OLDER WOMAN

Background factors

11.33 What is the intrinsic fertility of older women, above age 40?

The available evidence suggests, as shown at the bottom of *Table 1.2* (p. 14), that the intrinsic fertility of such women is reduced to about half what it was at the age of 25, with a further decline above 45. An unknown part of this is due to reduced frequency of intercourse. Whatever the explanation, the conclusion is that a method with an accidental pregnancy rate unacceptable in a younger woman might well be satisfactory for use in the 40s. For example, the POP in the Oxford/FPA study has a failure rate (0.3 per 100 woman-years) that is indistinguishable above age 45 from that to be expected in a younger woman using the combined pill. Another example is the recommendation to use the contraceptive sponge above 50 (*see Q 4.64*).

Some older women, however, might have actual or potential gynaecological morbidity to weigh up against the risks of the combined pill (*see Q 11.38*) and so might be better off because of its beneficial effects, although not really needing such a high efficacy method.

11.34 How can one normally diagnose physiological infertility after the menopause?

Despite much research, there is no simple answer to the question 'When can I stop all contraception?' Long spells of amenorrhoea in women under 45 can indicate the arrival of a premature menopause, but they might also be due to other spontaneously reversible causes. Even above that age, prolonged amenorrhoea does not rule out the chance of a later ovulation, although the risk is less if there are definite vasomotor symptoms.

We now know that FSH measurements alone are most misleading – they only mean reduced feedback of ovarian hormones on the pituitary at that time, the ovaries might well still have potentially fertile ova to release. Occasionally, women with many months of amenorrhoea, symptoms of the menopause and even elevated FSH levels subsequently ovulate and even conceive! As a rule of thumb, women above the age of 50 years who have had amenorrhoea for over 12 months, preferably also with vasomotor symptoms, can abandon alternative contraception. During the 1-year wait any simple method (e.g. contraceptive foam) is adequate. At a younger age there is a greater risk of spontaneous late ovulations, so 2 years' of amenorrhoea with extra precautions is recommended. Below 40 this is 'secondary amenorrhoea' and needs to be investigated fully by standard tests.

The classic rule is as above: 2 years' amenorrhoea are required for the diagnosis of final ovarian failure right up to age 50. This age limit seems to have been chosen arbitrarily, without any hard data. Lowering the 2-year requirement to under 45 in recent years has made life easier: minimally less safe, but perhaps acceptably so. But there still remains the problem that so many women have their menopause masked by the use of hormones (COC or HRT).

If FSH levels (preferably two) are performed it might be possible in some situations (*see Qs 7.63, 8.47, 11.44*) to shorten the time of use of other contraception after the apparently last period. But it must always be made clear that the risk of a later fertile ovulation cannot be completely excluded.

11.35 What are the medical risks associated with pregnancy above age 40?

Although it might be easier to prevent, pregnancy at this age is in many ways a greater catastrophe. Both maternal and perinatal mortality are much higher. There is also a steady increase in the risk of chromosome abnormalities with maternal age. Hence whereas we should certainly avoid using too 'strong' a method, the woman needs to be reassured that any chosen method will prove to be effective in her own case.

11.36 What is the 'best' method for women above 40?

There is no such thing as a single best method. Individualization is the key, as usual.

Hormonal methods

11.37 Is the term 'the contraceptive gap' now applicable to smokers only?

Yes: with modern pills, available epidemiology and the relevant authorities suggest that we can now legitimately continue the ordinary COC at a woman's request to the menopause, if she is an entirely healthy, migraine-free non-smoker. Age alone is no longer a contraindication.

For smokers, however, starting at age 35 we are left with a 'contraceptive gap' between that age and the menopause. It poses an acute problem for those many couples who have hitherto been 'spoilt' by non-intercourse-related methods. Many seek sterilization, some without being ready for so permanent a step: yet it would be unnecessary if they were non-smokers.

11.38 What are the desirable features of contraception at the climacteric?

Table 11.2 summarizes the desirable features. It is clear that only some appropriate combination of oestrogen with progestogen is capable of providing all the first six features in that table. What is appropriate? That depends on the need for contraception (*see Qs 11.39 and 11.40*).

TABLE 11.2 Desirable or 'ideal' features of any contraceptive for use during the climacteric (before and as required after the menopause)

1 Effective in this age group
2 Improves sex life by:
  (a) perceived effectiveness and reassuring period pattern, or amenorrhoea
  (b) not being an intercourse-related method
  (c) oestrogenic slowing of skin ageing, improved body image and libido, and treatment of vaginal dryness
3 Controls climacteric symptoms (especially vasomotor and psychological symptoms, and the urethral syndrome)
4 Controls symptoms of 'normal' cycle (especially the premenstrual syndrome, and irregular, heavy or painful periods)
5 Reduces incidence or manifestations of gynaecological pathology. This potential benefit applies to pelvic infection, extrauterine pregnancy, fibroids, dysfunctional haemorrhage, endometriosis, functional ovarian cysts, and above all carcinoma of the ovary and uterus
  (Consequent reduction in the risks of treatment for these conditions, especially hysterectomy)
6 Oestrogenic protection against osteoporosis
7 Absence of masking of the menopause
8 Absence of systemic adverse effects:
  (a) known serious conditions such as hypertension and cardiovascular disease
  (b) anxiety about possible effects on other serious conditions, for example, breast cancer, especially with long duration of use

Note: Only a combination of oestrogen and progestogen is capable of providing all the above desirable features (*excepting* numbers (7) and (8)). The remaining options chiefly act as contraceptives – usually without a positive benefit on the conditions shown.

Over and above the reassurance of regular bleeds, it is now clear that there is often some symptomatic loss of ovarian function starting 5–10 years before the actual menopause. Women in these years would derive additional non-contraceptive benefits if (upon their request) they were allowed by their physicians to use some form of combined therapy. Many of the desirable features listed in *Table 11.2* would then be provided, at least in theory. There is the potential to improve sexual harmony by avoiding intercourse-related methods, and by preventing oestrogen deficiency with associated skin ageing, poor vaginal lubrication and loss of libido. The first manifestations of climacteric symptoms can be suppressed. Many women suffer preventable hot flushes and in some osteoporosis might begin before they see their last period. Symptoms of the so-called 'normal' menstrual cycle (premenstrual syndrome, heavy and painful periods) are often controlled.

Perhaps most important is the reduced risk of those gynaecological disorders that are related to the menstrual cycle, listed at (5) in the table. It follows that use of an appropriate COC – or of course the LNG-IUS, without or as indicated with added oestrogen – will often eliminate the need for and risk of other medical or surgical treatments.

11.39 *Table 11.2* suggests that the benefits of the COC are greater in the older age group and so still outweigh the risks even if they – especially the circulatory ones of *Table 5.8* (p. 169) – are increased somewhat with age. But which pill should be used?

First, this increased permissiveness *re* the COC applies only to completely arterial and venous risk-factor-free women. Second, enthusiasm for the COC must also be tempered with caution as regards breast cancer risk, which does go up with age (*see Qs 5.91 and 5.92*), by probably about 30 in 10 000 added cases for use to age 45 (see *Table 5.6*, p. 156), although this is balanced by even greater protection against (particularly) ovarian cancer. Third, the COC is not the only oestrogen/progestogen combined option anyway.

Ideally, the minimum acceptable dose of any progestogen and the oestrogen should always be used, to produce the fewest possible metabolic effects on both lipids and clotting factors. At present, the first choice normally lies between Mercilon™, Femodette™ and Loestrin-20™, as the only 20-µg combined products available in the UK.

11.40 Is it ever appropriate to give a cyclical HRT regimen before the menopause? And might this suffice for contraception?

Not for contraception – none of those giving oestrogen alone at some time in their cycle is reliable. There are new modalities for the perimenopause being devised, which do use natural oestrogens by various routes plus continuous progestogen and are contraceptive but only the LNG-IUS plus HRT is usable before final ovarian failure without causing (usually) unacceptable bleeding.

Otherwise standard HRT products, although medically even safer (*see Q 11.41*), are best reserved (and then usefully) for those with oestrogen deficiency symptoms who are not at risk of pregnancy. They might be abstaining, relying on sterilization or vasectomy, or happily using some other contraceptive.

11.41 So what is the real difference between the COC and HRT? How is it we can recommend HRT to smokers of any age, whereas smokers must stop the COC at 35?

Synthetic oestrogen (ethinylestradiol, EE), even at the lowest practical dose for contraception plus acceptable cycle control, has a long half-life and does create significant prothrombotic changes in the blood. The fear is that these might facilitate superimposed arterial thrombosis in an important artery, if its wall has already been affected by atheroma. These arterial wall changes are much more likely among smokers, who also have enhanced platelet aggregation and impaired fibrinolysis. So: no COC remains the rule for older smokers.

After the menopause – or leading up to it if birth control is not an issue (*see Q 11.40*) – the 'gentler' natural oestrogens are sufficient as oestrogen replacement. Blocking ovulation is no longer an issue and along with intermittent progestogen they can and do give good control of endometrial shedding, especially when no longer competing with the woman's own hormones. Moreover, the possibility that after ovarian failure they have beneficial effects on atherogenesis in the vessel walls has, in my opinion, *not* been refuted by the negative results of 2002 WHI study report. (This study recruited too old an age group of women – in their 60s – many with arterial risk factors, to be truly seen as a primary prevention study. We await more data!)

11.42 Why, then, do we not use natural oestrogens for contraception in all women, with or without risk factors, before the menopause?

Mainly because of the need for contraception and cycle control, which EE does so well. Because natural oestrogens are less completely or predictably absorbed and have lower potency, they have so far not proved so effective in either capacity. This might change with further research.

Natural (opposed) oestrogens can be used for women, especially smokers, for example using sterilization or vasectomy but needing HRT before the menopause: in synchrony with their own cycle, and with forewarning about breakthrough bleeding. But in risk-factor-free women a

COC with only 20 µg of EE is usually preferable because it 'removes' the menstrual cycle and then replaces it with a (usually) well-controlled artificial cycle.

11.43 If the combined pill or cyclical HRT products are used in a woman's late 40s, will they not mask the menopause?

Yes. The 'standard' teaching has been to switch to a non-hormonal method and only discontinue all contraception after the occurrence of complete amenorrhoea for 12 months (or 2 years if under age 45). But this precludes use of HRT (whose withdrawal bleeds like those of the combined pill will indefinitely mask the menopause, and which is not safely contraceptive) at the very time when vasomotor symptoms might be most pronounced.

11.44 How can infertility at the menopause be diagnosed in women still using the COC?

The 'standard' teaching at Q 11.34 is impossible to follow with increasing use at this age of (cyclical) HRT and, for healthy non-smokers, of a 20 µg COC (because the withdrawal bleeds will indefinitely mask the true menopause). The former is not safely contraceptive and, if it can be avoided, the defined risks of the latter make it better not to use it unnecessarily when fertility is extremely low or absent.

The following is a possible protocol for COC-users. We normally use it when the woman reaches about age 51 (the average age of the menopause):

1 Measure FSH at the end of the pill-free week.
2 If it is normal, she still needs contraception. Above 50 the risks of the COC would in most cases be thought unjustifiable, there is no need for such a powerful contraceptive and an alternative should be offered; foam (*see Q 4.64*) or any POP can be ideal (*see Qs 11.46 and 7.62*).
3 If the FSH is high – above the 'menopausal' level specified by the laboratory – there are preliminary data that such a woman has begun – as a consequence of ovarian failure – to rely totally on the COC for her oestrogen. Therefore when it is stopped, even for just 7 days, the FSH climbs rapidly. She might even report 'hot flushes' at the end of each pill-free week, the situation being comparable to sudden loss of ovarian oestrogen by oophorectomy. She now switches to a simple barrier contraceptive (or just Delfen™ foam or the Today™ sponge, which is adequate at this age) or the POP for about 6 weeks, and reports any subsequent bleeds and vasomotor symptoms. If all four of the following are true it is very suggestive of ovarian failure:
(a) a second high FSH result
(b) no spontaneous bleeds after stopping the COC

(c)   definite 'hot flushes' occurring

(d)   above age 51.

4   After advice that the risk of later ovulation can even so not be completely excluded, the woman might then elect to discontinue contraception, whether or not she also chooses to commence HRT.

5   Or, for greater peace of mind, she might elect to continue contracepting for 6–12 months with, for example, any POP (*see Q 11.46*) or foam.

11.45 How can infertility due to ovarian failure be diagnosed in women who were started on HRT before their menopause?

A similar protocol at about age 51 is as follows:

1   Measure FSH: theoretically this should have the best chance of being high in the oestrogen-only phase.

2   A level above 25 IU/L, which is somewhat raised despite the HRT feedback on the pituitary, is suggestive of ovarian failure. But this should definitely be confirmed, exactly as for the COC above, after stopping the exogenous hormones for 6 weeks. The same four criteria – (a) to (d) in *Q 11.44* – should apply before all contraception is maybe stopped (with no guarantees given). Again, for greater peace of mind she might elect to continue some form of contraception for 6–12 months.

3   If the woman has a normal FSH result and/or ever later menstruates while off either COC or HRT, she should assume some residual fertility and (continue to) use a contraceptive – again, whether or not she decides to take HRT.

11.46 How can infertility due to ovarian failure be diagnosed in POP-users?

Women can, if they so choose, use this ultra-low dose contraceptive well beyond age 50. There is no particular need to use Cerazette™, indeed an old-type POP makes it easier to identify failing ovaries. Also there is no rush, the POP is safe enough to use well into the 60s!

Unlike with Cerazette™ or DMPA (although I would not advise DMPA being continued anyway, above 45, *see Q 7.16*), if prolonged amenorrhoea occurs in an old-type POP-user, as a new phenomenon along with symptoms suggestive of the menopause, the woman can have her FSH measured while still using the method. If it is low, she still needs the POP. If it is high, the same criteria (presence and persistence of vasomotor symptoms, amenorrhoea and a repeat high FSH value 6 weeks after stopping the treatment, plus age above 51) mean that her chances of a further fertile ovulation are extremely low, and possibly nil. With all the caveats above, she can therefore discontinue contraception (*see Q 7.63*).

In all these cases (COC, HRT or POP) younger women and any who want more complete reassurance can, if preferred, continue using a simple method, as usual until 1 year after the last non-hormonally-induced bleed (or 2 years if under 45).

The answers to the last three questions make it abundantly clear that we still do not have (and badly need) a simple test of complete and final ovarian failure at the menopause!

11.47 Is it always important to establish precisely when the menopause takes/took place?

No, not in my opinion. If contraception is not an issue and the woman is on any form of HRT with natural oestrogen, the diagnosis of the precise time of the menopause can be considered to be of academic interest only. The woman simply continues seeing artificial 'periods' for as long as she chooses to use that HRT. The management of any irregular bleeding is the same, and she will have essentially 100% certainty of ovarian failure if she stops at age 58.

Users of POP, Implanon™, IUDs and IUS might all (because their methods have no known excess risks with age) prefer simply to continue their method until they reach that age of presumed zero fertility.

For reasons of risk, the COC is different: it is not recommended after the menopause, or normally at all above age 51, because fertility is so low that a very simple contraceptive will suffice. Any who abandon contraception without having followed the strict rules of *Q 11.34* (with or without being on HRT), have to be prepared to take responsibility for their decision: a guarantee that ovulation will not occur again cannot be given.

11.48 Aside from a low-dose COC, while we await new developments, what contraceptive forms of combination hormone therapy might be given – especially in smokers above age 35 who hate barrier methods?

This essentially means using natural oestrogens in some form. It is already not uncommon for some doctors to prescribe an oestrogen preparation by any of the standard routes (e.g. percutaneously) in the years leading up to the menopause, and combine it with old type POPs. But we do not know whether enough protection is given to the endometrium this way, and the failure rate is also unknown – probably similar to that of the POP alone, although some have argued it might be higher due to interference by the oestrogen with the mucus effect of the POP.

Now that Cerazette™ is available, pending more data (ideally a proper trial) I would be prepared to use it along with HRT on a named patient basis (see *Appendix A, see also Q 11.49*).

Alternatives to the oestrogen/progestogen combinations for older women

Most of these are simply contraceptives. They do not provide the gynaecological benefits, the control over climacteric symptoms or the potential prophylaxis against osteoporosis that are given by the combined pill or (not always with contraception) other HRT oestrogen–progestogen regimens. Yet they remain valid options when hormones are not desired or are contraindicated.

11.49 Do many older women get on well with the progestogen-only pill?

Yes, in this age group this is highly effective and deservedly popular (*see Qs 7.1–7.78*) – and acceptable if desired even beyond age 51.

The problems (*see Q 7.32*) include erratic bleeding patterns with fear of pregnancy; and how to treat low-oestrogen symptoms when they arrive. One option then is the Cerazette™ plus HRT combination mentioned in *Q 11.48*. If any such combination with a POP is used as a contraceptive and hopefully endometrial protective form of HRT, in the absence of very good data it would certainly be wise to follow the full named patient routine in *Appendix A*.

See also *Qs 7.63 and 11.44* regarding diagnosis of the menopause.

11.50 What about injectables and implants (see *Chapter 8*)?

These have similar problems to the POP, related both to amenorrhoea and to irregular bleeding. Moreover, most women are looking for added oestrogen at this age, hence various (not always licensed) combinations are sometimes tried by prescribers: therefore *Appendix A* would again apply). DMPA is best not used above 45 anyway (*see Qs 8.23–8.27*) – even WHO calls this WHO 2.

11.51 Is the copper IUD underutilized at this age?

Yes, definitely (*see Q 9.20*). It is suitable not only because the banded IUDs are as effective as sterilization, especially when combined with reduced fertility, but also because infection and expulsion rates decline with age and are lowest in the 40s. In the absence of intermenstrual or very heavy bleeding it can be highly acceptable. There is no need routinely to change any copper intrauterine device fitted after the 40th birthday, until after the menopause (*see Q 9.138*).

11.52 How about the levonorgestrel-releasing IUS (see *Qs 9.145–9.151*)?

This is a fantastic option. Not only can protection against most of the gynaecological problems be expected, especially menorrhagia, which is so common in this age group, even due to fibroids, but also it provides local progestogen protection against endometrial hyperplasia and cancer. This also permits oestrogen hormone replacement to be given later when it is indicated, systemically, on a named patient basis (see *Appendix A*) while almost completely avoiding the side-effects of systemic progestogens. It is PMS-free, contraceptive, 'no-period HRT', usable before proof of ovarian failure!

11.53 What about the condom and vaginal contraceptives?

These options are as appropriate at this as any other age, and have their own obvious advantages. But in my experience they (especially the condom) are not sufficiently 'user-friendly' to be accepted for the first time by couples who have not used them regularly earlier in their reproductive life. Many women introduced to the diaphragm, however, are surprised by its ease and convenience.

The use of spermicides alone is not recommended in the younger older years. But Delfen™ foam is, in my experience, sufficient contraception and very acceptable:

- above the age of 50, and
- at any age for that necessary time following what appears to be the menopause (*see Qs 11.34, 11.44–11.46*) – which can only ever be finally diagnosed in retrospect.

11.54 Can the methods based on fertility awareness be recommended leading up to the climacteric?

No. At present for those whose views make this the only acceptable approach, the mucus and cervical assessment methods (*see Qs 2.24 and 2.35*), or Persona™, all require a lot of unnecessary abstinence by older women. This is because during the climacteric there is follicular activity with oestrogenic mucus and estrone-3-glucuronide in the urine – but without necessarily being followed by a fertile ovulation.

In an older woman who ovulates only (say) once every 4 months, a most useful new technology would be a means to predict each actual ovulation, far enough ahead to allow for sperm survival. Just three short spells of abstinence per year and she could avoid all the risks of the artificial methods of birth control.

11.55 Isn't postcoital contraception (as in *Chapter 10*) best avoided in this age group?

Not so, it might be entirely justifiable. There should be no hesitation in using either hormonal method even above the age of 45, so long as there is actually a finite pregnancy risk.

11.56 Surely either male or female sterilization is the ideal answer, for many older couples above age 35?

It certainly can be, for many; 210 million couples worldwide rely on female sterilization (WHO 2003). According to recent surveys around 45% of couples above age 40 in the UK rely on sterilization of one or other partner. The methods are effective and highly convenient, free of all proven long-term risks after the initial operation.

Yet female sterilization, specifically, is likely to be used much less in developed countries in the future. This is because of what I term a 'push' and a 'pull'. The 'push' is that we now know it doesn't work very well (CREST study, *see* Q 11.57) and is prone to late failures; the 'pull' is from all the new reversible methods that are at least as effective (*see* Q 11.58).

Most authorities consider any association of bleeding problems with female sterilization by tubal occlusion using clips or rings is coincidental, not causal. The principal explanation is that after sterilization the woman discontinues the COC, or other hormonal contraceptive, that had been controlling the pain and bleeding of her 'normal' or abnormal menstrual cycle for years without her knowing it. This is how I can ask medical students my catch question: how is it that vasectomy might be able to cause both menorrhagia and dysmenorrhoea?!

Female sterilization appears to give a so-far unexplained protection against ovarian cancer.

There are many traps for the unwary clinician, however. An infrequent but real example is the sterilization-clip-induced ectopic in the cycle of the procedure, caused because the woman was not warned of the danger of less than perfectly protected intercourse in the 7 days before surgery.

More serious, because affecting far more people, is the problem of relationship/marriage breakdown, now that it is so frequent. Requests for reversal are more frequent after vasectomy because the man often remarries a younger woman. Careful counselling is therefore mandatory, including an assessment of both the general and the sexual relationship of the couple, and a consideration of relevant aspects of gynaecology even if vasectomy is the operation proposed. And then there is the late failure risk, now quantified as much higher than used to be thought (*see* Q 11.57).

11.57 What is the risk of late failure? Can total reassurance be given after say 1–2 years?

Unfortunately, no. Such late failures do occur, even after vasectomy with two subsequent negative sperm counts. Our estimate from the Elliot-Smith clinic in Oxford (at which I have operated since 1970) was around 1:2000. This still makes vasectomy much more effective than female sterilization: the American CREST study (in which over 10 000 women were followed-up for up to 10 years) showed a surprisingly high overall failure rate of 1.8% (*American Journal of Obstetrics and Gynecology* 1996 174:1161–1170). For every sterilization method assessed, at least 50% more failures were ascertained after 10 years as had been identified by the end of the first year.

They did not have the more effective Filshie clip, which is standard in the UK. However, on the CREST 'model', the 2-year failure rate of Filshie clips, which is now (2003) estimated as around 2:1000, would need increasing to about 3:1000 after 10 years. Currently, therefore, we should inform young women at counselling that the lifetime failure rate of Filshie clip sterilization is estimated at about 1:300 (contrast vasectomy: 1:2000) and that 1:3 of all sterilization failures is ectopic. Note: these numbers are rightly more positive about female sterilization, so long as done by the Filshie method, than those quoted in the last edition. The new (2003) outpatient hysteroscopic method Essure is also highly effective, but has other disadvantages (not always feasible; *completely* irreversible). Obviously all failure risks decline dramatically with diminishing fertility approaching the menopause.

For more on this operation in either sex I strongly recommend reading the RCOG evidence-based Guideline No 4 on *Male and female sterilisation*, available online from the RCOG website (*www.rcog.org.uk*) 2003.

11.58 Are the alternatives to sterilization offered often enough?

I think not. Many couples would actually prefer to avoid surgery and there are plenty of ways of doing so, as outlined above. Before referral for sterilization, especially of relatively young couples, in my experience three important choices are far too often not even mentioned. These are Implanon™, (*see* Q 8.64), the modern banded copper IUDs and the LNG-IUS. The gold standard among copper IUDs is the T-Safe Cu 380A™ (*see* Q 9.10). But GyneFIX™ and the LNG-IUS have their own merits.

Certainly, another method would be preferable to sterilization when the woman is past the age of about 48, because sterilization will not provide 'value for money'. (The chance of pregnancy is so low and her 'autosterilization' by the menopause is imminent.) Indeed, depending on the regularity or otherwise of her menstrual cycle and vasomotor symptoms, a simple method like Delfen™ foam or a contraceptive sponge might be adequate.

11.59 What about hysterectomy?

A hysterectomy is sometimes appropriate, and indeed might be essential gynaecological treatment. Hence the vital importance of diagnosing in the female partner large fibroids, adnexal masses and stress incontinence before even vasectomy is arranged.

However, even by the modern minimal access techniques, the morbidity and mortality greatly exceed those of the other options above.

11.60 Is transcervical resection or ablation of the endometrium for menorrhagia contraceptive?

Unfortunately, not so. After all, blastocysts can sometimes even implant in the ovary or on the peritoneum, so the absence of (most of) the endometrium is not enough. Younger women conceive with surprising ease. Moreover, important risks are emerging:

1. the pregnancy has a high chance of being a tubal ectopic
2. the fetus might have a major malformation
3. there might be serious intrauterine growth retardation
4. there might be varying degrees of placenta accreta.

11.61 So what contraception is recommended for a woman having endometrial resection/ablation?

It is normally preferable that laparoscopic sterilization is performed under the same anaesthetic. Otherwise one of the above effective methods could and should be initiated, not excluding an IUD. However, according to the experts in this field, IUDs are relatively contraindicated (WHO 3), and if used are best fitted immediately, with great care and antibiotic cover. And it must be understood that the device can sometimes be almost impossible to remove, stuck among adhesions in a shrunken uterine cavity. The LNG-IUS is a better option, WHO 2 (Alfred Cutner, personal communication, 2002).

The LNG-IUS (*see* Q 9.145), of course, might prevent the need for this surgery in the first place – especially as it often helps pain, which is not usually improved by the ablative techniques. Alternatively, the gynaecologist might insert it as an adjunct at the time of ablation, or after resection of submucous fibroids, or at follow-up hysteroscopy if the problems do not resolve.

11.62 So what is your conclusion – what practical guidelines are there regarding contraception for the older woman?

1. As usual, the choice will depend on the outcome of non-directive counselling, considering all the options discussed briefly here and more thoroughly earlier in this book. It begins to look as though no contraceptive method is absolutely contraindicated on the basis of age alone.
2. One of the very best modern options to emerge, though, is the levonorgestrel-releasing IUS – alone, or with oestrogen if needed for HRT to treat relevant symptoms.

11.63 What else is important in discussing contraception around the climacteric?

It is important to remember that contraception is often a 'ticket' to see the doctor. In reality there might be many basic anxieties concerned with sexuality, the woman's relationship to her partner, the 'empty nest' syndrome, new health problems, ageing, and low self-esteem with the 'finality' of the approaching menopause. Moreover, even if, as so often, the woman tries to assume sole responsibility, her partner's caring involvement should be sought and promoted if found! See also *Appendix B*.

THE FUTURE

11.64 Will we ever have a pill for men?

At long last, a marketed systemic male contraceptive looks promising within the next 5 years – although it will most probably not be a simple pill. The most promising approaches are a long-acting testosterone ester by injection or implant, coupled with an injectable or implanted progestogen.

The concept is one of suppressing spermatogenesis by pituitary suppression (similar to the effect of the COC in women) but maintaining masculinity and libido through the androgen content. A careful balance needs to be struck between efficacy and the risk of promoting aggression, prostatic hypertrophy and the already-present male susceptibility to arterial disease.

Although some women say they would never trust a man to use such methods effectively, I am confident they would in fact be a useful addition to choice in stable relationships. It would be good if I could be on the 'pill' for a while, then my wife perhaps also, sharing the risks and side-effects of contraception for a change! Better still if it could be an implant, as I might forget my pill!

11.65 What should be the direction of future contraceptive research?

Figure 11.2 displays elegantly, although simply, the primary sites of action both of the existing methods and those currently under study. Those that are most likely to become available within the next 10 years have been discussed in detail in the appropriate earlier chapters.

Inspection of the figure confirms an obvious fact: that the major scientific interest in birth control research has been directed at relatively high-technology, interventionist methods that have the potential or the reality of systemic side-effects. Returning to a theme with which we began the book (see *Table 11.1*, p. 490), the main choice for women is between the efficacy and convenience of systemic methods like the COC but the associated risk of both annoying and serious side-effects, and the relative lack of efficacy and inconvenience of methods like the diaphragm, coupled with their virtual absence of risk. ('Inconvenience' primarily indicates that the method is coitally related.)

Regrettably, most contraceptive researchers have concentrated on attempts to improve the existing pill and devising similar systemic agents; but they are always trying to make the effective, convenient but potentially

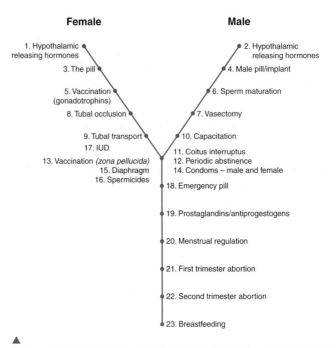

Female   **Male**

1. Hypothalamic
releasing hormones

2. Hypothalamic
releasing hormones

3. The pill

4. Male pill/implant

5. Vaccination
(gonadotrophins)

6. Sperm maturation

8. Tubal occlusion

7. Vasectomy

9. Tubal transport
17. IUD
13. Vaccination (zona pellucida)
15. Diaphragm
16. Spermicides

10. Capacitation
11. Coitus interruptus
12. Periodic abstinence
14. Condoms – male and female

18. Emergency pill

19. Prostaglandins/antiprogestogens

20. Menstrual regulation

21. First trimester abortion

22. Second trimester abortion

23. Breastfeeding

Fig. 11.2 Possible points of intervention to control fertility. Q 11.65. For existing methods, the figure shows the main sites of action of each (updated from *People* (IPPF) 1981 8(4):6–7).

dangerous methods safer. It is my view (and one that is shared by the majority of the women and their partners that I meet) that the researchers would do better to concentrate their resources on making the safe methods that also help to protect against STIs more effective and more independent of intercourse. This, indeed, is the orientation of the research programme at the Margaret Pyke Centre.

It is impossible to contradict the following statement: 'no chemical can be devised which, whether given to women or to men, and by whatever innovative route – whether oral, nasal, retinal, cutaneous, subcutaneous, rectal or vaginal – will be totally free of all risk'. Try as we will (and indeed must, because the urgency of world birth control demands research along every possible avenue) with new steroid compounds by slow-release and innovative routes, or using releasing hormone analogues, immune methods, or whatever; anything that gets into the bloodstream gets everywhere in the body and must therefore be capable of causing harmful effects, somewhere.

This is the heart of the problem to which Carl Djerassi drew attention in his classic book *The politics of contraception*. How do we prove that the unwanted effects of a systemic agent are acceptable or (hopefully) do not exist? It is because this process is so difficult, so expensive and so time consuming that Djerassi was so pessimistic about the future of contraceptive research.

Perhaps we should be starting somewhere else. Far more research should concentrate on producing a method, empowering women and men, which is as effective and 'user friendly' as the levonorgestrel IUS but as medically safe and STI-protective as the condom. This approach is surely at least as important as the conventional wisdom of the scientific establishment, which starts with current or innovative systemic methods (now for men as well as women) that are effective and convenient, and then strives diligently towards making them risk free.

Success down that road – although it must be travelled as well – will be nearly as impossible to prove as it ever will be to achieve! And even then, in view of the world shortage of monogamy … for safer sex many couples will still need to use a condom or equivalent as well.

FURTHER READING

Main sources of references* and quotations

Carter Y, Moss C, Weyman A 1998 RCGP handbook of sexual health in primary care. RCGP, London

Filshie M, Guillebaud J 1989 Contraception: science and practice. Butterworths, London

Guillebaud J 2000 Contraception today. A pocketbook for general practitioners. Martin Dunitz, London

*Guillebaud J 2003 Contraception. In: McPherson A, Waller D (eds) Women's Health (formerly Women's problems in general practice), 5th edn. Oxford University Press, Oxford

*Kubba A, Sanfilippo J, Hampton N (eds) 1999 Contraception and office gynecology: choices in reproductive healthcare. WB Saunders, London

*Potts M, Diggory P 1983 Textbook of contraceptive practice. Cambridge University Press, Cambridge

Sapire E 1990 Contraception and sexuality in health and disease. McGraw-Hill, Isando

*WHO 2000 Medical eligibility criteria for contraceptive use. WHO/RHR/00.02. WHO, Geneva

*WHO 2002 Selected practice recommendations for contraceptive use. WHO, Geneva

Important background reading – plus titles for a general readership

Cooper A, Guillebaud J 1999 Sexuality and disability. Radcliffe Medical Press, London

Djerassi C 1981 The politics of contraception: birth control in the year 2001, 2nd edn. Freeman, Oxford

Ehrlich P, Ehrlich A 1991 The population explosion. Arrow Books, London

Guillebaud J 1997 The pill, 5th edn. Oxford University Press, Oxford

Montford H, Skrine R 1993 Psychosexual medicine series 6. Contraceptive care: meeting individual needs. Chapman & Hall, London

*Population reports (various years to 2003) [Excellent comprehensive reviews of the literature on developments in population, contraceptives and sterilisation. Obtainable from the Population Information Program, Johns Hopkins School of Public Health, 111 Market Place, Suite 310, Baltimore, MD 21202, USA. Website: www.jhuccp.org]

Skrine R, Montford H 2001 Psychosexual medicine – an introduction. Edward Arnold, London

Szarewski A, Guillebaud J 2000 Contraception – a user's handbook, 3rd edn. Oxford University Press, Oxford

BELIEVABLE WEBSITES IN REPRODUCTIVE HEALTH

www.ippf.org.uk
Access to on-line Directory of Hormonal Contraception: the names and
formulation of the products used in every country! Note: This very
effectively replaces Appendix A4 of last edition: the world directory of
pill names.

www.margaretpyke.org
Training courses on offer and a useful search engine for most of your FAQs.

www.who.int/reproductive-health
WHO's Eligibility criteria and new Practice recommendations.

www.rcog.org.uk
Access to excellent evidence-based clinical guidelines on menorrhagia,
infertility, male and female sterilization and induced abortion. Newly
revised 2003, plus parallel patient information.

www.ffprhc.org.uk
Provides Faculty guidance on important topics, notably emergency
contraception (April 2003); also access to FACT reviews and the *Journal of
Family Planning and Reproductive Health Care*.

www.fpa.org.uk
Patient information plus those essential leaflets! Also an invaluable
telephone helpline for clients (tel: 0845 310 1334).

www.jhuccp.org
Website of Johns Hopkins School of Public Health Information Program:
produces the excellent Population Reports (see Further reading).

www.fertilityuk.org
The fertility awareness and natural family planning service, including
teachers available locally.

www.the-bms.org
Website of the British Menopause Society.

www.ipm.org.uk
Website of the Institute of Psychosexual Medicine.

www.teenagepregnancyunit.gov.uk
The Teenage Pregnancy Unit's site for all publications, FAQs, helplines (Sexwise line: 0800 282930).

www.likeitis.org.uk
Reproductive health for lay persons by Marie Stopes – fronted by Geri Halliwell.

www.ruthinking.co.uk
The Teenage Pregnancy Unit's site for teens. Catchphrase 'Sex, are you thinking about it enough!' Gives places/times of UK local services, in both sexual and reproductive health.

www.playingsafely.co.uk
Website for the DoH's safer sex campaign for under-30s.

www.teenagehealthfreak.com
FAQs as asked by teens, on all health subjects, from anorexia to zits!.

www.ecotimecapsule.com; www.elephantintheroom.com;
www.optimumpopulation.org; www.peopleandplanet.net
Websites *re* the 'Apology to the Future' project and related issues.

APPENDIX A
Use of licensed products in an unlicensed way

Whenever licensing procedures have not yet caught up with what is widely held to be the best evidence-based practice, such use is quite often necessary to provide optimal contraceptive care. It is legitimate, medically and legally, providing certain criteria are observed. These are well established (Mann R 1991 In: Goldberg A, Dodds-Smith I (eds) *Pharmaceutical medicine and the law.* London: Royal College of Physicians, p 103–110).

The prescribing physician must accept full liability and also:

- Adopt an evidence-based practice, endorsed by a responsible body of professional opinion.
- Ensure good practice, including follow-up, to comply with professional indemnity requirements. *Note*: This will often mean the doctor *providing dedicated written materials because the manufacturer's insert (PIL) does not apply.*
- *Explain to the individual that it is an unlicensed prescription.*
- *Give a clear account of the risks and the benefits.*
- *Obtain informed (verbal) consent and record this and the discussion in full.*
- *Keep a separate record of the patient's details.*

This is generally called 'named patient prescribing'.

Some common examples … but there are certainly others that you might identify in your own contraceptive practice

- Advising the use of more than one pill per day: when enzyme-inducers are being used with COC (*Qs 5.37–5.38*), POP (*Q 7.28*) or hormonal EC (*Q10.30*).
- Use of 'add-back' oestrogen along with Depo Provera™ (*Qs 8.27 (Box 8.1) and 8.38(10)*), in selected cases to treat diagnosed hypo-oestrogenism.
- Use of *banded* copper IUDs for longer than licensed under age 40 (T-Safe Cu 380A™ for more than 8 years, GyneFIX™ (until the licence changes) for more than 5 years), and above age 40 any copper device used until the menopause (*Qs 9.136 and 9.138*).
- Use of the LNG-IUS above age 40 for more than 5 years for contraception (*never* HRT), at a patient's fully informed request (*Q 9.137 and 9.138*).

■ Use (until licensed) of the LNG-IUS as part of HRT (*Qs 9.151 and 11.52*)

■ Use of any hormonal EC beyond 72 h after the earliest exposure or more than once in a cycle (*Q 10.9*).

■ Use of the POP with HRT together – as contraception in the older woman (*Q 11.49*).

■ Long-term omission or shortening of the pill-free interval as in the bicycle/tricycle regimens of pill-taking – for any reason (*Q 5.31*).

NB At any time in the currency of this edition, future updates to the relevant licence and the summary of product characteristics may remove the need to follow the above 'named patient' protocol in some of these examples – indeed, hopefully, all of them in due course.

APPENDIX B
Factors to be considered in giving contraceptive advice

Some notes in a handout prepared by Dr Elphis Christopher for the Margaret Pyke Centre Doctors' Courses in Basic Family Planning, edited and used here with her kind permission.

The factors wheel (see *Fig. 11.1*, Q 11.1)

INTRODUCTION
Although divided into equal segments in *Fig. 11.1*, the different factors are not compartmentalized but rather overlapping and interlocking. Some factors are obviously more important than others and individuals, couples and societies will vary over time: changing with increasing knowledge and experience both about contraception and abortion and the reality of pregnancy, child-rearing and population pressures. Altered socioeconomic circumstances and changing relationships (separation, divorce) will also have differing consequences for the use of contraception. Running like a *leitmotif* through all the aspects of family planning is the status of women and how their role is perceived – whether they are seen principally as child-bearers and child-rearers.

Attitudes towards sexuality and its expression – whether regarded mainly for procreation or pleasure – can have profound consequences for the sustained use of contraception and the planning of families.

Sexual activity is often impulsive and not planned for, tied up as it is with powerful and often overwhelming drives and emotions (*sex is hot*) whereas the use of contraception requires forethought and conscious effort (*contraception is cold*).

At some level most couples would really prefer *not* to be bothered about contraception …

1. SOCIETY, CULTURE AND RELIGION
Societal attitudes towards reproduction, fertility, sexuality and family planning are important in so far as they create the general climate in which arise the decisions about whether to have children, how many and whether to use contraception.

All religions are pronatalist and antiabortion; some might allow a pregnancy to be terminated for specific reasons, e.g. where the woman's life is at risk.

Religions might not be adverse to planning or limiting one's family but might be divided as to the means to do it, e.g. restricted to abstinence or natural family planning for strict Roman Catholics.

There is a notion shared by some Catholics and some from an Afro-Caribbean background that there are a certain number of souls/children waiting 'out there' and it would be wrong to prevent their arrival …

Orthodox Jews believe that the man must not impede the sperm, hence male methods are not used, although the woman can use contraception.

For Muslims, both husband and wife must agree to the use of birth control; abortion is allowed to prevent a handicapped child. Strict Muslim women can be examined only by female doctors and can touch their own vulva with the left hand. Somewhat of a problem for female barrier users!

Both Jews and Muslims must avoid sexual relations during and for a specified time after any menstrual bleeding – a major perceived obstacle to intrauterine and some hormonal methods.

Cultural factors rather than religious ones appear more significant among Caribbean women. Birth outside of wedlock is not considered a social stigma. Fertility (or the proof of it) is considered very important.

How seriously people take their religion and their perception and knowledge of what it actually says with regard to family planning obviously varies. Some might have rejected their background. Thus, in giving contraceptive advice it is essential to ascertain the particular person's views (today) and to avoid making assumptions about their beliefs and attitudes.

Treat the person not the culture.

SOME ASPECTS OF 'SUBCULTURE'

Feelings of:

- Apathy: those for whom birth control is fate.
- Anathema: may feel they have little control over other areas of their lives. Their sexual relationships are the one free area of their lives.
- God's will.

Especially among the socially deprived (of whatever ethnic background) in the inner cities, such vulnerable individuals find it difficult to seek advice about sexual or contraceptive matters because of a fear of professional attitudes; they are highly suspicious about loss of confidentiality. Sex, however, is free and available within a relationship; it is private and satisfying. Sex might provide a positive counterbalance to the idleness of unemployment and low self-esteem. Motherhood might seem the only source of fulfilment in an otherwise gloomy picture.

They often lead chaotic disordered lifestyles with frequent change of partners and might be poorly motivated to sustain their use of contraception and need much support, e.g. by a domiciliary family planning service.

2. CLASS, EDUCATION AND KNOWLEDGE

Generally speaking, those in long-term education and from a higher socioeconomic class tend to have similar family sizes, regardless of cultural/societal/religious influences, and are more motivated to use contraception.

Included in education is sex education. For years there has been a belief that teaching teenagers about contraception will be giving them a licence to have sex. Sexual ignorance is seen as bliss. The adolescent is often caught in a double bind. There is a loss of face for a teenager to admit to ignorance on sexual matters, although he/she might desperately need help.

There is considerable anxiety about sex education and its effects among certain ethnic groups in the UK, particularly the Cypriot and Asian minorities.

3. FAMILY, PARENTS, PEER GROUP

In patriarchal cultures, such as Asian and Cypriot, marriages are arranged or semi-arranged. A marriage is not considered a true one unless there are children, especially sons, who increase the status of women within those societies.

Peer group pressure can be significant among certain teenage groups, especially girls, who have been in local authority care.

4. THE COUPLE

The balance and quality of the relationship can affect the use of contraception. Consider:

- Trust, mutuality, sharing good communication.
- Humour.
- Consideration and care, which can cope with the vicissitudes of contraception.

Erratic use of contraception

- Anger, disappointment, resentment with the partner: the woman might stop the pill and try to withhold sex.
- The question of who is in control – who is in charge – can get acted out in whether contraception is used and who is the one who uses it.

- Resentment of the other's sexuality demands/needs.
- Conflict about pregnancy: where one partner wants a pregnancy but the other does not and sabotages the use of the method (pills thrown away, IUDs removed without telling the partner).
- A pregnancy might be 'arranged' to hold on to the partner.
- When relationships are beginning or ending this often leads to erratic or non-use of contraception.

The sexual relationship – attitudes to sex itself

Whether attitudes are positive or negative, and whether there is a degree of sexual self-confidence, can be revealed at the contraceptive consultation. Vaginal examination is very pertinent here – it can reveal a lot.

Sexual problems can present covertly, and can be shown by:

Ambivalence towards contraceptive methods

- Nothing is suitable; reluctance to be examined.
- Sex is really for procreation.
- Giving in to sexual desires – losing control – might not fit in with image of nice clean upright woman.
- Inability to give oneself permission to enjoy sex.

Sexual abuse can lead to

- Promiscuity ('acting out').
- Masochistic behaviour.
- Repeated terminations.
- Repeated sexually transmitted infections.
- Person being cold, unresponsive.
- Vaginismus.
- Avoidance of vaginal examination.
- 'Sex made good by having babies'.

Sexual problems

These can influence the use and choice of contraception. If the man has premature ejaculation or the woman has no sexual desire, or if there is infrequent sex, the couple might feel the use of contraception is pointless. Or the methods themselves might cause sexual problems, e.g. the man might lose his erection with the condom.

5. THE INDIVIDUAL

Attitudes to the concepts of male/female, femininity/masculinity. These might be equated with the possibility of having children. Sexual identity and self-esteem might be obtained from this (especially pertinent for teenage girls with nothing else in their lives). For the man who feels inadequate and unable to compete with other men, getting a woman pregnant might satisfy a need to prove himself.

Unconscious factors
- The need for a baby.
- Testing the relationship.
- Unresolved conflict about the future of the relationship.
- Sex is 'disgusting', although consciously saying it is a good thing.
- After birth 'mothers can't be lovers' (altered body image; real and imagined damage).
- Bad birth experience.
- Abnormal birth, stillbirth.
- After abortion – grief and dismay about the need for a termination might lead to erratic use of contraception despite consciously saying she does not want to get pregnant.
- After diagnosis of sexually transmitted disease or abnormal cervical smear/colposcopy (feelings of anger, grief, shame, past secrets, sexual abuse might all be revealed; woman might not want to continue with her sexual relationship but be unable to talk about it, she might complain of loss of libido, blaming the pill).

6. CHILDREN
Importance and value of children. Confer adult status, carry on the family name, insurance for old age, keep you young, ensure some kind of immortality, keep the marriage or relationship together, prevent boredom and loneliness, provide interest/entertainment, satisfy the need to be needed, define a role in life and provide stability.

- They can be used as a bastion against an unfriendly world 'me and my baby' (certain teenage mothers), or as creating one's own tribe (can be seen in families with social problems).
- Can lead to non-use or poor use or fault finding with all contraceptive methods.

7. METHODS THEMSELVES AND SERVICES
Truism – we do not have the perfect method = MAGIC.

8. ABORTION SERVICES
Need for good abortion service as a supplement to family planning services because methods fail, couples fail to use methods conscientiously and women should not have to have a child they feel they cannot care for properly. But abortion interacts in many ways, e.g. with conscientiousness of use of methods, effects of guilt feelings, etc.

How are emotional factors revealed?
- Ambivalence about methods.
- Dissatisfaction with methods.
- Reluctance to be examined – psychosomatic examination, vaginismus, always menstruating.
- Belief that the vagina is a private area, frightening, vulnerable dangerous, dirty, messy, blood and discharge comes from it, not owned as a nice pleasurable place, symbol of messy sexual desires, exposure is shameful.
- Reluctance to involve partner.
- Not keeping subsequent appointments.
- Running out of supplies.

Vulnerable groups who need special support
- The young.
- The young single mother.
- Where there are different fathers for pregnancies/children.
- Chaotic lifestyle, unstable relationships.
- Mentally and physically handicapped.
- Mental illness.
- Families with children 'in care' and/or on the non-accidental injury register.
- Women who have repeated abortions.
- Women with five or more children, especially with poor spacing and achieved by a young age.

Some defences
- Chaos creator in waiting room. Diverts you from the problem. Patient wants you to get rid of her at one level; at another, a cry for help.
- Hostility, aggression, hides anxiety.
- Chatty, friendly, doesn't let you get a word in, de-doctors you.
- Jokiness.
- Tears – real or imaginary – hostile 'keep out'.
- Sexualizes interview: 'Easier to relate to me sexually than work with me as a doctor'. Denial, avoidance, hidden communication – secret code you need to decipher; non-verbal clues.

Treatment
- Awareness on part of doctor about problems and how they present.
- Listen carefully (what lies behind patient's words) – overt, covert. Might need to confront: 'Nothing on offer seems right for you' or 'Perhaps you're angry that you have to take responsibility, perhaps you would prefer your partner to'.

■ Use of doctor's own feelings with this patient provides powerful clues, for example, anger, sympathy or seduced, feeling put down (or on a pedestal), preening with pride 'only you can help, doctor.'

Above all:

■ Reactions to suggestion of vaginal examination and to the actual examination.

GLOSSARY

AIDS– acquired immune deficiency syndrome
ALO – *Actinomyces*-like organisms
AMI – acute myocardial infarction
AUC – area under the curve – in pharmacokinetic studies
BBD – benign breast disease
BBT – basal body temperature
BICH – benign intracranial hypertension
BME – bimanual examination
BMI – body mass index (weight in kg ÷ height in metres squared)
BNF – British National Formulary
BP – blood pressure
BTB – breakthrough bleeding
BV – bacterial vaginosis
CASH Study – Cancer and Sex Hormones Study
CDC – Centers for Disease Control
CGHFBC – Collaborative Group on Hormonal Factors in Breast Cancer
CIC – combined injectable contraceptive
CIN – cervical intraepithelial neoplasia
COC – combined oral contraceptive
CPA – cyproterone acetate
CSF – cerebrospinal fluid
CSM – Committee on Safety of Medicines
CVS – cardiovascular system
D&C – dilatation and curettage (superseded by hysteroscopy)
DES – diethylstilboestrol
DM – diabetes mellitus
DMPA – depot medroxyprogesterone acetate
DoH – Department of Health (DH)
DSG – desogestrel
DVT – deep venous thrombosis
E-3-G – estrone-3-glucuronide
EC – emergency contraception
EE – ethinylestradiol
epinephrine – adrenaline (old name, still preferred!)
EVA – ethylene vinyl acetate
FDA – Food and Drug Administration
FFPRHC/Faculty of FPRHC – Faculty of

Family Planning and Reproductive Health Care (a faculty of the RCOG since 1995)
FH – family history
FNH – focal nodular hyperplasia
FOC – functional ovarian cyst
FPA – Family Planning Association
FSH – follicle stimulating hormone
GA – general anaesthesia
GSD – gestodene
GUM – genitourinary medicine
h – hour
hCG – human chorionic gonadotrophin
HDL – high-density lipoprotein
HDL-C – high-density lipoprotein cholesterol
HELLP – hypertension, elevated liver enzymes, low platelets
HIV – human immunodeficiency virus
HPV – human papilloma virus (certain types can act as cervical carcinogens)
HRT – hormone replacement therapy
i.m – intramuscular (injection)
I.U.D. – intrauterine death
i/c – intercourse
IARC – International Agency for Research on Cancer
IHD – ischaemic heart disease
IMB – intermenstrual bleeding
INR – international normalised ratio (blood test for adequate anticoagulation with warfarin)
IPPF – International Planned Parenthood Federation
IU – international unit
IUD – intrauterine device
IUS – intrauterine system
JCC – Joint Committee on Contraception (predecessor body to Faculty of FPRHC)
L – litre
LA – local anaesthesia
LAM – lactational amenorrhoea method
LDL – low-density lipoprotein
LH – luteinizing hormone
lidocaine – lignocaine
LMP – last menstrual period

LNG – levonorgestrel
LNG-IUS – levonorgestrel-releasing intrauterine system
LSCS – lower segment caesarean section
min – minute
MHRA – Medicines and Healthcare products Regulatory Agency. New body which has taken over roles of the MDA and MCA
MPA – medroxyprogesterone acetate
MPC – Margaret Pyke Centre (for study and training in family planning, London)
MRI – magnetic resonance imaging
N-9 – nonoxynol-9
NAFPD – National Association of Family Planning Doctors
NET EN – norethisterone oenanthate
NET – norethisterone (norethindrome in the US)
NFP – natural family planning
NGM – norgestimate
NICE – National Institute of Clinical Excellence
NMR – nuclear magnetic resonance (imaging technique)
OC – oral contraceptive
PC – postcoital
PCOS – polycystic ovary syndrome
PD – peak day
PFI – pill-free interval
PG – prostaglandin
PGD – patient group directions (equates to protocols for nurse practitioners)
PGSI – prostaglandin synthetase inhibitor
PID – pelvic inflammatory disease
PIL – patient information leaflet (as produced by a manufacturer and officially approved)

PMS – premenstrual syndrome
POEC – progestogen-only emergency contraception
POP – progestogen-only pill
PPA – 'post-pill amenorrhoea' (not a true entity!)
RCGP – Royal College of General Practitioners
RCOG – Royal College of Obstetricians and Gynaecologists
RCT – randomized controlled trial
SAH – subarachnoid haemorrhage
SEM – scanning electron microscope
SHBG – sex hormone binding globulin
SLE – systemic lupus erythematosus
SPC – summary of product characteristics (as produced by a manufacturer, equates to datasheet)
SRE – sex and relationships education
STI – sexually transmitted infection
SVT – superficial venous thrombosis
TIA – transient ischaemic attack
TSS – toxic shock syndrome
UC – ulcerative colitis
UPSI – unprotected sexual intercourse
US – ultrasound
US FDA – US Food and Drug Administration
VTE – venous thromboembolism
VVs – varicose veins
WHO 1, WHO 2, WHO 3, WHO 4 – WHO categories for contraindications, explained at Q 5.119
WHO – World Health Organization
WTB – withdrawal bleeding

QUESTIONS FREQUENTLY ASKED BY USERS

LIST OF FIGURES

LIST OF TABLES

INDEX

A

Abdominal pain
  emergency contraception, 484 (PQ)
  POPs and, 311
  severe, due to COCs, 240
    differential diagnosis, 252
Abortion
  defences, 540
  emergency contraception, 484 (PQ)
  emotional factors, 540
  infections following, 393
  IUDs and
    insertion after, 416, 511
    removal, 378–379
  POPs and, 312 (PQ)
  postseptic, 406
  rate, 492
  safety, 3
  services, 539–541
  vulnerable groups, 540
Acetazolamide, 209
Acne, 145
  COCs and, 139, 258
  management, 199, 260–261
Acquired immune deficiency syndrome
    (AIDS) see HIV/AIDS
Acquired thrombophilia, 181
Actinomyces-like organisms (ALO) in IUD
    users, 399–402
  action, 400–401
    in asymptomatic women, 401–402
  detection, 399–402
  follow-up, 401, 402
  frequency, 399–400
  investigations, 400–401
  serious consequences, 400
  treatment, 401
Actinomycosis, 400
  counselling, 401

Africa, condom use, 47
Age
  cancer risk, 153, **153**, 155, **156**, 267
  cardiovascular disease, 173–174
    haemorrhagic stroke, 171
    ischaemic stroke, 170
  COCs and, **192**
    prescribing, 265–267
  condom failure rate, 48
  contraception choice, 489, **490**
  contraception usage, **16–17**
  IUDs and, 429
    effectiveness, 372
    expulsion rate, 387
    PID, 391, **391**
  POP effectiveness, 287–288, **288**
  see also Older women; Young
    people/teenagers
AIDS *see* HIV/AIDS
Airport security, IUDs and, 448 (PQ)
Alcohol
  COCs and, 274–275 (PQ)
  compliance, 495
  unprotected sex, 468
Allergic rhinitis, COCs and, 253
Allergy
  COC, **165**, 204, **263**, 263–264
    promoting, 253
  emergency contraception, 471
  IUD, 406, 408, 446 (PQ)
    insertion, 423
Allis forceps, 420
Altitude, COCs and, 208–209
Amenorrhoea
  COCs and, 146, 205
  fertility, 86
  guilt, 143
  history, 146–147
  injections/implants, 339, 341
    management, 343–344
  investigation, 144
  low body weight, 145–146
  normal oestrogenization, 146
  POPs and, 284–285, 308, 309
  'post-pill,' 143–144
  prolonged, risks, 144–146
  treatment, 144–146
  weight-related, 145–146
American Tips, 54
Ampicillin
  COC efficacy, **126**
  IUD insertion, 409

C

R

T

W